Essential Concepts in
CLINICAL RESEARCH

RANDOMISED CONTROLLED TRIALS AND OBSERVATIONAL EPIDEMIOLOGY

SECOND EDITION

KENNETH F. SCHULZ PhD MBA
Distinguished Scientist, FHI 360, Durham, NC, USA
Clinical Professor, Department of Obstetrics and Gynecology
University of North Carolina School of Medicine
Chapel Hill, NC, USA

DAVID A. GRIMES MD
Clinical Professor, Department of Obstetrics and Gynecology
University of North Carolina School of Medicine
Chapel Hill, NC, USA

Foreword by
RICHARD HORTON FRCP FRCPCH FMedSci
Editor-in-Chief, *The Lancet*

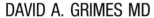

ELSEVIER
Edinburgh   London   New York   Oxford   Philadelphia   St Louis   Sydney   2019

ELSEVIER

First edition 2006
Second edition 2019

The right of Kenneth F. Schulz and David A. Grimes to be identified as authors of this work has been asserted by them in accordance with the Copyright, Designs and Patents Act 1988.

Notices

ISBN: 978-0-7020-7394-6

Executive Content Strategist: Laurence Hunter
Content Development Specialist: Carole McMurray
Project Manager: Nayagi Athmanathan
Design: Renee Duenow
Illustration Manager: Karen Giacomucci
Illustrator: Jade Myers at Matrix Art Services
Marketing Manager: Deborah Watkins

Printed in China
Last digit is the print number: 9 8 7 6 5 4 3 2 1

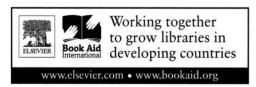

Working together
to grow libraries in
developing countries

www.elsevier.com • www.bookaid.org

Essential Concepts in
CLINICAL RESEARCH

CONTENTS

Publishing

FOREWORD

It all began on a beach in Florida. Unlikely, but true. A course in epidemiology. The venue: Captiva Island. Ken Schulz and David Grimes had honed their course with care and precision. They made the basic science of clinical medicine and public health exciting and enjoyable. We would start early—before dawn. Having captured the best of our brains, Ken and David moved us to the beach in the afternoon for competitive volleyball. Our minds refreshed daily, the velocity of our understanding accelerated. The course was carefully timed. The week of the Super Bowl. Never has epidemiology been so entertaining. The memory remains ingrained. This book records those moments, although maybe not all of them, with elan and vigour. If you read carefully, you might even be able to taste the salty air of the Florida coastline.

Medicine is an art and a science. But these qualities are not distinct domains. An art without numerical literacy is quackery. Science without conceptual underpinnings is philosophically bankrupt. Ken and David marry the clinical and the quantitative with impressive success. It's perhaps too common to proclaim a text as 'essential'. If one were to compose a canon for clinicians, many books would deserve a place. Novels with penetrating human insight. Histories exploring the contingencies of scientific discovery. Biographies displaying gifts of endeavour and courage, humility and opportunity. I would include *Essential Concepts in Clinical Research* in my personal canon. Not only because Ken and David have been my teachers but also because I have seen them first-hand inspire generations of young clinical scientists. Now let yourself be inspired too.

Richard Horton
richard.horton@lancet.com

We designed this book for two audiences—busy clinicians and active clinical researchers.

Providing digestible chapters for clinicians to read the medical literature more critically was a major goal. Clinical practice should be inspired by compassion and guided by science. Regrettably, despite long years of academic training, many clinicians report that they struggle to read medical science critically. We hope this book will provide helpful tools to critique articles and derive satisfaction, indeed fun, from clinical science. Importantly, more critical and thoughtful consumers of research make better clinicians.

Clinical researchers comprise our other major audience. We hope our chapters help to eliminate bias in medical research. Methodological research studies routinely reveal extensive deficiencies in the medical literature, both in conduct and reporting. Not surprisingly, many clinical researchers have poor formal training in research methods. Indeed, meagre research training represents a major failing of medical, nursing, and other clinical education. Knowledge of clinical research essentials, however, bolsters clinical researchers with a methodological background that enhances the quality of their research. The needs of researchers overlap with those of clinicians.

Of course, these short chapters cannot cover the full breadth of clinical research, an enterprise spanning many study designs and disciplines. Our view of clinical research incorporates both observational and experimental designs. Just as Sir Austin Bradford Hill in the late 1940s and early 1950s used retrospective case-control, long-term prospective cohort, and randomised trial designs, researchers gain from having a broad range of tools at their disposal. Moreover, we also encourage the cross-fertilisation from other disciplines that enriches research. Clinical researchers benefit by incorporating, for example, epidemiologists, biostatisticians, physician assistants, nurses, microbiologists, and behavioural scientists into their research team.

Our book is not another introductory text in biostatistics, medical statistics, or epidemiology. Many such excellent books exist, and we do not replicate their approach. Our focus is not on statistics but on providing readable, approachable guidance to the elimination of bias in study design. While both validity and precision are important in clinical research, the former takes precedence. Valid studies with some imprecision are preferable to large database studies that are precise yet replete with bias.

This book is our second edition. The first edition, published in 2006, contained 16 chapters, each representing a peer-reviewed article published in *The Lancet* from 2002 to 2005. We have used our first edition in teaching clinical research to physicians in the United States as well as researchers in Africa, Asia, and South America. We are gratified by the positive comments on its readability and helpfulness. Yet books have a shelf life, and we realised our book would benefit from updating. In this second edition, all the original chapters have been updated to incorporate additional topics and recent references.

This second edition features six new chapters. These address Limitations of Observational Epidemiology (Chapter 7), Boosting Recruitment to Randomised Controlled Trials (Chapter 10), Implementation of Treatment Blinding in Randomised Trials (Chapter 17), Surrogate Endpoints and Composite Outcomes: Shortcuts to Unknown Destinations (Chapter 18), Conducting a Randomised Trial as Part of a Prospective Meta-Analysis (Chapter 21), and Reporting Studies in Medical Journals: CONSORT and Other Reporting Guidelines (Chapter 22).

As mentioned, our book focuses on the essential concepts in study design that eliminate bias. For some topics, such as cohort studies (Chapter 4), the chapter is straightforward. We distil basic concepts into engaging, approachable material. Not all the chapters are at an introductory level, however. For other topics, such as generating allocation sequences in non–double-blinded randomised trials (Chapter 13) and allocation concealment (Chapter 14), the chapters are more complex. We present concepts that are not found in many other textbooks. Other chapters describe the fundamentals but also address ongoing controversy, such as whether underpowered trials are unethical (Chapter 11) and the limitations of observational epidemiology (Chapter 7). In every chapter, we share insights from our combined research experience of over 80 years.

We cover descriptive studies, cohort studies, case-control studies, controls in case-control studies, bias, screening tests, and likelihood ratios, but we devote 12 chapters to randomised controlled trials. This disproportion is intentional, as trials are the gold standard in clinical research. Moreover, we can emphasise certain methods because research has identified the important methodological elements of randomised trials that minimise bias. Finally, because clinicians might be more likely to act on trial results than on those of observational studies, investigators need to ensure that trials are implemented and reported well. We hope readers will benefit from this detailed coverage of randomised trials.

We thank Richard Horton, Editor-in-Chief of *The Lancet*, for inviting the initial series of essays. He inspired us to take pen to paper (nowadays, fingers to keyboard). We thank The Foundation for Exxcellence in Women's Health (indeed, the correct spelling contains "xx", as in the female chromosome) for supporting our clinical research courses in recent years. Our new chapters stem from discussions held in these courses.

All chapters in the first edition were skilfully reviewed by the late Ward Cates and David Sackett. We are indebted to these two visionaries for their wisdom and insights, and we dedicate this second edition to their memory.

Fortunately, our wives, Susan Schulz and Corey Grimes, are not only supportive and tolerant of our work, but they are also excellent writers and editors. They have corrected and clarified our writing throughout this second edition. We deeply appreciate their help. Any errors or omissions are, of course, ours.

Finally, we thank Laurence Hunter, Carole McMurray and Nayagi Athmanathan of Elsevier for guiding us through the publishing experience.

Kenneth F. Schulz
David A. Grimes

CHAPTER 1

An Overview of Clinical Research: The Lay of the Land

Many clinicians report that they cannot read the medical literature critically. To address this difficulty, we provide a primer of clinical research for clinicians and researchers alike. Clinical research falls into two general categories: experimental and observational, based on whether the investigator assigns the exposures or not. Experimental trials can also be subdivided into two: randomised and nonrandomised. Observational studies can be either analytical or descriptive. In this book, we distinguish between the two by this criterion: analytical studies feature a comparison (control) group, whereas descriptive studies do not. Within analytical studies, cohort studies track people forward in time from exposure to outcome. By contrast, case-control studies work in reverse, tracing back from outcome to exposure. Cross-sectional studies are like a snapshot, which measures both exposure and outcome at one time point. Descriptive studies cannot examine associations, a fact often forgotten or ignored. Measures of association, such as relative risk or odds ratio, are the preferred way of expressing results of dichotomous outcomes (e.g., sick versus healthy). Confidence intervals around these measures indicate the precision of these results. Measures of association with confidence intervals reveal the strength, direction, and plausible range of an effect, as well as the likelihood of chance occurrence. By contrast, p values address only chance. Testing null hypotheses at a p value of 0.05 has no basis in medicine and should be discouraged.

Clinicians today are in a bind. Increasing demands on their time are squeezing out opportunities to stay abreast of the literature, much less read it critically. PubMed currently catalogues 30,000 journals, and its citations include more than 27 million entries. Results of several studies indicate an inverse relation between quality of care and time since graduation from medical school;[1] older clinicians consistently have a harder time keeping up.[2] In many jurisdictions, attendance at a specified number of hours of continuing medical education (CME) courses is mandatory to maintain a licence to practice. Continuing medical education courses have at best a modest effect on the quality of care, and such courses alone appear unlikely to affect complex clinical behaviours.[3] This deficiency of traditional CME offerings emphasises the importance of self-directed learning through reading. However, many clinicians lack the requisite skills to read the medical literature critically.[4,5] Scientific illiteracy[6] and innumeracy[5] remain major failings of medical education.

This book on research methods is designed for busy clinicians and active researchers. The needs of clinicians predominate; hopefully, this primer will produce more critical and thoughtful consumers of research, and thus better practitioners. The needs of clinicians overlap with those of researchers throughout the chapters, but that overlap becomes most pronounced in the discussion of randomised controlled trials. For readers to assess randomised trials accurately, they should understand the relevant guidelines on the conduct of trials; these guidelines have been derived from empirical methodological research.

The disproportionate coverage of randomised controlled trials is intentional; randomised controlled trials are the gold standard in clinical research. Randomised controlled trials help to eliminate bias, and research has identified the important methodological elements of trials that minimise bias.[7,8] Finally, because trials are deemed more credible than observational studies,[9,10] clinicians might be more likely to act on their results than on those of other study types; hence, investigators need to ensure that trials are done well and reported well. To start, we provide a brief overview of research designs and discuss some of the common measures used.

A Taxonomy of Clinical Research

Analogous to biological taxonomy, a simple hierarchy can be used to categorise most studies (Panel 1.1).[11] To do so, however, the study design must be known. As in biology, anatomy dictates physiology. The anatomy of a study determines what it can and cannot do. A difficulty that readers encounter is that authors sometimes do not report the study type or provide sufficient detail to figure it out. A related problem is that authors sometimes incorrectly label the type of research done. Examples include calling nonrandomised controlled trials randomised,[12] and labelling nonconcurrent cohort studies case-control studies.[13-15] The adjective 'case-controlled' is also sometimes (inappropriately) applied to any study with a comparison group. The media compound the confusion by implying causation[16] (when researchers cautiously reported only an association).[17]

Biology has animal and plant kingdoms. Similarly, clinical research has two large kingdoms: experimental and observational research. Fig. 1.1 shows that one can quickly decide the research kingdom by noting whether the investigators assigned the exposures (e.g., treatments) or whether they observed

---

PANEL 1.1 ■ Rating Clinical Evidence: Assessment System of the US Preventive Services Task Force[11]

Quality of Evidence

I   Evidence from at least one properly designed randomised controlled trial.

II-1   Evidence obtained from well-designed controlled trials without randomisation.

II-2   Evidence from well-designed cohort or case-control studies, preferably from more than one centre or research group.

II-3   Evidence from multiple time series with or without the intervention. Important results in uncontrolled experiments (such as the introduction of penicillin treatment in the 1940s) could also be considered as this type of evidence.

III   Opinions of respected authorities, based on clinical experience, descriptive studies, or reports of expert committees.

Strength of Recommendations

A   Strongly recommends

B   Recommends

C   Makes no recommendation for or against

D   Recommends against

I   Concludes evidence insufficient to recommend for or against

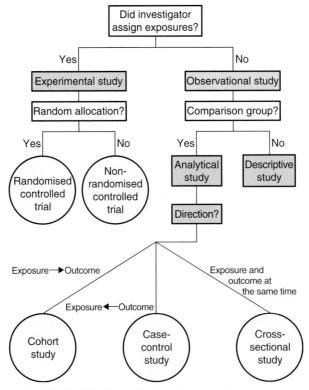

Fig. 1.1   Algorithm for classification of types of clinical research.

usual clinical practice.[18-20] At the top of the hierarchy, for experimental studies one needs to distinguish whether the exposures were assigned by a truly random technique (with concealment of the upcoming assignment from those involved) or whether some other allocation scheme was used, such as alternate assignment.[21] Many reports fail to include this critical information.[22]

With observational studies, which dominate the literature, especially in lower-impact journals,[23] the next step is to ascertain whether the study has a comparison or control group. If so, the study is termed analytical.[24] If not, it is a descriptive study (see Fig. 1.1). If the study is analytical, the temporal direction needs to be identified. If the study determines both exposures and outcomes at one time point, it is termed cross-sectional. An example would be measurement of serum cholesterol of patients admitted to a hospital with myocardial infarction versus that of their next-door neighbour. This type of study provides a snapshot of the population of sick and well at one time point.[25] A weakness of cross-sectional studies is that the temporal sequence may be unclear: did the exposure precede the outcome? In addition, cross-sectional studies are inappropriate for rare diseases or those that resolve quickly; severe diseases causing early death can mean that those studied are not representative of all those with a given disease.[19]

If the study begins with an exposure (e.g., oral contraceptive use) and follows women for years to measure outcomes (e.g., ovarian cancer), then it is deemed a cohort study. Cohort studies can be either concurrent or nonconcurrent. By contrast, if the analytical study begins with an outcome (e.g., ovarian cancer) and looks back in time for an exposure, such as use of oral contraceptives, then the study is a case-control study.

Studies without comparison groups are called descriptive studies.[24] At the bottom of the research hierarchy is the case report. Indeed, the literature is replete with reported oddities.[26]

When more than one patient is described, it becomes a case-series report. Some new diseases first appear in the literature this way.[27]

What Studies Can and Cannot Do

DESCRIPTIVE STUDY

Starting at the bottom of the research hierarchy, descriptive studies are often the first foray into a new area of medicine, a first 'toe in the water'. Investigators do descriptive studies to describe the frequency, natural history, and possible determinants of a condition.[18,19] The results of these studies show how many people develop a disease or condition over time, describe the characteristics of the disease and those affected, and generate hypotheses about the cause of the disease. These hypotheses can be assessed through more rigorous research, such as analytical studies or randomised controlled trials. An example of a descriptive study would be the early reports of legionnaires' disease[28] and toxic-shock syndrome.[29] An important caveat (often forgotten or intentionally ignored) is that descriptive studies, which do not have a comparison group, do not allow assessment of associations.[30] Only comparative studies (both analytical and experimental) enable assessment of possible causal associations.

CROSS-SECTIONAL STUDY: A SNAPSHOT IN TIME

Sometimes termed a frequency survey or a prevalence study,[24] cross-sectional studies are done to examine the presence or absence of disease and the presence or absence of an exposure at a particular time. Thus prevalence, not incidence, is the focus. As both outcome and exposure are ascertained at the same time (Fig. 1.2), the temporal relation between the two can be unclear. For example, assume that a cross-sectional study finds obesity to be more common among women with arthritis than among those without this condition. Did the extra weight load on joints lead to arthritis, or did women with arthritis become involuntarily inactive and then obese? This 'chicken-egg' question is unanswerable in a cross-sectional study.

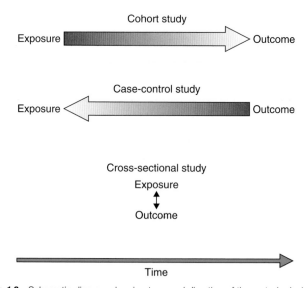

Fig. 1.2   Schematic diagram showing temporal direction of three study designs.

COHORT STUDY: LOOKING FORWARD IN TIME

Cohort studies proceed in a logical sequence from exposure to outcome (see Fig. 1.2). Hence, this type of research is easier to understand than case-control studies. Investigators identify a group with an exposure of interest and another group or groups without the exposure. The investigators then follow the exposed and unexposed groups forward in time to determine outcomes. If the exposed group develops a higher incidence of the outcome than the unexposed, then the exposure is associated with an increased risk of the outcome, and vice versa.

Cohort studies can be prospective, retrospective, or both. In a prospective cohort study, the exposed and unexposed are identified and followed forward in time to outcomes. In a retrospective cohort study, the investigator goes back in time through medical records to identify exposure groups, then tracks them to outcomes through existing medical records. In some disciplines, retrospective cohort studies are more common than prospective cohort studies. As described in Chapter 4, ambidirectional cohort studies look backward and forward in time.

The cohort study has important strengths and weaknesses. Because exposure is identified at the outset, one can usually determine that the exposure preceded the outcome. Recall bias is less of a concern than in the case-control study. The cohort study enables calculation of true incidence rates, relative risks, and attributable risks. However, for the study of rare events or events that take years to develop, this type of research design can be slow to yield results and thus prohibitively expensive. Nonetheless, several famous, large cohort studies[31,32] continue to provide important information.

CASE-CONTROL STUDY: THINKING BACKWARDS

Case-control studies work backwards. Because thinking in this direction is not intuitive for clinicians, case-control studies are widely misunderstood. Indeed, in one sample from the rehabilitation literature, 97% of research articles designated 'case-control' were mislabelled.[33]

Starting with an outcome, such as disease, this type of study looks backward in time for exposures that might be related to the outcome. As shown in Fig. 1.2, investigators define a group with an outcome (e.g., ovarian cancer) and a group without the outcome (controls). Then, through chart reviews, interviews, electronic medical records, or other means, the investigators ascertain the prevalence (or amount) of exposure to a risk factor (e.g., oral contraceptives, ovulation-induction drugs) in both groups. If the prevalence of the exposure is higher among cases than among controls, then the exposure is associated with an increased risk of the outcome.

Case-control studies are especially useful for outcomes that are rare or that take a long time to develop, prototypes being cardiovascular disease and cancer. These studies often require less time, effort, and money than would cohort studies. The Achilles heel of case-control studies is choosing an appropriate control group, discussed further in Chapter 6. Controls should be similar to cases in all important respects except for not having the outcome in question. Inappropriate control groups have ruined many case-control studies and caused much harm. Additionally, recall bias (better recollection of exposures among the worried cases than among the healthy controls) is inevitable in studies that rely on memory. Because the case-control study samples on cases and controls, not on exposures, investigators cannot calculate incidence rates, relative risks, or attributable risks. Instead, odds ratios are the measure of association used; when the outcome is uncommon (e.g., most cancers) the odds ratio provides a good proxy for the true relative risk.[34]

Investigations of outbreaks of food-borne diseases often use case-control studies. On a cruise ship, the entire universe of those at risk is known. Those with vomiting and diarrhoea (cases) are asked about food exposures, as are a sample of those not ill (controls). If a higher proportion of those who are ill reports having eaten a specific food than those who are well, the food becomes suspect. In 50 outbreaks associated with cruise ships from 1970 to 2003, the most common culprit was found to be seafood (28% of outbreaks).[35]

VARIATIONS ON THESE THEMES

Nested Case-Control Studies

Here, a group of persons being studied is followed forward in time until outcomes occur. Instead of analysing everyone in the group in usual cohort fashion, those with the outcome are deemed cases, and a sample of those without the disease become controls.[36] Then, the analysis proceeds in typical case-control fashion. The smaller case-control study is 'nested' within a larger cohort under scrutiny.[24]

Why analyse a cohort study this way? This approach may be useful when determining the exposure involves an expensive, painful, invasive test or ponderous interview. Determining exposure information for all participants might be impractical or prohibitively expensive. All cases have exposure determined, but only a small sample of all healthy persons (controls) need this done. A study of inflammatory markers and postpartum depression is illustrative. A prospective cohort of women being followed through pregnancy had blood samples collected and banked at specified times. Sixty-three women with depression had a sophisticated protein panel run on their blood sample to examine 92 inflammation markers. The same panel was run on blood from 228 controls without depression.[37] Performing this extensive testing on all women in the cohort would have been costly.

Case-Cohort Studies

In this modification of a case-control study, '…controls are drawn from the same cohort as the cases regardless of their disease status. Cases of the disease of interest are identified, and a sample of the entire starting cohort (regardless of their outcomes) forms the controls'[24] Here, one control group can be used for multiple groups of cases, increasing the efficiency of the exploration. Controls are randomly selected from the population at risk; these controls are called the 'reference subcohort'.[38] In a traditional case-control study, researchers would need to recruit a different control group for each group of cases being studied; here, one control group can be recycled repeatedly.

A case-cohort study examined risk factors for hospitalisation after dog-bite injury.[39] The cohort consisted of 1384 dog-bite patients (Fig. 1.3) seen at one hospital emergency department; 111 of these who were admitted formed the case group. A simple random sample of the other patients

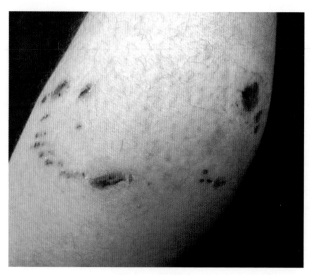

Fig. 1.3 Dog bite.

comprised the control subcohort (221 patients). As noted previously, controls were selected independent of their disease status; by chance, 21 patients randomly chosen as controls were themselves cases (admitted to the hospital). Infected bites and bites to multiple sites were most strongly related to the risk of being hospitalised.

Case-Crossover Studies

This study type can be used to assess adverse drug reactions or events rapidly triggered by an exposure. For example, a case with an adverse event is queried about exposures in the prior hour, deemed the hazard window.[25] The control interval might be the same time window in the same patient 1 day earlier. This helps to control for confounding by indication, because each study participant serves as both the case and the control.[40] An example would be studying the association between sedatives and car wrecks.[41]

The possibility that chiropractic manipulation might precipitate carotid artery stroke prompted a case-crossover study in Canada.[42] All incident strokes over a 9-year period were the cases; each served as his or her own control. The exposure windows used were 1, 3, 7, and 14 days before the stroke. No significant differences in risk between visits to chiropractors and primary care providers were evident, suggesting no role of spinal manipulation in triggering stroke.

Case-Time-Control Studies

This approach is a variant of the case-crossover design in which a traditional control group provides the background exposure history. This type of study is defined as 'a study in which exposure of cases and controls during one period is compared in matched-pair analyses to their own exposure during another period of similar length'.[24] This approach is used in pharmacological studies to study brief exposures with acute effects, such as nonsteroidal antiinflammatory drugs and cardiac arrest outside of a hospital.[43] This approach helps to control for time trends in exposures.[40]

NONRANDOMISED TRIAL: PENULTIMATE DESIGN?

Some experimental trials do not randomly allocate participants to exposures (e.g., treatments or prevention strategies). Instead of using truly random techniques, investigators may use methods that fall short of the mark (e.g., alternate assignment).[44] The US Preventive Services Task Force[11] designates this research design as class II-1, indicating less scientific rigour than randomised trials, but more than analytical studies (see Panel 1.1).

After the investigators have assigned participants to treatment groups, the way a nonrandomised trial is done and analysed resembles that of a cohort study. The exposed and unexposed are followed forward in time to ascertain the frequency of outcomes. Advantages of a nonrandomised trial include use of a concurrent control group and uniform ascertainment of outcomes for both groups. However, selection bias can occur, because allocation concealment may be impossible to maintain.

RANDOMISED CONTROLLED TRIAL: GOLD STANDARD

The randomised controlled trial is the only known way to avoid selection and confounding biases in clinical research. This design approximates the controlled experiment of basic science. It resembles the cohort study in several respects, with the important exception of randomisation of participants to exposures (see Fig. 1.2).

The hallmark of randomised controlled trials is assignment of participants to exposures (e.g., treatments) purely by the play of chance. When properly implemented, random allocation precludes selection bias. Randomised controlled trials reduce the likelihood of bias in determination of outcomes. Trials feature uniform diagnostic criteria for outcomes and, often, blinding of treatment assignment, thus reducing the potential for information bias. A unique strength of this study design is that it eliminates confounding bias, both known and unknown (discussed in Chapter 3). Trials tend to be statistically efficient. If properly designed and done, a randomised controlled trial is likely to be free of bias and is thus especially useful for examination of small or moderate effects. In observational studies, bias can easily account for weak associations (i.e., small differences).[45]

Randomised controlled trials have drawbacks, too. External validity is a concern. Whereas the randomised controlled trial, if properly done, has internal validity (i.e., it measures what it sets out to measure), it might not have external validity. This term indicates the extent to which results can be generalised to the broader community.[20] Unlike the observational study, the randomised controlled trial includes only volunteers who pass through a screening process before inclusion. Those who volunteer for trials tend to be different from the population of those with the condition; only a tiny fraction of those with a condition find their way into trials.[46] Another limitation is that a randomised controlled trial cannot be used in some instances, because intentional exposure to harmful substances (e.g., toxins, bacteria, or other noxious substances) would be unethical. As with cohort studies, the randomised controlled trial can be prohibitively expensive. Indeed, the cost of large trials can run into the hundreds of millions of US dollars.[47]

Measurement of Outcomes

CONFUSING FRACTIONS

Identification and quantification of outcomes is the business of research. However, slippery terminology often complicates matters for investigators and readers alike. For example, the term 'rate' (as in 'maternal mortality rate') has been misused in textbooks and journal articles for decades. Additionally, 'rate' is often used interchangeably with proportions and ratios.[24] Fig. 1.4 presents a simple approach to classification of these common terms.

A ratio is a value obtained by dividing one number by another.[24] These two numbers can be either related or unrelated. This feature (i.e., relatedness of numerator and denominator) separates ratios into two groups: those in which the numerator is included in the denominator (e.g., rate and proportion) and those in which it is not.

A rate measures the frequency of an event in a population, usually over a period of time. As shown in Fig. 1.4, the numerator (those with the outcome) of a rate must be contained in

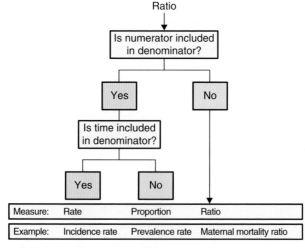

Fig. 1.4 Algorithm for distinguishing rates, proportions, and ratios.

the denominator (those at risk of the outcome). Although all ratios feature a numerator and denominator, rates have two distinguishing characteristics: time and a multiplier. Rates indicate the time during which the outcomes occur and a multiplier, commonly to a base ten, to yield whole numbers. For example, the age-adjusted incidence of all unprovoked seizures in Minnesota is 61 per 100,000 person-years. In contrast, the prevalence of epilepsy there is 6.8 per 1000 population.[48] The latter measure is the total number of persons with a condition at a point in time divided by the population at risk at that point in time (or midway in the time interval).[24]

Proportion is often used synonymously with rate, but the former does not have a time component. Like a rate, a proportion is a ratio with the numerator contained in the denominator.[24] Because the numerator and denominator have the same units, these divide out, leaving a dimensionless quantity (a number without units). An example of a proportion is prevalence (e.g., 27 of 100 at risk have hay fever). This number indicates how many of a population at risk have a condition at a particular time (here, 27%); as documentation of new cases over time is not involved, prevalence is more properly considered a proportion than a rate.

Although all rates and proportions are ratios, the opposite is not true. In some ratios, the numerator is not included in the denominator. The most notorious example may be the venerable maternal mortality ratio. The definition includes women who die of pregnancy-related causes in the numerator, and women with live births (usually 100,000) in the denominator. However, not all those in the numerator are included in the denominator (e.g., a woman who dies of an ectopic pregnancy at 7 weeks' gestation cannot be in the denominator). Thus this 'rate' is actually a ratio, not a rate, a fact still not widely understood.[49]

MEASURES OF ASSOCIATION: RISKY BUSINESS

Relative risk (also termed the risk ratio) is another useful ratio: the frequency of outcome in the exposed divided by the frequency of outcome in the unexposed. If the frequency of the outcome is the same in both groups, then the ratio is 1.0, indicating no association between exposure and outcome. By contrast, if the outcome is more frequent in those exposed, then the ratio will be greater than 1.0, implying an increased risk associated with exposure. Conversely, if the frequency of disease is less among the exposed, then the relative risk will be less than 1.0, implying a protective effect.

Also known as the cross-products ratio or relative odds,[24] the odds ratio has different meanings in different settings. In case-control studies, this ratio is the usual measure of association. It indicates the odds of exposure among the case group divided by the odds of exposure among controls. If cases and controls have equal odds of having the exposure, the odds ratio is 1.0, indicating no association. If the cases have a higher odds of exposure than the controls, then the ratio is greater than 1.0, implying an increased risk associated with exposure. Conversely, odds ratios less than 1.0 indicate a protective effect.

An odds ratio can also be calculated for cross-sectional, cohort, and randomised controlled studies. Here, the disease-odds ratio is the ratio of the odds in favour of disease in the exposed versus that in the unexposed. In this context, the odds ratio has some appealing statistical features when studies are aggregated in meta-analysis, but the odds ratio does not indicate the relative risk when the proportion with the outcome is greater than 5% to 10%.[34] Stated alternatively, the odds ratio is always a valid measure of association, but it is not a good proxy for the relative risk unless the outcome is uncommon ('rare disease assumption').

The confidence interval (CI) reflects the precision of study results. The interval provides a range of plausible values for a point estimate, such as a proportion, relative risk, or odds ratio. The confidence interval has a specified probability of containing the true value for the entire population from which the study sample was taken. Although 95% CIs are the most commonly used, others, such as 90%, are sometimes seen.[50] The wider the confidence interval, the less precision exists in the result, and vice versa. For relative risks and odds ratios, when the 95% CI does not include 1.0, the difference is significant at the usual 0.05 level. However, use of this feature of confidence intervals as a back-door means of hypothesis testing is inappropriate.[51]

Conclusion

Understanding what kind of study has been done is a prerequisite to thoughtful reading of research. Clinical research can be divided into experimental and observational; observational studies are further categorised into those with and without a comparison group. Only studies with comparison groups allow investigators to assess possible causal associations, a fact often forgotten or ignored. Dichotomous outcomes of studies should be reported as measures of association with confidence intervals; testing null hypotheses at arbitrary p values of 0.05 has no basis in medicine.

References

1. Goulet, F., Hudon, E., Gagnon, R., Gauvin, E., Lemire, F., Arsenault, I., 2013. Effects of continuing professional development on clinical performance: results of a study involving family practitioners in Quebec. Can. Fam. Physician 59, 518–525.
2. Decker, S.L., Jamoom, E.W., Sisk, J.E., 2012. Physicians in nonprimary care and small practices and those age 55 and older lag in adopting electronic health record systems. Health Aff. (Millwood) 31, 1108–1114.
3. Forsetlund, L., Bjorndal, A., Rashidian, A., et al., 2009. Continuing education meetings and workshops: effects on professional practice and health care outcomes. Cochrane Database Syst. Rev. CD003030.
4. Windish, D.M., Huot, S.J., Green, M.L., 2007. Medicine residents' understanding of the biostatistics and results in the medical literature. JAMA 298, 1010–1022.
5. Rao, G., Kanter, S.L., 2010. Physician numeracy as the basis for an evidence-based medicine curriculum. Acad. Med. 85, 1794–1799.
6. Hadley, J.A., Wall, D., Khan, K.S., 2007. Learning needs analysis to guide teaching evidence-based medicine: knowledge and beliefs amongst trainees from various specialities. BMC Med. Educ. 7, 11.
7. Schulz, K.F., Altman, D.G., Moher, D., 2010. CONSORT 2010 statement: updated guidelines for reporting parallel group randomised trials. BMJ 340, c332.
8. Moher, D., Hopewell, S., Schulz, K.F., et al., 2010. CONSORT 2010 explanation and elaboration: updated guidelines for reporting parallel group randomised trials. J. Clin. Epidemiol. 63, e1–37.
9. Martinez, M.E., Marshall, J.R., Giovannucci, E., 2008. Diet and cancer prevention: the roles of observation and experimentation. Nat. Rev. Cancer 8, 694–703.
10. Albert, R.K., 2013. "Lies, damned lies …" and observational studies in comparative effectiveness research. Am. J. Respir. Crit. Care Med. 187, 1173–1177.
11. Harris, R.P., Helfand, M., Woolf, S.H., et al., 2001. Current methods of the US Preventive Services Task Force: a review of the process. Am. J. Prev. Med. 20, 21–35.
12. Wu, T., Li, Y., Bian, Z., Liu, G., Moher, D., 2009. Randomized trials published in some Chinese journals: how many are randomized? Trials 10, 46.
13. Grimes, D.A., 2009. "Case-control" confusion: mislabeled reports in obstetrics and gynecology journals. Obstet. Gynecol. 114, 1284–1286.
14. Hellems, M.A., Kramer, M.S., Hayden, G.F., 2006. Case-control confusion. Ambul. Pediatr. 6, 96–99.
15. Caro, J.J., Huybrechts, K.F., 2009. Case-control studies in pharmacoeconomic research: an overview. Pharmacoeconomics 27 (8), 627–634.
16. Rossman S. Diet soda can increase risk of dementia and stroke, study finds. https://www.usatoday.com/story/news/nation-now/2017/04/21/diet-soda-can-increase-risk-dementia-and-stroke-study-finds/100736786/, accessed 23 April 2017.
17. Pase, M.P., Himali, J.J., Beiser, A.S., et al., 2017. Sugar- and artificially sweetened beverages and the risks of incident stroke and dementia: a prospective cohort study. Stroke 48, 1139–1146.
18. Meyer, A.M., Wheeler, S.B., Weinberger, M., Chen, R.C., Carpenter, W.R., 2014. An overview of methods for comparative effectiveness research. Semin. Radiat. Oncol. 24, 5–13.
19. DiPietro, N.A., 2010. Methods in epidemiology: observational study designs. Pharmacotherapy 30, 973–984.

20. Stang, A., 2008. Appropriate epidemiologic methods as a prerequisite for valid study results. Eur. J. Epidemiol. 23, 761–765.
21. Hill, C.L., LaValley, M.P., Felson, D.T., 2002. Discrepancy between published report and actual conduct of randomized clinical trials. J. Clin. Epidemiol. 55, 783–786.
22. Strech, D., Soltmann, B., Weikert, B., Bauer, M., Pfennig, A., 2011. Quality of reporting of randomized controlled trials of pharmacologic treatment of bipolar disorders: a systematic review. J. Clin. Psychiatry 72, 1214–1221.
23. Kuroki, L.M., Allsworth, J.E., Peipert, J.F., 2009. Methodology and analytic techniques used in clinical research: associations with journal impact factor. Obstet. Gynecol. 114, 877–884.
24. Porta, M., 2014. A Dictionary of Epidemiology. Oxford University Press, New York.
25. Hartung, D.M., Touchette, D., 2009. Overview of clinical research design. Am. J. Health Syst. Pharm. 66, 398–408.
26. Goldberg, H.R., Allen, L., Kives, S., 2017. Fetiform teratoma in the ovary of a 7-year-old girl: a case report. J. Pediatr. Adolesc. Gynecol. 30, 256–258.
27. Pneumocystis pneumonia—Los Angeles, 1981. MMWR Morb. Mortal. Wkly Rep. 30, 250–252.
28. Keys, T.F., 1977. A sporadic case of pneumonia due to legionnaires disease. Mayo Clin. Proc. 52, 657–660.
29. McKenna, U.G., Meadows 3rd, J.A., Brewer, N.S., Wilson, W.R., Perrault, J., 1980. Toxic shock syndrome, a newly recognized disease entity. Report of 11 cases. Mayo Clin. Proc. 55, 663–672.
30. Caillouette, J.C., Koehler, A.L., 1987. Phasic contraceptive pills and functional ovarian cysts. Am. J. Obstet. Gynecol. 156, 1538–1542.
31. Wei, E.K., Colditz, G.A., Giovannucci, E.L., et al., 2017. A comprehensive model of colorectal cancer by risk factor status and subsite using data from the nurses' health study. Am. J. Epidemiol. 185, 224–237.
32. Iversen, L., Sivasubramaniam, S., Lee, A.J., Fielding, S., Hannaford, P.C., 2017. Lifetime cancer risk and combined oral contraceptives: the Royal College of General Practitioners' Oral Contraception Study. Am. J. Obstet. Gynecol. 216, 580.e1–580.e9.
33. Mayo, N.E., Goldberg, M.S., 2009. When is a case-control study not a case-control study? J. Rehabil. Med. 41, 209–216.
34. Grimes, D.A., Schulz, K.F., 2008. Making sense of odds and odds ratios. Obstet. Gynecol. 111, 423–426.
35. Rooney, R.M., Cramer, E.H., Mantha, S., et al., 2004. A review of outbreaks of foodborne disease associated with passenger ships: evidence for risk management. Public Health Rep. 119, 427–434.
36. Etminan, M., 2004. Pharmacoepidemiology II: the nested case-control study—a novel approach in pharmacoepidemiologic research. Pharmacotherapy 24, 1105–1109.
37. Brann, E., Papadopoulos, F., Fransson, E., et al., 2017. Inflammatory markers in late pregnancy in association with postpartum depression—A nested case-control study. Psychoneuroendocrinology 79, 146–159.
38. Checkoway, H., Pearce, N., Kriebel, D., 2007. Selecting appropriate study designs to address specific research questions in occupational epidemiology. Occup. Environ. Med. 64, 633–638.
39. Rhea, S., Weber, D.J., Poole, C., Cairns, C., 2014. Risk factors for hospitalization after dog bite injury: a case-cohort study of emergency department visits. Acad. Emerg. Med. 21, 196–203.
40. Schneeweiss, S., Sturmer, T., Maclure, M., 1997. Case-crossover and case-time-control designs as alternatives in pharmacoepidemiologic research. Pharmacoepidemiol. Drug Saf. 6 (Suppl 3), S51–S59.
41. Lu, C.Y., 2009. Observational studies: a review of study designs, challenges and strategies to reduce confounding. Int. J. Clin. Pract. 63, 691–697.
42. Cassidy, J.D., Boyle, E., Cote, P., Hogg-Johnson, S., Bondy, S.J., Haldeman, S., 2017. Risk of carotid stroke after chiropractic care: a population-based case-crossover study. J. Stroke Cerebrovasc. Dis. 26, 842–850.
43. Sondergaard, K.B., Weeke, P., Wissenberg, M., et al., 2017. Non-steroidal anti-inflammatory drug use is associated with increased risk of out-of-hospital cardiac arrest: a nationwide case-time-control study. Eur. Heart J. Cardiovasc. Pharmacother. 3, 100–107.
44. Sharma, P.K., Yadav, T.P., Gautam, R.K., Taneja, N., Satyanarayana, L., 2000. Erythromycin in pityriasis rosea: A double-blind, placebo-controlled clinical trial. J. Am. Acad. Dermatol. 42, 241–244.
45. Grimes, D.A., Schulz, K.F., 2012. False alarms and pseudo-epidemics: the limitations of observational epidemiology. Obstet. Gynecol. 120, 920–927.

46. Rothwell, P.M., 2005. External validity of randomised controlled trials: "to whom do the results of this trial apply?". Lancet 365, 82–93.

47. Roth, J.A., Etzioni, R., Waters, T.M., et al., 2014. Economic return from the Women's Health Initiative estrogen plus progestin clinical trial: a modeling study. Ann. Intern. Med. 160, 594–602.

48. Logroscino, G., Hesdorffer, D.C., 2005. Methodologic issues in studies of mortality following epilepsy: measures, types of studies, sources of cases, cohort effects, and competing risks. Epilepsia 46 (Suppl 11), 3–7.

49. MacDorman, M.F., Declercq, E., Cabral, H., Morton, C., 2016. Recent increases in the U.S. maternal mortality rate: disentangling trends from measurement issues. Obstet. Gynecol. 128, 447–455.

50. Catton, C.N., Lukka, H., Gu, C.S., et al., 2017. Randomized trial of a hypofractionated radiation regimen for the treatment of localized prostate cancer. J. Clin. Oncol. 35, 1884–1890.

51. Sterne, J.A., Smith, G.D., 2001. Sifting the evidence—what's wrong with significance tests? BMJ 322, 226–231.

Descriptive Studies: What They Can and Cannot Do

Descriptive studies often represent the first scientific toe in the water in new areas of inquiry. A fundamental element of descriptive reporting is a clear, specific, and measurable definition of the disease or condition in question. Like newspapers, good descriptive reporting answers the five basic 'W' questions: who, what, why, when, where … and a sixth: so what? Case reports, case-series reports, cross-sectional studies, and surveillance studies deal with individuals, whereas ecological correlational studies examine populations. The case report is the least publishable unit in medical literature. Case-series reports aggregate individual cases in one publication. Clustering of unusual cases in a short period often heralds a new epidemic, as happened with AIDS. Cross-sectional (prevalence) studies describe the health of populations. Surveillance can be thought of as watchfulness over a community; feedback to those who need to know is an integral component of surveillance. Ecological correlational studies look for associations between exposures and outcomes in populations (e.g., per capita cigarette sales and rates of coronary artery disease) rather than in individuals. Three important uses of descriptive studies include trend analysis, healthcare planning, and hypothesis generation. A frequent error in reports of descriptive studies is overstepping the data; studies without a comparison group allow no inferences to be drawn about associations, causal or otherwise. Hypotheses about causation from descriptive studies are often subsequently tested in rigorous analytical studies.

Descriptive studies play several important roles in medical research. They are often the first foray into a new disease or area of inquiry—the first scientific 'toe in the water'.[1] They document the health of populations and often prompt more rigorous studies. Because descriptive studies are common,[2,3] clinicians need to know their uses, strengths, and weaknesses.

A descriptive study is 'concerned with and designed only to describe the existing distribution of variables without much regard to causal relationships or other hypotheses'.[4] The key qualifier about causal hypotheses is sometimes forgotten by investigators, resulting in erroneous conclusions.[5]

Here, we provide an overview of the advantages and disadvantages of descriptive studies, provide examples of several types of descriptive study, examine their clinical uses, and show how they can be misinterpreted.

The Descriptive Triad—Or Pentad?

FIVE 'W' QUESTIONS

Traditional descriptive epidemiology has focused on three key features: person, place, and time,[6] or, in the infectious disease model, agent, host, and environment.[7] An alternative way of thinking about descriptive epidemiology is newspaper coverage. Good descriptive research, like good newspaper reporting, should answer five basic 'W' questions—who, what, why, when, and where—and an implicit sixth question: so what?

Who Has the Disease in Question?

Age and sex are universally described, but other characteristics might be important too, including race, occupation, or recreational activities. The risk of venous thromboembolism, for example, increases progressively with age.[8] Breast cancer is rare in men, who account for only 1% of cases. However, Klinefelter syndrome (47,XXY chromosome complement) increases the risk more than 20-fold.[9] Black women have two to three times the risk of leiomyomas of the uterus as do white women.[10] Percival Pott's discovery of the association between chimney sweeps and scrotal cancer related to soot is a classic in occupational epidemiology.[11] The phrase 'mad as a hatter' stems from mercury-induced psychosis in workers with occupational exposure to this heavy metal in the hat industry.[12] Commercial fishing remains a dangerous occupation,[13] and driving all-terrain vehicles[14] or snowmobiles[15] while drunk is a dangerous way to have fun.

What Is the Condition or Disease Being Studied?

Development of a clear, specific, and measurable case definition is an essential step in descriptive epidemiology. Without such a description, the reader cannot interpret the report. Some conditions, such as fractures, can be overt. Other diagnoses might be challenging: multiple sclerosis, systemic lupus erythematosus, and pelvic inflammatory disease (salpingitis), for example. By use of the consensus or Delphi panel approach rather than empirical evidence, some organisations have promulgated case definitions[16] that have subsequently been shown to be invalid.[17,18]

Stringent criteria for case definitions are desirable. Admittedly, if only the more severe cases of disease are targeted, milder or earlier cases will be missed. Although this approach inevitably leads to some underreporting,[19] the trade-off is better specificity; severe cases of a disease are less likely to be confused with other conditions than are mild cases. An example would be the stringent case definition used for toxic shock syndrome, which requires involvement of multiple organ systems. In recent decades, the Centers for Disease Control and Prevention has repeatedly revised its case definition of HIV infection, which in turn influences the reported incidence and prevalence of the disease.[20]

Why Did the Condition or Disease Arise?

Descriptive studies often provide clues about cause that can be pursued with more sophisticated research designs (Panel 2.1).

When Does the Condition Occur?

Time provides important clues about health events. The prototype might be the outbreak of food poisoning within hours after ingestion of staphylococcal toxin. Some temporal relations can be long, such as mesothelioma decades after asbestos exposure.[22] Furthermore, cervical and other epithelial cancers develop decades after infection with human papillomavirus, and births and infections such as pneumonia and influenza have regular seasonal patterns. Iatrogenic morbidity in teaching

PANEL 2.1 ■ Examples of Early Leads From Descriptive Studies	
Clinical Observation	*Underlying Association*
Hepatocellular adenoma in young women	Exposure to high-dose oral contraceptives
Blindness in newborn infants	High ambient oxygen concentrations in incubators
Kaposi sarcoma in young men	Infection with HIV-1
Angiosarcoma of the liver in employees	Industrial exposure to vinyl chloride
Cataracts, heart defects, and deafness in newborns	Maternal infection with rubella during pregnancy
Gout	Lead nephropathy among plumbers and painters[21]

hospitals has seasonal variation as well, when new trainees arrive in July.[23] (Readers should try to schedule illnesses later in the academic year.)

Where Does or Does Not the Disease or Condition Arise?

Like age, geography influences health. Proximity to rodents and insects (and their parasites) has shaped both medical and political history (e.g., the Black Plague). Despite high levels of public hygiene in ancient Rome, including public baths and toilets (Fig. 2.1), gastrointestinal parasites were common in the population.[24] Living downwind from a smelter[25] or drinking city water in Flint, Michigan,[26] can lead to lead poisoning. The prevalence of malaria is inversely related to elevation above sea level,[27] and Zika virus infection has emerged as another mosquito-borne illness of importance; weather patterns may influence its spread.[28]

So What?

The implicit 'W' relates to the public health effect.[29,30] Is the condition a current and timely one? Is it serious? Are large numbers involved? Are its societal implications broad? Has it been studied before? Although many descriptive reports herald new illnesses or monitor health, the net effect of others might be only thicker curricula vitae at the expense of thinner forests.

Types of Descriptive Studies

Descriptive studies consist of two major groups: those that deal with individuals and those that relate to populations. Studies that involve individuals are the case report, the case-series report, cross-sectional studies, and surveillance, whereas ecological correlational studies examine populations.

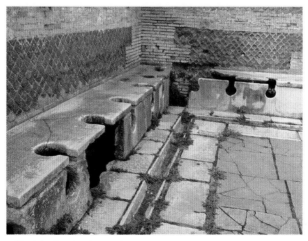

Fig. 2.1 Public toilets in Ostia Antica, the seaport of ancient Rome.

CASE REPORT

The case report is the least publishable unit in the medical literature. Often, an observant clinician reports an unusual disease or association, which prompts further investigations with more rigorous study designs (see Panel 2.1). For example, clinicians reported benign hepatocellular adenomas, a rare tumour, in women who had taken oral contraceptives.[31] A large case-control study pursued this lead and confirmed a strong association between long-term use of high-dose pills and this rare, but sometimes deadly, tumour.[32] Not all case reports deal with serious health threats, however; some simply enliven the generally bland medical literature. Examples include joggers' nipples,[33] chicken bones in the uterus,[34] and scrotal burn from a laptop computer.[35]

Some journals refuse to publish case reports, perhaps because they can drag down the journal's impact factor.[36] In response, the number of journals devoted to case reports is increasing exponentially.[37] Because of inconsistent and incomplete reporting of unusual cases, the **Ca**se **Re**port (CARE) reporting guidelines[38] have been developed, analogous to CONSORT[39] and STROBE[40] guidelines. The CARE guidelines have a 13-point checklist for necessary elements of a case report. Similarly, the **Su**rgical **Ca**se **Re**port (SCARE) guidelines[41] were developed by consensus for surgical case reports. The effect of these new guidelines will need evaluation in the years ahead. Suggestions have been made for standardising the peer review of submitted case reports as well.[42]

CASE-SERIES REPORT

A case series aggregates individual cases in one report. It is defined as 'a collection of subjects (usually patients) with common characteristics used to describe some clinical, pathophysiological, or operational aspect of a disease, treatment, exposure, or diagnostic procedure. Some are similar to the larger case reports and share their virtues'.[4] Sometimes, the appearance of several similar cases in a short period heralds an epidemic.[43] For example, a cluster of homosexual men in Los Angeles with a similar clinical syndrome alerted the medical community to the AIDS epidemic in North America.[44] Whereas a report of a single unusual case might not trigger further investigation, a case series of several unusual cases (in excess of what might typically be expected) adds to the concern. A convenient feature of case-series reports is that they can constitute the case group for a case-control study, which can then explore hunches about causes of disease.

The distinction between case-series reports and cohort studies is murky. Dekkers et al.[45] and Esene et al.[46] have suggested that a case series samples participants based on an **outcome** (with or without regard to exposure); absolute risks cannot be determined. A cohort study chooses participants based on **exposure**, follows them to outcome, and calculates absolute risks. However, in their view, inclusion of a comparison group is not essential to be deemed a cohort study. Others continue to advocate the definitions we use in this book.[47,48] Analogous to the SCARE guidelines[41] described previously, the **P**referred **R**eporting **O**f **Ca**se **S**eries in **S**urgery (PROCESS) guidelines[49] have been promulgated for case-series reports in the surgical disciplines.

CROSS-SECTIONAL (PREVALENCE) STUDIES

Prevalence studies describe the health of populations. The definition is 'a study that examines the relationship between disease (or other health outcomes) and other variables of interest as they exist in a defined population at one particular time'.[4] Synonyms include 'prevalence study' and 'disease-frequency survey'. Cross-sectional studies can be considered a snapshot of the population at one moment of time; prevalence is the measure, as opposed to incidence. For example, in the United States, periodic surveys of the health status of the population are done by the federal government (e.g., the Health Interview Survey and the Health and Nutrition Examination Survey).

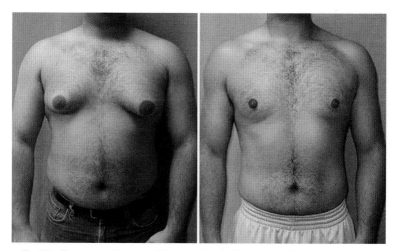

Fig. 2.2 Gynaecomastia, a condition associated with drugs and liver disease in men.

Analogous to the decennial census, these studies provide an assessment of the population at a particular time.

Prevalence studies can be done in smaller populations as well. For example, a survey done in a Puerto Rican pharmaceutical factory indicated a high prevalence of gynaecomastia among employees (Fig. 2.2). This finding led to the hunch that exposure to ambient oestrogen dust in the plant might be the cause; serum concentrations of oestrogen lent support to the hypothesis. After improvements in dust control in the factory, the epidemic disappeared.[50] Gynaecomastia can be either endogenous from abnormal hormonal status or exogenous from drugs or herbs.[51,52]

Although generally distinguished from cohort and case-control studies, the cross-sectional study can be thought of as a hybrid, the case-control analogue of a population cohort study. Because both exposure and outcome are ascertained at the same time (the defining feature of a cross-sectional study), costs are small and loss to follow-up is not a problem. However, because exposure and outcome are identified at one time point, the temporal sequence is often impossible to work out. An exception would be long-standing exposures, such as sex or blood type, which unquestionably preceded the outcome.

SURVEILLANCE

Surveillance is another important type of descriptive study. Surveillance can be thought of as watchfulness over a community. A more formal definition is 'systematic and continuous collection, analysis, and interpretation of data, closely integrated with the timely and coherent dissemination of the results and assessment to those who have the right to know so that action can be taken'.[4] The key feature here is feedback, as in a servomechanism. Prevention and control of the problem are fundamental parts of the feedback loop.

Surveillance can be either active or passive. Passive surveillance relies on data generally gathered through traditional channels, such as death certificates. By contrast, active surveillance searches for cases. Active surveillance can improve sensitivity. Investigators in the Philippines compared the incidence rate of dengue fever in a prospective seroepidemiological cohort study (active surveillance) with the incidence rate derived from the city health department (passive surveillance). The cumulative incidence rate was five times higher with active surveillance.[53]

Active surveillance can improve specificity as well. For example, septic transfusion reactions remain a problem in hospitals. Active surveillance by culturing aliquots of transfused platelets over 7 years found a prevalence of bacterially contaminated products of $389/10^6$ (20 of 51,440 units). Five neutropenic patients had septic transfusion reactions, and none was identified through passive surveillance. In contrast, 284 septic transfusion reactions were reported through passive surveillance, but none had received contaminated platelets.[54] Passive surveillance had poor sensitivity and specificity.

Epidemiological surveillance has made important contributions to health, but none more impressive than smallpox eradication. Surveillance and containment were in part responsible for the elimination of smallpox from the world, an extraordinary public-health achievement.[55] Without a nonhuman vector, the virus died out. Surveillance indicated that by 2014, four of six World Health Organization regions had been declared free of polio, and work continues towards its elimination.[6] Rinderpest, a disease of cattle, was declared eradicated in 2011, and dracunculiasis (guinea worm disease) may be the next important disease to be wiped off the planet.[56]

ECOLOGICAL CORRELATIONAL STUDIES

Correlational studies look for associations between exposures and outcomes in populations rather than in individuals.[4] Because the data might already have been collected, correlational studies can be a convenient initial search for hypotheses. The measure of association between exposure and outcome is the correlation coefficient r, which indicates how linear is the relation between exposure and outcome. US counties at high elevation have lower rates of heart disease than do counties at low altitude.[57] What this means is unclear. Another ecological study found no correlation between statin use and coronary mortality in Western Europe.[58] In contrast, an inverse relationship between oral contraceptive use and ovarian cancer incidence has been documented in several countries, which is plausible, based on analytic study results.[59]

Correlational studies have important limitations (i.e., the inability to link exposure to outcome in individuals and to control for confounding, a mixing or blurring of effects). A particular trap of ecological studies is an error in logic termed 'ecological fallacy', 'an erroneous inference that may occur because an association observed between variables on an aggregate level does not necessarily represent or reflect the association that exists at an individual level…'.[4] For example, an ecological correlation study compared nighttime light levels (judged by satellite imaging) and breast-cancer rates by census tract in Connecticut. Cancer rates came from the state tumour registry. The report implied causality in its results that '…support the possibility that electric light at night accounts for a portion of the breast cancer burden in high-risk societies'.[60] Really? Before turning off street lights to protect women's breasts, better evidence will be required. Like case reports and case-series reports, ecological studies can generate hypotheses but not definitive answers.[61]

Uses of Descriptive Studies

TREND ANALYSIS

Descriptive studies play several useful roles. Being able to monitor the health of populations is important to healthcare administrators. Trend analysis is often provided by ongoing surveillance. Examples include the epidemic of syphilis and HIV infection in Russia,[62] multiple births from assisted reproductive technologies,[63] and obesity across the United States.[64] Each of these epidemics raises troubling societal issues.

PLANNING

A second use is healthcare planning. For example, the introduction of laparoscopy, coupled with bad press about oral contraceptives and intrauterine devices, tripled US rates of tubal sterilisation in the 1970s.[65] Hospitals and ambulatory surgery centres had a surge in demand for operations, yet less need for hospital beds. Between 1981 and 1995, inpatient interval tubal sterilisation completely migrated to outpatient procedures.[66] The growing use of long-acting reversible methods of contraception may be decreasing reliance on tubal sterilisation procedures as well.[67]

CLUES ABOUT CAUSE

A third (and most fun) use of descriptive studies is to develop hypotheses about cause[68] (see Panel 2.1). Observant clinicians noted an association between high concentrations of oxygen in incubators and blindness in babies; this finding led to analytical studies, then a randomised controlled trial, confirming the association.[69] Few fans of singer Stevie Wonder, born prematurely in 1950, know that he became blind from his time in an incubator.[70] The link between intrauterine exposure to thalidomide and limb-reduction defects was first chronicled in correspondence with *The Lancet*.[71] Case reports and case-series reports have highlighted dangers associated with homoeopathy.[72] Today's bisphosphonate-induced osteonecrosis of the jaw[73] had an earlier manifestation—'phossy jaw' (Fig. 2.3)—in the late 19th century among factory workers exposed to yellow phosphorus, a key component of 'strike-anywhere' matches.[74] Case reports and case-series reports published in *The Lancet* have prompted randomised controlled trials to evaluate promising leads.[75]

Advantages and Disadvantages

Descriptive studies have both strengths and weaknesses. Often, the data are already available and thus inexpensive and efficient to use. Furthermore, few ethical difficulties exist because no new intervention is involved. However, descriptive studies have important limitations. Temporal

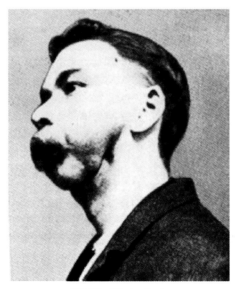

Fig. 2.3 'Phossy jaw'.

associations between putative causes and effects might be unclear. A dangerous pitfall is that the investigators might draw causal inferences when none is possible.

OVERSTEPPING THE DATA

A common mistake in inference is *post hoc ergo propter hoc* reasoning (after the thing, therefore on account of the thing), an example of a false cause. This illogic often prevails in courts of law but should not in science.[76] In other words, a temporal association is incorrectly inferred to be a causal one. In one egregious example, seven women in Pasadena, California, created controversy around the world in the late 1980s. Seen in one physician's office, the women had developed functional ovarian cysts while taking the new multiphasic oral-contraceptive pills.[5] Based on this case-series report, the report warned that phasic pills might pose a threat to patient health and safety. The media carried the story, and unknown numbers of women around the world stopped taking their pills, because they did not understand the difference between functional cysts and ovarian cancer. Because the report had no comparison group (e.g., women using monophasic pills or those using other contraceptives), the authors could not draw any conclusions about cause of disease.

In the wake of this report, damage-control efforts started quickly. Within 2 years, a publication showed no temporal association between the marketing of multiphasic pills and the number of women admitted to hospital for treatment of benign ovarian cysts.[77] However, 5 years elapsed before cohort[78] and case-control studies[79] confirmed no association between multiphasic pills and ovarian cysts. By this time, the public-health damage had been done; pill scares led to unplanned pregnancies and preventable abortions.[80] The unjustified causal implication from this case-series report was both unwarranted and unethical.[81,82]

Another sad example in which misinterpretation of descriptive studies hurt public health is routine electronic foetal monitoring in labour. A quarter of a century ago, temporal associations between the introduction of electronic foetal monitoring and falling perinatal mortality rates led to the conclusion that continuous foetal heart-rate monitoring was beneficial. (One could make an equally robust claim for hand-held calculators and pet rocks.)

Based on this rosy assessment from prominent obstetricians, this expensive and intrusive technology took obstetrics by storm. However, the initial upbeat assessment did not survive scientific scrutiny. Randomised controlled trials showed that, by comparison with routine intermittent auscultation, routine electronic foetal monitoring confers no lasting benefit to infants, but it significantly increases operative deliveries, thus harming women.[83] Despite this evidence, most births in the United States include electronic foetal monitoring. Failure to appreciate the limitations of descriptive studies caused lasting harm and squandered billions of dollars, a massive and ongoing public-health blunder. The contemporary analogy in women's health is the explosion of robotic surgery, for which there is no established indication at the time of this writing.[84] The medical-industrial complex endangers patient health.[85]

Conclusion

Descriptive studies are often the first, tentative approach to a new event or condition. These studies generally emphasise features of a new disease or assess the health status of communities. Health administrators use descriptive studies to monitor trends and plan for resources. By contrast, epidemiologists and clinicians generally use descriptive reports to search for clues of cause of disease (i.e., generation of hypotheses). In this role, descriptive studies are often a springboard into more rigorous studies with comparison groups. Common pitfalls of descriptive reports include an absence of a clear, specific, and reproducible case definition, and interpretations that overstep the data. Studies without a comparison group do not allow conclusions about cause of disease.

References

1. Hulley, S.B., Cummings, S.R., Browner, W.S., Grady, D., Newman, T.B., 2013. Designing Clinical Research, fourth ed. Lippincott Williams & Wilkins, Philadelphia.
2. Kuroki, L.M., Allsworth, J.E., Peipert, J.F., 2009. Methodology and analytic techniques used in clinical research: associations with journal impact factor. Obstet. Gynecol. 114, 877–884.
3. Kocak, F.U., Unver, B., Karatosun, V., 2011. Level of evidence in four selected rehabilitation journals. Arch. Phys. Med. Rehabil. 92, 299–303.
4. Porta, M., 2014. A Dictionary of Epidemiology. Oxford University Press, New York.
5. Caillouette, J.C., Koehler, A.L., 1987. Phasic contraceptive pills and functional ovarian cysts. Am. J. Obstet. Gynecol. 156, 1538–1542.
6. Maes, E.F., Diop, O.M., Jorba, J., Chavan, S., Tangermann, R.H., Wassilak, S.G., 2017. Surveillance systems to track progress toward polio eradication—worldwide, 2015-2016. MMWR Morb. Mortal. Wkly Rep. 66, 359–365.
7. Garbelli, A., Riva, V., Crespan, E., Maga, G., 2017. How to win the HIV-1 drug resistance hurdle race: running faster or jumping higher? Biochem. J. 474, 1559–1577.
8. Puurunen, M.K., Gona, P.N., Larson, M.G., Murabito, J.M., Magnani, J.W., O'Donnell, C.J., 2016. Epidemiology of venous thromboembolism in the Framingham Heart Study. Thromb. Res. 145, 27–33.
9. Brinton, L.A., Cook, M.B., McCormack, V., et al., 2014. Anthropometric and hormonal risk factors for male breast cancer: male breast cancer pooling project results. J. Natl. Cancer Inst. 106, djt465.
10. Stewart, E.A., Cookson, C., Gandolfo, R.A., Schulze-Rath, R., 2017. Epidemiology of uterine fibroids: a systematic review. BJOG 124, 1501–1512.
11. Azike, J.E., 2009. A review of the history, epidemiology and treatment of squamous cell carcinoma of the scrotum. Rare Tumors 1, e17.
12. Levin, P., 2007. From mad hatters to dental amalgams: heavy metals: toxicity and testing. MLO Med. Lab. Obs. 39, 20, 2, 4.
13. Byard, R.W., 2013. Commercial fishing industry deaths—forensic issues. J. Forensic Legal Med. 20, 129–132.
14. Bethea, A., Samanta, D., Willis, J.A., Lucente, F.C., Chumbe, J.T., 2016. Substance exposure and helmet use in all-terrain vehicle accidents: nine years of experience at a level 1 trauma center. J. Saf. Res. 59, 61–67.
15. Vanlaar, W., McAteer, H., Brown, S., Crain, J., McFaull, S., Hing, M.M., 2015. Injuries related to off-road vehicles in Canada. Accid. Anal. Prev. 75, 264–271.
16. Hager, W.D., Eschenbach, D.A., Spence, M.R., Sweet, R.L., 1983. Criteria for diagnosis and grading of salpingitis. Obstet. Gynecol. 61, 113–114.
17. Hadgu, A., Westrom, L., Brooks, C.A., Reynolds, G.H., Thompson, S.E., 1986. Predicting acute pelvic inflammatory disease: a multivariate analysis. Am. J. Obstet. Gynecol. 155, 954–960.
18. Risser, J.M., Risser, W.L., 2009. Purulent vaginal and cervical discharge in the diagnosis of pelvic inflammatory disease. Int. J. STD AIDS 20, 73–76.
19. DeVries, A.S., Lesher, L., Schlievert, P.M., et al., 2011. Staphylococcal toxic shock syndrome 2000-2006: epidemiology, clinical features, and molecular characteristics. PLoS One 6, e22997.
20. Schneider, E., Whitmore, S., Glynn, K.M., Dominguez, K., Mitsch, A., McKenna, M.T., 2008. Revised surveillance case definitions for HIV infection among adults, adolescents, and children aged <18 months and for HIV infection and AIDS among children aged 18 months to <13 years—United States, 2008. MMWR Recomm. Rep. 57, 1–12.
21. Chow, K.M., Liu, Z.C., Szeto, C.C., 2006. Lead nephropathy: early leads from descriptive studies. Intern. Med. J. 36, 678–682.
22. Plato, N., Martinsen, J.I., Sparen, P., Hillerdal, G., Weiderpass, E., 2016. Occupation and mesothelioma in Sweden: updated incidence in men and women in the 27 years after the asbestos ban. Epidemiol. Health 38, e2016039.
23. Inaba, K., Recinos, G., Teixeira, P.G., et al., 2010. Complications and death at the start of the new academic year: is there a July phenomenon? J. Trauma. 68, 19–22.
24. Mitchell, P.D., 2017. Human parasites in the Roman World: health consequences of conquering an empire. Parasitology 144, 48–58.
25. Soto-Jimenez, M.F., Flegal, A.R., 2011. Childhood lead poisoning from the smelter in Torreon, Mexico. Environ. Res. 111, 590–596.

26. Campbell, C., Greenberg, R., Mankikar, D., Ross, R.D., 2016. A case study of environmental injustice: the failure in Flint. Int. J. Environ. Res. Public Health 13, 951.
27. Betuela, I., Maraga, S., Hetzel, M.W., et al., 2012. Epidemiology of malaria in the Papua New Guinean highlands. Tropical Med. Int. Health 17, 1181–1191.
28. Caminade, C., Turner, J., Metelmann, S., et al., 2017. Global risk model for vector-borne transmission of Zika virus reveals the role of El Nino 2015. Proc. Natl. Acad. Sci. U. S. A. 114, 119–124.
29. Rogawski, E.T., Gray, C.L., Poole, C., 2016. An argument for renewed focus on epidemiology for public health. Ann. Epidemiol. 26, 729–733.
30. Chapman, P.M., Guerra, L.M., 2005. The "so what?" factor. Mar. Pollut. Bull. 50, 1457–1458.
31. Schenken, J.R., 1976. Letter: Hepatocellular adenoma: relationship to oral contraceptives? JAMA 236, 559.
32. Rooks, J.B., Ory, H.W., Ishak, K.G., et al., 1979. Epidemiology of hepatocellular adenoma. The role of oral contraceptive use. JAMA 242, 644–648.
33. Levit, F., 1977. Jogger's nipples [letter]. N. Engl. J. Med. 297, 1127.
34. Hunger, C., Ring, A., 2001. Chicken bones in the uterus—an exceptional reason for sterility. Zentralbl. Gynakol. 123, 604–606.
35. Ostenson, C.G., 2002. Lap burn due to laptop computer. Lancet 360, 1704.
36. Carey, J.C., 2010. The importance of case reports in advancing scientific knowledge of rare diseases. Adv. Exp. Med. Biol. 686, 77–86.
37. Akers, K.G., 2016. New journals for publishing medical case reports. J. Med. Libr. Assoc. 104, 146–149.
38. Gagnier, J.J., Kienle, G., Altman, D.G., Moher, D., Sox, H., Riley, D., 2014. The CARE guidelines: consensus-based clinical case report guideline development. J. Clin. Epidemiol. 67, 46–51.
39. Schulz, K.F., Altman, D.G., Moher, D., 2010. CONSORT 2010 statement: updated guidelines for reporting parallel group randomised trials. BMJ 340, c332.
40. von Elm, E., Altman, D.G., Egger, M., Pocock, S.J., Gøtzsche, P.C., Vandenbroucke, J.P., 2007. The Strengthening the Reporting of Observational Studies in Epidemiology (STROBE) statement: guidelines for reporting observational studies. Lancet 370, 1453–1457.
41. Agha, R.A., Fowler, A.J., Saeta, A., Barai, I., Rajmohan, S., Orgill, D.P., 2016. The SCARE Statement: consensus-based surgical case report guidelines. Int. J. Surg. 34, 180–186.
42. Ramulu, V.G., Levine, R.B., Hebert, R.S., Wright, S.M., 2005. Development of a case report review instrument. Int. J. Clin. Pract. 59, 457–461.
43. Yang, L.J., Chang, K.W., Chung, K.C., 2012. Methodologically rigorous clinical research. Plast. Reconstr. Surg. 129, 979e–988e.
44. Centers for Disease Control and Prevention (CDC), 1996. Pneumocystis pneumonia—Los Angeles. 1981. MMWR Morb. Mortal. Wkly Rep. 45 (34), 729–733.
45. Dekkers, O.M., Egger, M., Altman, D.G., Vandenbroucke, J.P., 2012. Distinguishing case series from cohort studies. Ann. Intern. Med. 156, 37–40.
46. Esene, I.N., Ngu, J., El Zoghby, M., et al., 2014. Case series and descriptive cohort studies in neurosurgery: the confusion and solution. Childs Nerv. Syst. 30, 1321–1332.
47. Kooistra, B., Dijkman, B., Einhorn, T.A., Bhandari, M., 2009. How to design a good case series. J. Bone Joint Surg. Am. 91 (Suppl 3), 21–26.
48. Carey, T.S., Boden, S.D., 2003. A critical guide to case series reports. Spine (Phila Pa 1976) 28, 1631–1634.
49. Agha, R.A., Fowler, A.J., Rajmohan, S., Barai, I., Orgill, D.P., 2016. Preferred reporting of case series in surgery; the PROCESS guidelines. Int. J. Surg. 36, 319–323.
50. Harrington, J.M., Stein, G.F., Rivera, R.O., de Morales, A.V., 1978. The occupational hazards of formulating oral contraceptives—a survey of plant employees. Arch. Environ. Health 33, 12–15.
51. Ladizinski, B., Lee, K.C., Nutan, F.N., Higgins 2nd, H.W., Federman, D.G., 2014. Gynecomastia: etiologies, clinical presentations, diagnosis, and management. South. Med. J. 107, 44–49.
52. Nuttall, F.Q., Warrier, R.S., Gannon, M.C., 2015. Gynecomastia and drugs: a critical evaluation of the literature. Eur. J. Clin. Pharmacol. 71, 569–578.
53. Undurraga, E.A., Edillo, F.E., Erasmo, J.N., et al., 2017. Disease burden of dengue in the Philippines: adjusting for underreporting by comparing active and passive dengue surveillance in Punta Princesa, Cebu City. Am. J. Trop. Med. Hyg. 96, 887–898.
54. Hong, H., Xiao, W., Lazarus, H.M., Good, C.E., Maitta, R.W., Jacobs, M.R., 2016. Detection of septic transfusion reactions to platelet transfusions by active and passive surveillance. Blood 127, 496–502.

55. Henderson, D.A., Klepac, P., 2013. Lessons from the eradication of smallpox: an interview with D. A. Henderson. Philos. Trans. R. Soc. Lond. B Biol. Sci. 368, 20130113.

56. The Lancet Infectious Diseases, 2016. Guinea worm disease nears eradication. Lancet Infect. Dis. 16, 131.

57. Hart J. Heart disease death rates in low versus high land elevation counties in the U.S. Dose-Response 2015, 13, https://doi.org/10.2203/dose-response.

58. Vancheri, F., Backlund, L., Strender, L.E., Godman, B., Wettermark, B., 2016. Time trends in statin utilisation and coronary mortality in Western European countries. BMJ Open 6, e010500.

59. Iversen, L., Sivasubramaniam, S., Lee, A.J., Fielding, S., Hannaford, P.C., 2017. Lifetime cancer risk and combined oral contraceptives: the Royal College of General Practitioners' Oral Contraception Study. Am. J. Obstet. Gynecol. 216, 580.e1–580.e9.

60. Portnov, B.A., Stevens, R.G., Samociuk, H., Wakefield, D., Gregorio, D.I., 2016. Light at night and breast cancer incidence in Connecticut: an ecological study of age group effects. Sci. Total Environ. 572, 1020–1024.

61. Sedgwick, P., 2014. Ecological studies: advantages and disadvantages. BMJ 348, g2979.

62. Shakarishvili, A., Dubovskaya, L.K., Zohrabyan, L.S., et al., 2005. Sex work, drug use, HIV infection, and spread of sexually transmitted infections in Moscow, Russian Federation. Lancet 366, 57–60.

63. Luke B., 2017. Pregnancy and birth outcomes in couples with infertility with and without assisted reproductive technology: with an emphasis on US population-based studies. Am. J. Obstet. Gynecol. 217, 270–281.

64. Flegal, K.M., Kruszon-Moran, D., Carroll, M.D., Fryar, C.D., Ogden, C.L., 2016. Trends in obesity among adults in the United States, 2005 to 2014. JAMA 315, 2284–2291.

65. Peterson, H.B., Greenspan, J.R., DeStefano, F., Ory, H.W., Layde, P.M., 1981. The impact of laparoscopy on tubal sterilization in United States hospitals, 1970 and 1975 to 1978. Am. J. Obstet. Gynecol. 140, 811–814.

66. Chan, L.M., Westhoff, C.L., 2010. Tubal sterilization trends in the United States. Fertil. Steril. 94, 1–6.

67. Finer, L.B., Jerman, J., Kavanaugh, M.L., 2012. Changes in use of long-acting contraceptive methods in the United States, 2007-2009. Fertil. Steril. 98, 893–897.

68. Lennon, P., Fenton, J.E., 2011. The case for the case report: refine to save. Ir. J. Med. Sci. 180, 529–532.

69. Silverman, W.A., 1991. Memories of the 1953-54 Oxygen Trial and its aftermath. The failure of success. Control. Clin. Trials 12, 355–358.

70. Fanaroff, J.M., 2013. Ethical support for surfactant, positive pressure, and oxygenation randomized trial (SUPPORT). J. Pediatr. 163, 1498–1499.

71. Riley, D., 2013. Case reports in the era of clinical trials. Glob. Adv. Health Med. 2 (2), 10–11. https://doi.org/10.7453/gahmj.2013.012. PMID: 24416660.

72. Posadzki, P., Alotaibi, A., Ernst, E., 2012. Adverse effects of homeopathy: a systematic review of published case reports and case series. Int. J. Clin. Pract. 66, 1178–1188.

73. de Boissieu, P., Gaboriau, L., Morel, A., Trenque, T., 2016. Bisphosphonate-related osteonecrosis of the jaw: data from the French national pharmacovigilance database. Fundam. Clin. Pharmacol. 30, 450–458.

74. Marx, R.E., 2008. Uncovering the cause of "phossy jaw" Circa 1858 to 1906: oral and maxillofacial surgery closed case files-case closed. J. Oral Maxillofac. Surg. 66, 2356–2363.

75. Albrecht, J., Meves, A., Bigby, M., 2005. Case reports and case series from Lancet had significant impact on medical literature. J. Clin. Epidemiol. 58, 1227–1232.

76. Brent, R.L., 1995. Bendectin: review of the medical literature of a comprehensively studied human non-teratogen and the most prevalent tortogen-litigen. Reprod. Toxicol. 9, 337–349.

77. Grimes, D.A., Hughes, J.M., 1989. Use of multiphasic oral contraceptives and hospitalizations of women with functional ovarian cysts in the United States. Obstet. Gynecol. 73, 1037–1039.

78. Lanes, S.F., Birmann, B., Walker, A.M., Singer, S., 1992. Oral contraceptive type and functional ovarian cysts. Am. J. Obstet. Gynecol. 166, 956–961.

79. Holt, V.L., Daling, J.R., McKnight, B., Moore, D., Stergachis, A., Weiss, N.S., 1992. Functional ovarian cysts in relation to the use of monophasic and triphasic oral contraceptives. Obstet. Gynecol. 79, 529–533.

80. Goodyear-Smith, F., Arroll, B., 2002. Termination of pregnancy following panic-stopping of oral contraceptives. Contraception 66, 163–167.

81. Altman, D.G., 1994. The scandal of poor medical research. BMJ 308, 283–284.

82. von Elm, E., Egger, M., 2004. The scandal of poor epidemiological research. BMJ 329, 868–869.
83. Alfirevic, Z., Devane, D., Gyte, G.M., Cuthbert, A., 2017. Continuous cardiotocography (CTG) as a form of electronic fetal monitoring (EFM) for fetal assessment during labour. Cochrane Database Syst. Rev. 2, CD006066.
84. Liu, H., Lawrie, T.A., Lu, D., Song, H., Wang, L., Shi, G., 2014. Robot-assisted surgery in gynaecology. Cochrane Database Syst. Rev. 12, CD011422.
85. Relman, A.S., 1980. The new medical-industrial complex. N. Engl. J. Med. 303, 963–970.

CHAPTER 3

Bias and Causal Associations in Observational Research

Readers of medical literature need to consider two types of validity, internal and external. Internal validity means that the study measured what it set out to; external validity is the ability to generalise from the study to the reader's patients. Bias is a systematic distortion of the truth. With respect to internal validity, all observational research has some degree of selection bias, information bias, and confounding bias. Selection bias stems from an absence of comparability between groups being studied. The effect of information bias depends on its type. If information is gathered differently for one group than for another, bias results. By contrast, nondifferential misclassification (noise) tends to obscure real differences. Confounding is a mixing or blurring of effects: a researcher attempts to relate an exposure to an outcome but actually measures the effect of a third factor (the confounding variable). Confounding can be controlled in several ways: restriction, matching, stratification, multivariable techniques, and propensity scores. If a reader cannot explain away study results on the basis of selection, information, or confounding bias, then chance might be another explanation. Chance should be examined last, however, as these biases can account for significant, though bogus, results. Differentiation between spurious, indirect, and causal associations can be difficult. Considerations such as temporal sequence, strength and consistency of an association, and evidence of a dose–response effect lend support to a causal link. Unlike the physical sciences, the biological sciences lack absolute truths. In clinical research, all we have are hypotheses. Observational epidemiology is a young science and a blunt tool; its findings should always be viewed as tentative.

Clinicians face two important questions as they read medical research: is the report believable and if so, is it relevant to my practice? Uncritical acceptance of published research has led to serious errors and squandered resources.[1] Based on observational studies, the American Heart Association used to recommend menopausal oestrogen therapy for prevention of heart disease. Taking vitamins B, C, E, and beta-carotene was thought to prevent heart disease. Fibre and folate intake were thought to protect against colorectal cancer. All these hypotheses were refuted by randomised controlled trials.[2] In this chapter, we will discuss two types of validity, describe a simple checklist for readers, and offer some considerations by which to judge reported associations.

Internal and External Validity

Analogous to a laboratory test, a study should have internal validity (i.e., the ability to measure what it sets out to measure). Internal validity is 'the degree to which a study is free from bias or systematic error'.[3] Errors stemming from random, not systematic error, relate to precision. Given the choice between internal validity and precision, the former usually deserves priority. A valid study result with some imprecision is preferable to a precisely wrong answer due to a huge sample size and inadequate control of bias.[4,5] Internal validity is the *sine qua non* of clinical research; extrapolation of invalid results to the broader population is not only worthless but potentially dangerous.

A second important concern is external validity: can results from study participants be extrapolated to the reader's patients? External validity is defined as 'the degree to which results of a study may apply, be generalised, or be transported to populations or groups that did not participate in the study'.[3] Because a total enumeration or census approach to medical research is usually impossible, the customary tactic is to choose a sample, study it, and, hopefully, extrapolate the result to one's practice. Gauging external validity is necessarily more subjective than is assessment of internal validity.

Internal and external validity entail important trade-offs. For example, randomised controlled trials are more likely than observational studies to be free of bias,[6] but because they usually enrol selected participants, external validity can suffer. This problem of atypical participants is also termed distorted assembly. Participants in randomised controlled trials tend to be different (including being healthier)[7,8] than those who choose not to take part, in part due to eligibility criteria.[9] The filtering process for admission to randomised trials might, therefore, result in an eclectic population no longer representative of the general public.

Bias

Bias undermines the internal validity of research. Unlike the conventional meaning of the word (i.e., prejudice), bias in research denotes a systematic, rather than random, deviation from the truth. All observational studies have built-in bias; the challenge for investigators, editors, and readers is to ferret these out and judge how they might have affected results. Regrettably, randomised controlled trials that do not follow the rules of conduct are vulnerable to bias,[10] and the methodological quality of trials is related to the observed results.[11-13]

A simple checklist, such as that shown in Panel 3.1, can be helpful when reading observational study reports.

Several glossaries have catalogued biases in clinical research. Sackett's original compilation included 35 different biases.[14] Since that early effort, the list of potential biases has grown. More recent lists include 69[15] to 74.[16] We are lumpers, not splitters, and prefer to group all these possible biases into three widely accepted categories: selection, information, and confounding.[16,17] The common theme for all three is 'different'.[17] Something 'different' systematically distorts the planned comparison.

PANEL 3.1 ■ What to Look for in Observational Studies

Is Selection Bias Present?

- In a cohort study, are participants in the exposed and unexposed groups similar in all important respects except for the exposure?
- In a case-control study, are cases and controls similar in all important respects except for the disease in question?

Is Information Bias Present?

- In a cohort study, is information about outcome obtained in the same way for those exposed and unexposed?
- In a case-control study, is information about exposure gathered in the same way for cases and controls?

Is Confounding Present?

- Could the results be accounted for by the presence of a factor (e.g., age, smoking, sexual behaviour, diet) associated with both the exposure and the outcome but not directly involved in the causal pathway?

If the Results Cannot Be Explained By These Three Biases, Could They Be the Result of Chance?

- Is the difference statistically significant, and, if not, did the study have adequate power to find a clinically important difference?
- What are the relative risk or odds ratio and 95% CI?
- Does the size of the treatment effect warrant attention, or is it likely due to bias (Chapter 7)?

Selection Bias

ARE THE GROUPS SIMILAR IN ALL IMPORTANT RESPECTS?

Selection bias stems from a disparity between groups being studied. For example, in a cohort study, the exposed and unexposed groups differ in some important respect aside from the exposure. Some use the term 'selection bias' to indicate that a nonrepresentative sample has been chosen for study.[18] Because this problem would not affect the internal validity of an analytic study, choosing a non-representative sample should be considered a problem with external validity and not a type of bias.[3]

Membership bias is a type of selection bias: people who choose to be members of a group (e.g., joggers) might differ in important respects from others. For instance, both cohort and case-control studies initially suggested that exercising after myocardial infarction prevented repeat infarction. However, a randomised controlled trial failed to confirm this benefit.[14] Those who chose to exercise might have differed in other important ways from those who did not exercise, such as diet, smoking, and presence of angina.

The protective effect of menopausal oestrogen therapy against coronary heart disease consistently found in observational studies was likely due to membership bias: women who chose to be oestrogen takers were healthier in other ways than those who did not. While the Women's Health Initiative trial[19] has been widely criticised for methodological flaws, the lack of cardioprotection from oestrogen in women more than 10 years into menopause has been corroborated in other trials.[20] However, women who started oestrogen within a decade of menopause enjoyed a reduction in both coronary heart disease and death.[20] Timing made a big difference, a feature missed in the original analysis.[19]

In case-control studies, selection bias implies that cases and controls differ importantly aside from the disease in question. Two types of selection bias have earned eponyms: Berkson and Neyman bias. Also known as an admission-rate bias, Berkson bias (or paradox) results from differential rates of hospital admission for cases and controls. The formal definition is 'a form of selection bias that arises when the variables whose association is under study affect selection of subjects into the study'.[3] Alternatively, knowledge of the exposure of interest might lead to an increased rate of admission to hospital. For example, doctors who care for women with salpingitis might be more likely to hospitalise those with a telltale IUD string noted on pelvic examination than those without.[21] In a hospital-based case-control study, this would stack the deck (or gynaecology ward) with a high proportion of intrauterine device (IUD)-exposed cases, spuriously increasing the odds ratio.

Neyman bias is an incidence–prevalence bias. It arises when a gap in time occurs between exposure and selection of study participants. This bias crops up in studies of diseases that are quickly fatal, transient, or subclinical. Neyman bias creates a case group not representative of cases in the community. For example, a hospital-based case-control study of myocardial infarction and snow shovelling (the exposure of interest) would miss individuals who died in their driveways and thus never reached a hospital; this might lower the odds ratio of infarction associated with this exposure.

Other types of selection bias include unmasking (detection signal) and nonrespondent bias. An exposure might lead to a search for an outcome, as well as the outcome itself. For example, women with leg pain and known to be taking oral contraceptives are more likely to get a diagnostic workup than are other women.[22] In observational studies, nonrespondents are different from respondents. In Denmark, nonresponders to health surveys have higher mortality rates of alcohol morbidity and mortality than do responders.[23] In the Netherlands, adolescent responders to a survey smoked less, drank less alcohol, and had better health status than did nonresponders.[24]

Loss to follow-up can undermine cohort studies. If participants are lost at random, computer models suggest that even large proportions lost do not bias the results. However, when losses were not random (presumably the usual real-life situation), even small proportions of loss to follow-up introduced serious bias.[25] This underscores the importance of diligent procedures to minimise such losses.[26] Here, an ounce of prevention can be worth a ton of cure.

Information Bias
HAS INFORMATION BEEN GATHERED IN THE SAME WAY?

Information bias, also known as observation, classification, ascertainment, and measurement bias, is defined as 'a flaw in measuring exposure, covariate, or outcome variables that results in different quality (accuracy) of information between comparison groups'.[3] In a cohort study or randomised controlled trial, information about outcomes should be obtained the same way for those exposed and unexposed. In a case-control study, information about exposure should be gathered in the same way for cases and controls.

Information bias can arise in many ways. For example, an investigator might gather information about an exposure for a case by bedside interview, but by telephone interview for a community control. The presence of a disease might prompt a more determined search for the putative exposure of interest for cases than for controls. To minimise information bias, detail about exposures in case-control studies should preferably be gathered by researchers unaware of whether the respondent is a case or a control. Similarly, in a cohort study with subjective outcomes, the observer should be unaware of the exposure status of each participant.

In case-control studies that rely on memory of remote exposures, recall bias is inescapable. Cases tend to search their memories to identify what might have caused their disease; healthy controls have no such motivation. Thus better recall among cases and underreporting among controls are routine. In a Swedish case-control study, the association between family history of cancer and lymphoma was consistently stronger based on self-report compared with registry data in Sweden.[27] Many case-control studies have reported an increase in cancer risk after abortion. However, when Swedish investigators compared histories of prior abortions obtained by personal interview with centralised medical records, they documented systematic underreporting of abortions among controls (but not among cases).[28] In cohort studies free from recall bias, induced abortion has had either a protective effect or no effect on risk of breast cancer.[29,30]

IS THE INFORMATION BIAS RANDOM OR IN ONE DIRECTION?

The effect of information bias depends on its type. If information is gathered differentially for one group than for another, then bias results, raising or lowering the relative risk or odds ratio dependent on the direction of the bias. By contrast, nondifferential misclassification (i.e., noise in the system) tends to obscure real differences. For example, an ambiguous questionnaire might lead to errors in data collection among cases and controls, shifting the odds ratio towards unity, meaning no association.

Confounding
IS AN EXTRANEOUS FACTOR BLURRING THE EFFECT?

Confounding is a mixing or blurring of effects. A researcher attempts to relate an exposure to an outcome but actually measures the effect of a third factor, termed a confounding variable. A confounding variable is associated with the exposure and it affects the outcome, but it is not an intermediate link in the chain of causation between exposure and outcome. More simply, confounding is a methodological fly in the ointment. Confounding is often easier to understand from examples than from definitions.

ORAL CONTRACEPTIVES AND MYOCARDIAL INFARCTION (AND SMOKING)

Early studies of the safety of oral contraceptives reported a pronounced increased risk of myocardial infarction. This association later proved to be spurious, because of the high proportion of cigarette smokers among users of birth control pills. Here, cigarette smoking confounded the relation between oral contraceptives and infarction. Women who chose to use birth control pills also chose, in large numbers, to smoke cigarettes, and cigarettes, in turn, increased the risk of myocardial infarction. Pill users who smoke have a dramatically increased risk of infarction; pill users without cardiovascular risk factors have no increased risk.[31] Although investigators thought they were measuring an effect of birth control pills, they were in fact measuring the confounding effect of smoking among pill users.

IUDs AND INFERTILITY (AND SEXUALLY TRANSMITTED DISEASE)

Case-control studies of IUDs and infertility nearly drove this highly effective contraceptive off the US market in the 1980s.[32,33] A reported doubling in the risk of tubal infertility related to IUD use led to dire warnings, a pharmaceutical company bankruptcy, an epidemic of lawsuits, and the disappearance of all copper IUDs.[34] Methodological flaws included failure to control adequately for the potentially confounding effect of sexually transmitted diseases.[35] However, nearly two decades passed until empirical evidence was available. A case-control study of tubal obstruction in Mexico City performed a chlamydia serology test on each case and control. Women who had used an IUD in the past had no increase in the risk of tubal obstruction; in contrast, nonusers with serological evidence of prior infection had a significant increase in risk (odds ratio 2.4; 95% CI 1.7–3.2).[36]

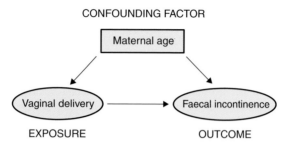

Fig. 3.1 Simple example of a directed acyclic graph. Here, age is a confounder for vaginal birth causing faecal incontinence. Maternal age is a cause of both childbirth and faecal incontinence, as indicated by the one-way arrow. To control for this confounding factor, the researcher would need to 'condition' (i.e., control for confounding by restriction, stratification, or multivariable methods) on the covariate maternal age. Conditioning is indicated by the box around the variable. By controlling for the confounder, the relationship between vaginal birth and faecal incontinence can be clarified.[77]

DIRECTED ACYCLIC GRAPHS

These causal diagrams, also termed causal graphs and path diagrams, are defined as 'a graphical display of causal relations among variables, in which each variable is assigned a fixed location on the graph (called a node), and in which each direct causal effect of one variable on another is represented by an arrow with its tail at the cause and its head at the effect'.[3] The descriptor 'acyclic' indicates no feedback loop; no variable can affect itself (Fig. 3.1). These graphs are sometimes used to help identify when to control for variables in the causal mix. Free software is available for creating directed acyclic graphs (DAGs).[37]

One of us (D.A.G.) regrets the lack of background research on 'DAG' before popularising the acronym: a 'dag' is matted faecal matter in wool around the perineum of a sheep.[38] Descriptions of DAGs in epidemiology are available for those interested.[39-41] Descriptions of dags in sheep are available as well.[42,43]

Control for Confounding

When important levels of selection bias or information bias exist in a study, the damage is done. Internal validity is doomed. By contrast, when confounding is present, this bias can be corrected, provided that confounding was anticipated and the requisite information gathered. Confounding can be controlled for either before or after a study is done. The purpose of these approaches is to achieve homogeneity between study groups concerning the confounding factor. Indeed, the ability to control for this bias is operationally what differentiates selection bias from confounding. In selection bias, unbalanced choice of participants and differential losses to follow-up pose incurable problems. The selection bias factors were either not measured or unmeasureable. In contrast, confounding bias can be remedied.[17] Despite guidelines for the reporting on confounding in observational research,[44] most reports do not handle this well.[45]

Confounding factors that are unsuspected or for which no information is available cannot be remedied. This problem of 'residual confounding'[46] plagues the analytic study literature, and quantitative methods have been proposed to estimate its effect.[47] Essentially, an unmeasured confounding bias becomes a selection bias. The only known way to control for unknown confounding is a randomised controlled trial.

RESTRICTION

The simplest approach is restriction (also called exclusion or specification).[48,49] For example, if cigarette smoking is suspected to be a confounding factor, a study can enrol only nonsmokers. Although this tactic avoids confounding, it reduces power and precludes extrapolation to smokers. Restriction might increase the internal validity of a study at the cost of poorer external validity. For these reasons, restriction is rarely used.

MATCHING

Another way to control for confounding is pairwise matching. In a case-control study in which smoking is deemed a confounding factor, cases and controls can be matched by smoking status. For each case who smokes, a control who smokes is found. This approach, although often used by investigators, has drawbacks. If matching is done on several potential confounding factors, the recruitment process can be cumbersome, and, by definition, one cannot examine the effect of a matched variable.[50] Sometimes a match cannot be found for a case if the pool of controls is small, and information is lost.

STRATIFICATION

Investigators can also control for confounding after a study has been completed. One approach is stratification.[51] Stratification is defined as 'the process of or result of separating a sample into several subsamples according to specified criteria, such as age groups, socioeconomic status, etc. The effect of confounding variable may be controlled by stratifying the analysis of results…'.[3] It can be considered a form of *post hoc* restriction, done during the analysis rather than during the accrual phase of a study. For example, results can be stratified by levels of the confounding factor. In the smoking example discussed previously, results are calculated separately for smokers and nonsmokers to see if the same effect arises independent of smoking.

The Mantel–Haenszel procedure[49] combines the various strata into a summary statistic that describes the effect. The strata are weighted inversely to their variance (i.e., strata with larger numbers contribute more than those with smaller numbers). If the Mantel–Haenszel adjusted effect differs substantially from the crude effect, then confounding is deemed present. In this instance the adjusted estimate of effect is considered the better estimate to use.

Stratification is appealing because of its simplicity: one can examine stratum-specific effects. In addition, researchers can look for effect modification (interaction), in which the result varies markedly depending on the presence of a third factor.[52] Stratification has limits: as the number of confounders examined grows, the number of strata grows exponentially. To examine 10 dichotomous variables, 2^{10} strata (>1000) would be required.[49] Needless to say, this can result in sparse or no data in some strata,[49] and thus loss of information.

Confounding is not always intuitive, as shown by the fictitious example in Fig. 3.2. In this hypothetical cohort of 2000 women, use of an IUD was strongly related to development of salpingitis (relative risk 3.0; 95% CI 1.7–5.4). However, the number of sexual partners was related to women's choice of contraception and to their risk of upper-genital-tract infection. Here, a disproportionate number of women with more than one sexual partner chose to use an IUD (700 versus 300 women with only one partner). The number of partners was also related to the risk of infection (6% among those with >1 partner versus 1% among those with only one partner). In each stratum by number of partners, the relative risk is 1.0, indicating no association between the IUD and salpingitis. The Mantel–Haenszel weighted relative risk, which controls for this confounding effect, is 1.0 (95% CI 0.5–2.0). In this fictitious example, the apparent three fold increase in risk associated with IUD use was all due to confounding bias.

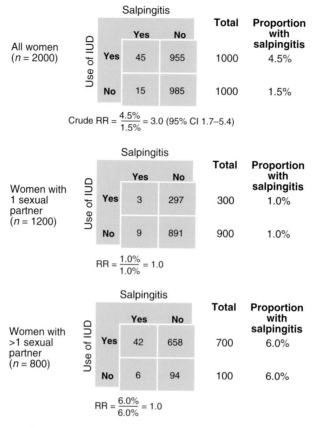

Fig. 3.2 Example of confounding in a hypothetical cohort study of intrauterine device use and salpingitis. When the crude relative risk (RR) is controlled for the confounding effect of number of sexual partners, the raised risk disappears.

MULTIVARIABLE ANALYSIS

In multivariable analysis, mathematical modelling examines the potential effect of one variable while simultaneously controlling for the effect of many other factors.[49] A major advantage of these approaches is that they can control for more factors than can simple stratification. For example, an investigator might use multivariate logistic regression to study the effect of oral contraceptives on ovarian cancer risk while simultaneously controlling for age, race, family history, parity, BRCA genes, etc. Another example would be use of a proportional hazards regression analysis for time to death; this method could control simultaneously for age, blood pressure, smoking history, serum lipids, and other risk factors.[53]

Disadvantages of multivariate approaches, for some researchers, include greater difficulty in understanding the results and loss of hands-on feel for the data. These techniques require expertise; when novices tackle logistic regression without training, strange outcomes are possible. Like surgeons, researchers should not dabble outside their area of expertise.

PROPENSITY SCORES

A propensity score is defined as 'the conditional probability of being exposed or treated given a certain set of measure covariates'.[3] When comparing outcomes for exposed and unexposed, the propensity score can help to adjust for differences in known covariates; the intended effect is to make the comparison groups more similar. This allows the research to balance the known and potentially important covariates between the groups being compared.[54]

Propensity scores are used in four general approaches: matching, stratification, covariance adjustment, and inverse probability of treatment weighting.[54] These methods are considered in detail elsewhere.[54-57] However, propensity score matching is often done incorrectly.[58] The bottom line seems to be that this complex approach is not demonstrably superior to well-accepted multivariable approaches.[59,60] Propensity scores are a current fad in epidemiological research. In general, we are wary of fads, especially when little empirical evidence supports their preferability. As evidence, both authors escaped the 1970s without owning a leisure suit.

SENSITIVITY ANALYSIS

Several other approaches to controlling for confounding are available. Sensitivity analysis, defined as 'a method to determine the robustness of an assessment by examining the extent to which results are affected by changes in methods, models, values of unmeasured variables, or assumptions'.[3] In this iterative process, the researcher looks at what effect varying assumptions have on the results—a set of 'what if' scenarios. For example, if changing value of a variable has little effect on the predicted result, then the variable probably does not explain variation in the outcome.[61] This technique can also explore the potential effect of hypothetical confounding factors. By inserting a factor into the model, the researcher would assign each participant an extreme value (e.g., all are male and then all are female) and see how that alters the weighting factors of the variables in the model.

INSTRUMENTAL VARIABLES

An instrumental variable is 'associated with the exposure, it affects the outcome only through the exposure, and it does not share any (uncontrolled) common cause with the outcome'.[3] The analysis separates the study population into strata according to the value of the instrumental variable; outcomes are examined by stratum. If the treatment rates vary by stratum but the outcome does not, then the exposure did not cause the outcome. On the other hand, if the outcomes differ by stratum, then this lends support to the exposure causing the outcome.[61]

In a pioneering study, the objective was to assess the effect of invasive technology (e.g., angioplasty) on survival 4 years after myocardial infarction.[62] Distance to a hospital was the instrumental variable. Those who lived distant from the hospital had less use of invasive technology but similar long-term outcomes, which suggests that any survival benefit from these invasive technologies is negligible.

Chance

If a reader cannot explain results on the basis of selection, information, or confounding bias, then chance might be another possibility. The reason for examining chance last in this sequence is that biases can easily cause statistically significant (though bogus) results. Alternatively, in huge data sets, the consideration of statistical significance is moot, because with a million participants,[52] every difference is statistically significant (though usually clinically meaningless). Regrettably, many readers (and some editors)[63] use the p value inappropriately: 'Yet fallacious and ritualistic use of tests continued to spread, including beliefs that whether P was above or below 0.05 was a universal arbiter of discovery'.[64]

Many clinicians are surprised to learn, however, that the p value of 0.05 as a threshold has no basis in medicine. Rather, it stems from agricultural and industrial experiments early in the 20th century.[63] Many 'negative' (better deemed 'indeterminate') studies simply have too few participants to do the job; conversely, in huge databases, nearly every difference is significant at a $p < 0.05$, a problem termed 'mass significance'. Investigators should use interval estimation with confidence intervals and not just hypothesis tests.[44,63,64]

Judging Associations
BOGUS, INDIRECT, OR REAL?

When statistical associations emerge from clinical research, the next step is to judge what type they are. Statistical associations do not necessarily imply causal associations. Indeed, a website and book are devoted to spurious statistical associations.[65] Examples include the correlation between the divorce rate in Maine and per capita consumption of margarine and, even more worrisome, between per capita cheese consumption and death from becoming tangled in bedsheets. Life is indeed a risky business, and none of us gets out alive.[66]

Although several classifications of associations are available, a simple approach includes just three types: spurious, indirect, and causal. Spurious associations are the result of selection bias, information bias, and chance. By contrast, indirect associations (which stem from confounding) are real but not causal. The risk of suicide increases in a dose-response relationship with cigarette smoking. This does not mean that smoking causes suicide. Instead, depressed persons are more likely to smoke; depression causes both smoking and suicide, so the association between cigarettes and smoking is due to the confounding effect of depression.[52]

Judgement of cause–effect relations can be tough. Few rules apply, but over the past half century, considerations first suggested by Hill[67] have received the most attention (Panel 3.2). The only iron-clad consideration is temporality: the cause must antedate the effect.[68] However, in many studies, especially with chronic diseases, answering this chicken–egg question can be daunting.

PANEL 3.2 ■ Considerations for Judging Causal Associations[67]

Temporal Sequence
- Did exposure precede outcome?

Strength of Association
- How strong is the effect, measured as relative risk or odds ratio?

Consistency of Association
- Has effect been seen by others?

Biological Gradient (Dose-Response Relation)
- Does increased exposure result in more of the outcome?

Specificity of Association
- Does exposure lead only to outcome?

Biological Plausibility
- Does the association make sense?

Coherence with Existing Knowledge
- Is the association consistent with other lines of available evidence (e.g., laboratory studies)?

Experimental Evidence
- Has a randomised controlled trial been done?

Analogy
- Is the association similar to others?

Strong associations support causation. How strong is strong? Hill's classic paper provided two examples: tainted water and cholera in the famous London epidemic, and smoking and death from lung cancer among British physicians. The smallest relative risks in these two examples were 14 and 8, respectively.[67] Observational research is adept at finding associations this large. However, these are seldom seen in contemporary research. Weak associations, which dominate in observational studies, can easily be due to bias,[68,69] and large amounts of bias readily produce strong (bogus) associations. Examples include the literature on IUDs and salpingitis[70] and abortion and breast cancer.[71] The 'world's record' may be a false 27-fold increase in ovarian cancer with fertility drugs.[52]

Consistent observation of an association in different populations and with different study designs also lends support to a real effect. For example, results of studies done around the world have consistently shown that oral contraceptives are associated with protection against ovarian cancer; a causal relation can, therefore, be argued.[72] Evidence of a biological gradient supports a causal association, too. For instance, protection against ovarian cancer is directly related to duration of use of oral contraceptives; the longer a woman takes birth control pills, the lower is her risk of this deadly cancer.[72] The risk of death from lung cancer is linearly related to years of cigarette smoking. In both of these examples, increasing exposure is associated with an increasing biological effect.

Other of Hill's considerations are less useful. Specificity is a weak one. With a few exceptions (perhaps the rabies virus), few exposures lead to only one outcome.[68] Should an association be highly specific, this provides support for causality. However, because many exposures (e.g., cigarette smoke or *Streptococcus pyogenes*) lead to numerous illnesses, lack of specificity does not argue against causation. Biological plausibility is another weak consideration, limited by our lack of knowledge.[73] Three hundred years ago, clinicians would have rejected the suggestion that citrus fruits could prevent scurvy or that mosquitoes were linked with blackwater fever (haemoglobinuria with malaria). The notion that bacteria could survive the acid environment of the stomach was unthinkable when we were in training.[74] Ancillary biological evidence that is coherent with the association might be helpful. For example, the effect of cigarette smoke on the bronchial epithelium of animals is coherent with an increased risk of cancer in human beings. Finally, experimental evidence is seldom available, and reasoning by analogy has sometimes caused harm. Because thalidomide can cause birth defects, for instance, some lawyers (successfully)[75] argued by analogy that Bendectin (an antiemetic widely used for nausea and vomiting in pregnancy) could also cause birth defects, despite evidence to the contrary.[76] After a lapse of several decades, the same drug is being marketed once again in the United States but with a different name. Same safe drug.

Conclusion

Studies need to have both internal and external validity: the results should be both correct and capable of extrapolation to the population. A simple checklist for bias (selection, information, and confounding) and then chance can help readers decipher research reports. When a statistical association appears in research, guidelines for judgement of associations can help a reader decide whether the association is bogus, indirect, or real.

References

1. Ioannidis, J.P., 2011. An epidemic of false claims. Competition and conflicts of interest distort too many medical findings. Sci. Am. 304, 16.
2. Shrank, W.H., Patrick, A.R., Brookhart, M.A., 2011. Healthy user and related biases in observational studies of preventive interventions: a primer for physicians. J. Gen. Intern. Med. 26, 546–550.
3. Porta, M., 2014. A Dictionary of Epidemiology. Oxford University Press, New York.
4. Grimes, D.A., 2010. Epidemiologic research using administrative databases: garbage in, garbage out. Obstet. Gynecol. 116, 1018–1019.

5. Dinger, J., Shapiro, S., 2012. Combined oral contraceptives, venous thromboembolism, and the problem of interpreting large but incomplete datasets. J. Fam. Plann. Reprod. Health Care 38, 2–6.

6. Ioannidis, J.P., Haidich, A.B., Pappa, M., et al., 2001. Comparison of evidence of treatment effects in randomized and nonrandomized studies. JAMA 286, 821–830.

7. Falagas, M.E., Vouloumanou, E.K., Sgouros, K., Athanasiou, S., Peppas, G., Siempos, I.I., 2010. Patients included in randomised controlled trials do not represent those seen in clinical practice: focus on antimicrobial agents. Int. J. Antimicrob. Agents 36, 1–13.

8. Uijen, A.A., Bakx, J.C., Mokkink, H.G., van Weel, C., 2007. Hypertension patients participating in trials differ in many aspects from patients treated in general practices. J. Clin. Epidemiol. 60, 330–335.

9. Carter, M.J., Fife, C.E., Walker, D., Thomson, B., 2009. Estimating the applicability of wound care randomized controlled trials to general wound-care populations by estimating the percentage of individuals excluded from a typical wound-care population in such trials. Adv. Skin Wound Care 22, 316–324.

10. Jadad, A.R., Enkin, M.W., 2008. Bias in randomized controlled trials. In: Randomized Controlled Trials: Questions, Answers, and Musings, Second ed. Blackwell Publishing Ltd, Oxford, pp. 29–47.

11. Schulz, K.F., Chalmers, I., Hayes, R.J., Altman, D.G., 1995. Empirical evidence of bias. Dimensions of methodological quality associated with estimates of treatment effects in controlled trials. JAMA 273, 408–412.

12. Moher, D., Pham, B., Jones, A., et al., 1998. Does quality of reports of randomised trials affect estimates of intervention efficacy reported in meta-analyses? Lancet 352, 609–613.

13. Savovic, J., Jones, H.E., Altman, D.G., et al., 2012. Influence of reported study design characteristics on intervention effect estimates from randomized, controlled trials. Ann. Intern. Med. 157, 429–438.

14. Sackett, D.L., 1979. Bias in analytic research. J. Chronic Dis. 32, 51–63.

15. Hartman, J.M., Forsen Jr., J.W., Wallace, M.S., Neely, J.G., 2002. Tutorials in clinical research: part IV: recognizing and controlling bias. Laryngoscope 112, 23–31.

16. Delgado-Rodriguez, M., Llorca, J., 2004. Bias. J. Epidemiol. Community Health 58, 635–641.

17. Schwartz, S., Campbell, U.B., Gatto, N.M., Gordon, K., 2015. Toward a clarification of the taxonomy of "bias" in epidemiology textbooks. Epidemiology 26, 216–222.

18. Sedgwick, P., 2014. Bias in observational study designs: prospective cohort studies. BMJ 349, g7731.

19. Writing Group for the Women's Health Initiative Investigators, 2002. Risks and benefits of estrogen plus progestin in healthy postmenopausal women: principal results From the Women's Health Initiative randomized controlled trial. JAMA 288, 321–333.

20. Boardman, H.M., Hartley, L., Eisinga, A., et al., 2015. Hormone therapy for preventing cardiovascular disease in post-menopausal women. Cochrane Database Syst. Rev. CD002229.

21. Kronmal, R.A., Whitney, C.W., Mumford, S.D., 1991. The intrauterine device and pelvic inflammatory disease: the Women's Health Study reanalyzed. J. Clin. Epidemiol. 44, 109–122.

22. Heinemann, L.A., Garbe, E., Farmer, R., Lewis, M.A., 2000. Venous thromboembolism and oral contraceptive use: a methodological study of diagnostic suspicion and referral bias. Eur. J. Contracept. Reprod. Health Care 5, 183–191.

23. Christensen, A.I., Ekholm, O., Gray, L., Glumer, C., Juel, K., 2015. What is wrong with nonrespondents? Alcohol-, drug- and smoking-related mortality and morbidity in a 12-year follow-up study of respondents and non-respondents in the Danish Health and Morbidity Survey. Addiction 110, 1505–1512.

24. Cheung, K.L., Ten Klooster, P.M., Smit, C., de Vries, H., Pieterse, M.E., 2017. The impact of nonresponse bias due to sampling in public health studies: a comparison of voluntary versus mandatory recruitment in a Dutch national survey on adolescent health. BMC Public Health 17, 276.

25. Kristman, V., Manno, M., Cote, P., 2004. Loss to follow-up in cohort studies: how much is too much? Eur. J. Epidemiol. 19, 751–760.

26. Dinger, J.C., Bardenheuer, K., Assmann, A., 2009. International Active Surveillance Study of Women Taking Oral Contraceptives (INAS-OC Study). BMC Med. Res. Methodol. 9, 77.

27. Chang, E.T., Smedby, K.E., Hjalgrim, H., Glimelius, B., Adami, H.O., 2006. Reliability of self-reported family history of cancer in a large case-control study of lymphoma. J. Natl. Cancer Inst. 98, 61–68.

28. Lindefors-Harris, B.M., Eklund, G., Adami, H.O., Meirik, O., 1991. Response bias in a case-control study: analysis utilizing comparative data concerning legal abortions from two independent Swedish studies. Am. J. Epidemiol. 134, 1003–1008.

29. Grimes, D.A., Brandon, L.G., 2014. Every Third Woman in America: How Legal Abortion Transformed Our Nation. Daymark Publishing, Carolina Beach, NC.
30. World Health Organization, 2000. Induced Abortion Does not Increase Breast Cancer Risk, Fact Sheet Number 240. World Health Organization, Geneva, Switzerland.
31. Hannaford, P., 2000. Cardiovascular events associated with different combined oral contraceptives: a review of current data. Drug Saf. 22, 361–371.
32. Cramer, D.W., Schiff, I., Schoenbaum, S.C., et al., 1985. Tubal infertility and the intrauterine device. N. Engl. J. Med. 312, 941–947.
33. Daling, J.R., Weiss, N.S., Metch, B.J., et al., 1985. Primary tubal infertility in relation to the use of an intrauterine device. N. Engl. J. Med. 312, 937–941.
34. Hubacher, D., Cheng, D., 2004. Intrauterine devices and reproductive health: American women in feast and famine. Contraception 69, 437–446.
35. Grimes, D.A., 1987. Intrauterine devices and pelvic inflammatory disease: recent developments. Contraception 36, 97–109.
36. Hubacher, D., Lara-Ricalde, R., Taylor, D.J., Guerra-Infante, F., Guzmán-Rodríguez, R., 2001. Use of copper intrauterine devices and the risk of tubal infertility among nulligravid women. N. Engl. J. Med. 345, 561–567.
37. Textor, J., Hardt, J., Knuppel, S., 2011. DAGitty: a graphical tool for analyzing causal diagrams. Epidemiology 22, 745.
38. Anonymous, 1999. Merriam-Webster's Collegiate Dictionary, 10th ed. Merriam-Webster, Inc., Springfield, MA
39. Greenland, S., Pearl, J., Robins, J.M., 1999. Causal diagrams for epidemiologic research. Epidemiology 10, 37–48.
40. Hernan, M.A., Hernandez-Diaz, S., Robins, J.M., 2004. A structural approach to selection bias. Epidemiology 15, 615–625.
41. Suttorp, M.M., Siegerink, B., Jager, K.J., Zoccali, C., Dekker, F.W., 2015. Graphical presentation of confounding in directed acyclic graphs. Nephrol. Dial. Transplant. 30, 1418–1423.
42. Pickering, N.K., Auvray, B., Dodds, K.G., McEwan, J.C., 2015. Genomic prediction and genome-wide association study for dagginess and host internal parasite resistance in New Zealand sheep. BMC Genomics 16, 958.
43. Byrne, B., Dunne, G., Lyng, J., Bolton, D.J., 2007. The development of a 'clean sheep policy' in compliance with the new Hygiene Regulation (EC) 853/2004 (Hygiene 2). Food Microbiol. 24, 301–304.
44. von Elm, E., Altman, D.G., Egger, M., Pocock, S.J., Gøtzsche, P.C., Vandenbroucke, J.P., 2007. The Strengthening the Reporting of Observational Studies in Epidemiology (STROBE) statement: guidelines for reporting observational studies. Lancet 370, 1453–1457.
45. Pouwels, K.B., Widyakusuma, N.N., Groenwold, R.H., Hak, E., 2016. Quality of reporting of confounding remained suboptimal after the STROBE guideline. J. Clin. Epidemiol. 69, 217–224.
46. Bavry, A.A., Bhatt, D.L., 2006. Interpreting observational studies—look before you leap. J. Clin. Epidemiol. 59, 763–764.
47. Groenwold, R.H., Hak, E., Hoes, A.W., 2009. Quantitative assessment of unobserved confounding is mandatory in nonrandomized intervention studies. J. Clin. Epidemiol. 62, 22–28.
48. Pourhoseingholi, M.A., Baghestani, A.R., Vahedi, M., 2012. How to control confounding effects by statistical analysis. Gastroenterol. Hepatol. Bed Bench 5, 79–83.
49. Kahlert, J., Gribsholt, S.B., Gammelager, H., Dekkers, O.M., Luta, G., 2017. Control of confounding in the analysis phase—an overview for clinicians. Clin. Epidemiol. 9, 195–204.
50. Hulley, S.B., Cummings, S.R., Browner, W.S., Grady, D., Newman, T.B., 2013. Designing Clinical Research, Fourth ed. Lippincott Williams & Wilkins, Philadelphia.
51. Gerhard, T., 2008. Bias: considerations for research practice. Am. J. Health Syst. Pharm. 65, 2159–2168.
52. Shapiro, S., 2008. Causation, bias and confounding: a hitchhiker's guide to the epidemiological galaxy Part 2. Principles of causality in epidemiological research: confounding, effect modification and strength of association. J. Fam. Plann. Reprod. Health Care 34, 185–190.
53. Lang, T.A., Secic, M., 2006. How to Report Statistics in Medicine: Annotated Guidelines for Authors, Editors, and Reviewers, Second ed. American College of Physicians, Philadelphia.

54. Deb, S., Austin, P.C., Tu, J.V., et al., 2016. A review of propensity-score methods and their use in cardiovascular research. Can. J. Cardiol. 32, 259–265.

55. Starks, H., Diehr, P., Curtis, J.R., 2009. The challenge of selection bias and confounding in palliative care research. J. Palliat. Med. 12, 181–187.

56. Concato, J., Lawler, E.V., Lew, R.A., Gaziano, J.M., Aslan, M., Huang, G.D., 2010. Observational methods in comparative effectiveness research. Am. J. Med. 123, e16–23.

57. Williamson, E.J., Forbes, A., 2014. Introduction to propensity scores. Respirology 19, 625–635.

58. Austin, P.C., 2008. A critical appraisal of propensity-score matching in the medical literature between 1996 and 2003. Stat. Med. 27, 2037–2049.

59. Sturmer, T., Joshi, M., Glynn, R.J., Avorn, J., Rothman, K.J., Schneeweiss, S., 2006. A review of the application of propensity score methods yielded increasing use, advantages in specific settings, but not substantially different estimates compared with conventional multivariable methods. J. Clin. Epidemiol. 59, 437–447.

60. Hlatky, M.A., Winkelmayer, W.C., Setoguchi, S., 2013. Epidemiologic and statistical methods for comparative effectiveness research. Heart Fail. Clin. 9, 29–36.

61. Sox, H.C., Goodman, S.N., 2012. The methods of comparative effectiveness research. Annu. Rev. Public Health 33, 425–445.

62. McClellan, M., McNeil, B.J., Newhouse, J.P., 1994. Does more intensive treatment of acute myocardial infarction in the elderly reduce mortality? Analysis using instrumental variables. JAMA 272, 859–866.

63. Sterne, J.A., Smith, G.D., 2001. Sifting the evidence—what's wrong with significance tests? BMJ 322, 226–231.

64. Greenland, S., Senn, S.J., Rothman, K.J., et al., 2016. Statistical tests, P values, confidence intervals, and power: a guide to misinterpretations. Eur. J. Epidemiol. 31, 337–350.

65. Spurious correlations. http://www.tylervigen.com/spurious-correlations, accessed 4 January 2016.

66. Newman, T.B., Browner, W.S., 1988. The epidemiology of life and death: a critical commentary. Am. J. Public Health 78, 161–162.

67. Hill, A.B., 1965. The environment and disease association or causation. Proc. R. Soc. Med. 58, 295–300.

68. Rothman, K.J., Greenland, S., 2005. Causation and causal inference in epidemiology. Am. J. Public Health 95 (Suppl 1), S144–S150.

69. Grimes, D.A., Schulz, K.F., 2012. False alarms and pseudo-epidemics: the limitations of observational epidemiology. Obstet. Gynecol. 120, 920–927.

70. Vessey, M.P., Yeates, D., Flavel, R., McPherson, K., 1981. Pelvic inflammatory disease and the intrauterine device: findings in a large cohort study. Br. Med. J. (Clin. Res. Ed.) 282, 855–857.

71. Bartholomew, L.L., Grimes, D.A., 1998. The alleged association between induced abortion and risk of breast cancer: biology or bias? Obstet. Gynecol. Surv. 53, 708–714.

72. Beral, V., Doll, R., Hermon, C., Peto, R., Reeves, G., 2008. Ovarian cancer and oral contraceptives: collaborative reanalysis of data from 45 epidemiological studies including 23,257 women with ovarian cancer and 87,303 controls. Lancet 371, 303–314.

73. Wakeford, R., 2015. Association and causation in epidemiology—half a century since the publication of Bradford Hill's interpretational guidance. J. R. Soc. Med. 108, 4–6.

74. Fennerty, M.B., 1994. Helicobacter pylori. Arch. Intern. Med. 154, 721–727.

75. Sanders, J., 1993. From science to evidence: the testimony on causation in the Bendectin cases. Stanford Law Rev. 46, 1–86.

76. Brent, R.L., 1995. Bendectin: review of the medical literature of a comprehensively studied human non-teratogen and the most prevalent tortogen-litigen. Reprod. Toxicol. 9, 337–349.

77. Sung, V.W., 2012. Reducing bias in pelvic floor disorders research: using directed acyclic graphs as an aid. Neurourol. Urodyn. 31, 115–120.

Cohort Studies: Marching Towards Outcomes

A cohort study tracks two or more groups forward from exposure to outcome. This type of study can be done by going ahead in time from the present (prospective cohort study) or, alternatively, by going back in time to comprise the cohorts and following them up to the present (retrospective cohort study). A cohort study is the best way to identify incidence and natural history of a disease and can be used to examine multiple outcomes after a single exposure. However, this type of study is less useful for examination of rare events or those that take a long time to develop. A cohort study should provide clear, specific, and measurable definitions of exposures and outcomes; determination of both should be as objective as possible. The control group (unexposed) should be similar in all important respects to the exposed, with the exception of not having the exposure. Observational studies, however, rarely achieve such a degree of similarity, so investigators need to measure and control for confounding factors. Avoiding loss to follow-up over time is a challenge, because differential losses introduce bias. Variations on the cohort theme include the before-after study and nested case-control study (within a cohort study). Strengths of a cohort study include the ability to calculate incidence rates, relative risks, and 95% confidence intervals (CIs). This format is the preferred way of presenting study results, rather than solely with p values.

The term 'cohort' has military, not medical, roots. The term was first used in research by Frost in a 1935 study examining mortality from tuberculosis.[1] A cohort was a 300- to 600-man unit in the Roman army; 10 cohorts formed a legion (Fig. 4.1). The etymology of the term provides a useful mnemonic: a cohort study consists of bands or groups of persons marching forward in time from an exposure to one or more outcomes.

This analogy might be helpful, because cohort studies have a bevy of confusing synonyms: incidence, longitudinal, panel, forward-looking, follow-up, concurrent, and prospective studies.[2] Although the terminology can seem daunting, the cohort study is easy for clinicians to understand,

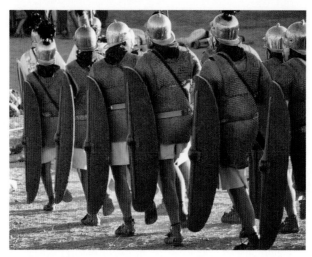

Fig. 4.1   Roman cohort on the march towards a battle outcome.

because it flows in a logical direction (unlike the case-control study). Here, we explain the terminology, describe the strengths and weaknesses of cohort studies, consider several logistical concerns,
mention two permutations of cohort studies, and summarise their analysis.

Data Collection: Forwards and Backwards

A cohort study follows two or more groups from exposure (or varying amounts of exposure) to outcome. In its simplest form, a cohort study compares the experience of a group exposed to some
factor with another group not exposed to the factor. If the former group has a higher or lower frequency of an outcome than the unexposed, then an association between exposure and outcome is
evident.

The defining characteristic of all cohort studies is direction: they track people forward in time
from exposure to outcome. Researchers doing this kind of study must, therefore, go forward in time
from the present or go back in time to choose their cohorts (Fig. 4.2). Either way, a cohort study
moves in the same direction, although gathering data might not. For example, an investigator who
wants to study the epidemic of multiple births stemming from assisted reproductive technologies[3]
could begin a cohort study now. Women exposed to these technologies and a similar group who
conceived naturally could be tracked forward through their pregnancies to monitor the frequency
of multiple births (a concurrent cohort study). Alternatively, the investigator might use existing
medical records and go back in time several years to identify women exposed and not exposed
to these technologies. The researcher would then track these women forward through records to
determine the birth outcomes. Again, the study moves from exposure to outcome, though the data
collection occurred after the fact (a retrospective cohort study). Other names for this approach
include historical cohort study, historical prospective study, nonconcurrent prospective study,
and (paradoxically) prospective study in retrospect.[2]

Yet a third variation exists: ambidirectional[4]. As the name implies, data collection goes in both
directions. This approach can be useful for exposures that have both short-term and long-term outcomes. In this hypothetical example, assisted reproductive technologies might be associated with
multiple births and with breast cancer later in life.[5] The investigator might, therefore, look back
through records for multiple births and also start to follow up these women into the future for breast

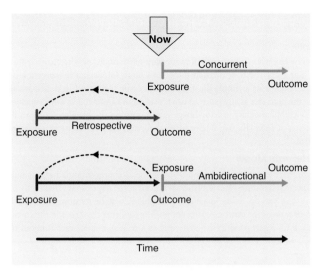

Fig. 4.2   Schematic diagram of concurrent, retrospective, and ambidirectional cohort studies.

cancer occurrence. Ambidirectional cohort studies include those that start after exposure has occurred but before the outcome has developed (e.g., smoking or asbestos exposure and later lung cancer).[4]

Advantages of Cohort Studies

Cohort studies have many appealing features. They are the best way to ascertain both the incidence and natural history of a disorder. The temporal sequence between putative cause and outcome is usually clear; the exposed and unexposed participants can often be confirmed free of the outcome at the outset.[6] By contrast, this chicken–egg question often frustrates cross-sectional and case-control studies. For example, cross-sectional studies indicate that chronic pain is associated with mental disorders, including depression.[7] Do mood and anxiety disorders increase perceived pain, or do patients with chronic pain develop mood and anxiety disorders because of their pain?

Cohort studies are useful in investigation of multiple outcomes that might arise after a single exposure. Stated alternatively, a cohort study of one exposure could examine many outcomes.[8] A prototype would be cigarette smoking (exposure) and stroke, emphysema, oral cancer, and heart disease (outcomes). Although assessment of many outcomes is often cited as a positive attribute of cohort studies, this feature can be abused.

P hacking, also known as data mining, snooping, fishing, and significance chasing, is defined as 'trying multiple things until you get the desired results'.[9] One review of observational study reports identified 10 articles that tested over 100 associations between exposure and outcome, the maximum being 264![10] Researchers commonly test associations between exposure and many outcomes but only report the significant ones, raising the likelihood of false-positive findings (alpha error). Investigators should have prespecified primary and secondary associations to examine (sometimes called hypothesis confirmation). Although investigators can look at other outcomes (hypothesis generation), they should report the findings of all tested associations, not just significant ones, so that readers can correctly interpret the results.

The cohort design is also useful in the study of rare exposures; a researcher can often recruit people with uncommon exposures (e.g., to ionising radiation or chemicals) in the workplace.[11] A hospital or factory might provide a large number of individuals with the exposure of interest,

---

PANEL 4.1 ■ Reporting Time-to-Event in Cohort Studies

Survival Analysis

Survival analysis is useful when lengths of follow-up vary substantially or when participants enter a study at different times. The Kaplan-Meier method provides a more sophisticated expression of the risk of the outcome over time than does a simple dichotomous outcome (e.g., alive or dead). It can determine the probability (p) of the outcome at any point in time; this result is graphed as a step function (which jumps at every event). A complementary, mirror-image graph portrays the likelihood of avoiding the outcome ($1 - p$) as a function of time (Kaplan-Meier survival curve). The log-rank test compares survival curves of different groups.[14]

Proportional Hazards Model

Another approach to different lengths of follow-up is the Cox proportional hazards model. It is a multivariable technique that has time-to-event (such as illness) as the dependent variable. By contrast, multiple logistic regression has 'yes–no' as the dependent variable. Coefficients from this model can be used to calculate the hazard ratio of the outcome, after controlling for other covariates in the equation. The hazard ratio (with 95% CIs) is interpreted in the same way as a relative risk for dichotomous outcomes.[14]

---

which would be rare in the general population. Also, with rare exposures, cohort studies facilitate sampling a high fraction of the exposed while sampling a small fraction of the unexposed. That leads to study efficiency. Unlike case-control studies (Chapter 5), which are useful for studying rare outcomes, cohort studies are adept at studying rare exposures.

Cohort studies also reduce the risk of survivor or prevalence–incidence bias, first described by Neyman.[12] Diseases that are rapidly fatal are difficult to study with a case-control design because of this. For example, a hospital-based case-control study of the link between snow shovelling and myocardial infarction would miss all cases who died in the driveway, shovel in hand. The most severe cases would be missed, and enrolled cases would not be representative of all infarct patients. A cohort study would be a less biased (but admittedly more cumbersome) approach: compare rates of myocardial infarction among those who shovel and those who do not shovel. Finally, cohort studies allow calculation of incidence rates, relative risks, and confidence intervals, the preferred measures for dichotomous outcomes.[13] Other outcome measures in cohort studies include life-table rates, survival curves, and hazard ratios (Panel 4.1).[14] In contrast, case-control studies cannot provide incidence rates; at best, odds ratios approximate relative risks only when the outcome is uncommon.[15]

Disadvantages of Cohort Studies

Cohort studies have important limitations, too. Selection bias is built into cohort studies. For example, in a cohort study investigating effects of jogging on cardiovascular disease, those who choose to jog probably differ in other important ways (such as diet and smoking) from those who do not exercise. In theory, both groups should be the same in all important respects, except for the exposure of interest (jogging), but this seldom occurs. The cohort design is challenging for rare diseases (e.g., scleroderma). Cohort studies of diseases that take a long time to develop (e.g., cancer) can be prohibitively expensive. However, several large long-term cohort studies have made landmark contributions to our knowledge of many diseases, both common and uncommon. Examples include the Royal College of General Practitioners' Oral Contraceptive Study,[16] the Framingham Heart Study, the Nurses' Health Study,[17] and the British Physicians' Study.[18]

Because the data already exist, retrospective cohort studies are popular. This feature is a double-edged sword: the quality of extant data is usually inferior—or incomplete—compared with information collected prospectively and targeted to the question at hand.[1,11] Moreover, privacy regulations make contacting patients for supplementary information difficult or impossible. Hence, data quality is usually better with prospective than retrospective cohort studies.[8]

Loss to follow-up can be a difficulty, particularly so with longitudinal studies that continue for decades. However, with multiple-stage follow-up procedures, high follow-up rates are achievable in large, contemporary cohort studies.[19,20] Differential losses to follow-up between those exposed and unexposed can bias results. Over time, the exposure status of study participants can change. For example, a proportion of women who use oral contraceptives will switch to an intrauterine device, and vice versa. Partitioning by duration of exposure to a method can avoid a blurring of exposure, sometimes termed 'contamination'.

What to Look for in Cohort Studies

WHO IS AT RISK?

All participants (both exposed and unexposed) in a cohort study must be at risk of developing the outcome.[1] For example, because women who have had a tubal sterilisation operation have almost no risk of salpingitis,[21] they should not be included in cohort studies of this disease. Similarly, women after hysterectomy have no risk of cervical cancer and should be excluded from studies of this cancer.

WHO IS EXPOSED?

Cohort studies need a clear, unambiguous definition of the exposure at the outset. This definition sometimes involves quantifying the exposure by degree, rather than just 'yes' or 'no'. For example, a large cohort study of smoking and nasopharyngeal cancer in China defined a daily smoker as 'one who smoked at least one cigarette per day for at least 6 months'.[22] Another large cohort study of the relationship between super-obesity and perinatal outcomes in Australia and New Zealand defined the exposure explicitly: any pregnant woman at ≥ 20 weeks' gestation with a body mass index >50 or a weight >140 kg.[23]

WHO IS AN APPROPRIATE CONTROL?

The key notion is that controls (the unexposed) should be similar to the exposed in all important respects, except for the lack of exposure. If so, the unexposed group will reveal the background rate of the outcome expected in the community. The unexposed group can come from either internal (persons from the same time and place, such as a hospital ward) or external sources. Internal comparisons are preferable. In a particular population, individuals segregate themselves (or through genetics or medical interventions) into exposure status (e.g., cigarette smoking, occupation, contraception). In a Scottish study of the potential effect of statins on prolonging breast cancer survival, the exposed were those who received a statin after breast cancer diagnosis, while the unexposed lacked this exposure; no association was found.[24]

If satisfactory internal controls are not available, researchers must look elsewhere. In a trial of an occupational exposure, finding an adequate number of employees in the factory without the exposure might be difficult. Hence, one might choose workers in a similar factory in the same community. This choice assumes that workers in the other factory have the same baseline risk of the outcome in question, which might not be the case. Even less desirable is use of population norms; disease-specific mortality rates are an example. A researcher might compare lung-cancer death rates among workers in the factory with rates of persons of the same age and sex in the population. Bias inevitably creeps into such comparisons because of the healthy-worker effect: those who work are healthier, in general, than those who do not (or cannot) work. Additionally, work has obvious economic benefits, which might further bias comparisons.

HAVE OUTCOMES BEEN ASSESSED EQUALLY?

Outcomes must be defined in advance; they should be clear, specific, and measurable. Identification of outcomes should be comparable in every way for the exposed and unexposed to avoid information bias. Failure to define objective outcomes leads to uninterpretable results. This challenge relates not only to subjective outcomes such as Gulf War[25] and chronic fatigue syndromes,[26] but also to more mundane diseases such as endometritis. Just how tender must a uterus be to merit this diagnosis? Because endometritis cannot be objectively defined, it cannot be studied; febrile morbidity may be a proxy. Similarly, the voluminous literature on the metabolic syndrome is currently unintelligible because of many different definitions.[27]

Keeping those who judge outcomes unaware of the exposure status of participants (blinding) in a cohort study is important for subjective outcomes, such as cellulitis or stiffness. By contrast, with objective outcome measures, such as fever or death, blinding the exposure status is less important.

Outcome information can come from many sources. For mortality studies, the death certificate is often used. Although convenient, the validity of the clinical information is highly variable. For nonfatal outcomes, sources include hospital charts, electronic medical records, insurance records, laboratory records, disease registries, hospital discharge logs, and physical examination and measurement of participants. Optimally, the person who judges outcomes should be unaware of the exposure. When diagnoses vary in their confidence, assignment of levels of assurance might be helpful, such as definite, probable, and suspect. A better approach is to have blinded adjudication of all possible important outcome measures reported by participants in a study.[28]

Tracking Participants Over Time
HAVE LOSSES BEEN MINIMISED?

Although loss of participants damages the power and precision of a study, differential loss to follow-up is worse. Participants quitting studies are not random events. If the likelihood of bailing out is related both to exposure and outcome, then bias can result. For example, some participants given a new antibiotic might have such poor outcomes that they are unable to complete questionnaires or to return for examination. Their disappearance from the cohort would make the new antibiotic look better than it is.

The best way of dealing with loss to follow-up is to avoid it. For example, restrict participation to only those judged likely to complete the study. Additionally, several safeguards are customary.[1] Obtaining the names of several family members or friends who do not live with the respondent is often helpful at the start of such studies. The participant's family doctor might also be helpful. Should the respondent move, these contacts would probably know his or her new address. Motor vehicle registration records can be useful, too. Furthermore, national vital statistics registries, such as the National Death Index in the United States, facilitate follow-up. Participants can be offered financial compensation for their time lost from work as a result of the study. Diligent tracking of participants is hard work and might require hiring personnel for this task alone, but high follow-up rates are possible.[19,20] Chapter 15 provides further hints on follow-up.

Reporting Cohort Studies

Many cohort studies are reported poorly (see Panel 4.2). Because of the importance of full, transparent reporting of observational studies, the STROBE guidelines[13] were published in 2007.

PANEL 4.2 ■ STROBE Statement—Checklist of Items That Should Be Included in Reports of Observational Studies[13]

	Item No	*Recommendation*
Title and Abstract	1	(*a*) Indicate the study's design with a commonly used term in the title or the abstract.
		(*b*) Provide in the abstract an informative and balanced summary of what was done and what was found.
Introduction		
Background/rationale	2	Explain the scientific background and rationale for the investigation being reported.
Objectives	3	State specific objectives, including any prespecified hypotheses.
Methods		
Study design	4	Present key elements of study design early in the paper.
Setting	5	Describe the setting, locations, and relevant dates, including periods of recruitment, exposure, follow-up, and data collection.
Participants	6	(*a*) *Cohort study*—Give the eligibility criteria and the sources and methods of selection of participants. Describe methods of follow-up.
		Case-control study—Give the eligibility criteria and the sources and methods of case ascertainment and control selection. Give the rationale for the choice of cases and controls.
		Cross-sectional study—Give the eligibility criteria and the sources and methods of selection of participants.
		(*b*) *Cohort study*—For matched studies, give matching criteria and number of exposed and unexposed.
		Case-control study—For matched studies, give matching criteria and the number of controls per case.
Variables	7	Clearly define all outcomes, exposures, predictors, potential confounders, and effect modifiers. Give diagnostic criteria, if applicable.
Data sources/ measurement	8*	For each variable of interest, give sources of data and details of methods of assessment (measurement). Describe comparability of assessment methods if there is more than one group.
Bias	9	Describe any efforts to address potential sources of bias.
Study size	10	Explain how the study size was arrived at.
Quantitative variables	11	Explain how quantitative variables were handled in the analyses. If applicable, describe which groupings were chosen and why.
Statistical methods	12	(*a*) Describe all statistical methods, including those used to control for confounding.
		(*b*) Describe any methods used to examine subgroups and interactions.
		(*c*) Explain how missing data were addressed.
		(*d*) *Cohort study*—If applicable, explain how loss to follow-up was addressed.
		Case-control study—If applicable, explain how matching of cases and controls was addressed.
		Cross-sectional study—If applicable, describe analytical methods taking account of sampling strategy.
		(*e*) Describe any sensitivity analyses.

Continued on following page

PANEL 4.2 ■ STROBE Statement—Checklist of Items That Should Be Included in Reports of Observational Studies (Continued)

	Item No	*Recommendation*
Results		
Participants	13*	(*a*) Report numbers of individuals at each stage of study (e.g., numbers potentially eligible, examined for eligibility, confirmed eligible, included in the study, completing follow-up, and analysed).
		(*b*) Give reasons for nonparticipation at each stage.
		(*c*) Consider use of a flow diagram.
Descriptive data	14*	(*a*) Give characteristics of study participants (e.g., demographic, clinical, social) and information on exposures and potential confounders.
		(*b*) Indicate number of participants with missing data for each variable of interest.
		(*c*) *Cohort study*—Summarise follow-up time (e.g., average and total amount).
Outcome data	15*	*Cohort study*—Report numbers of outcome events or summary measures over time.
		Case-control study—Report numbers in each exposure category or summary measures of exposure.
		Cross-sectional study—Report numbers of outcome events or summary measures.
Main results	16	(*a*) Give unadjusted estimates and, if applicable, confounder-adjusted estimates and their precision (e.g., 95% CI). Make clear which confounders were adjusted for and why they were included.
		(*b*) Report category boundaries when continuous variables were categorised.
		(*c*) If relevant, consider translating estimates of relative risk into absolute risk for a meaningful time period.
Other analyses	17	Report other analyses done (e.g., analyses of subgroups and interactions, and sensitivity analyses).
Discussion		
Key results	18	Summarise key results with reference to study objectives.
Limitations	19	Discuss limitations of the study, taking into account sources of potential bias or imprecision. Discuss both direction and magnitude of any potential bias.
Interpretation	20	Give a cautious overall interpretation of results considering objectives, limitations, multiplicity of analyses, results from similar studies, and other relevant evidence.
Generalisability	21	Discuss the generalisability (external validity) of the study results.
Other Information		
Funding	22	Give the source of funding and the role of the funders for the present study and, if applicable, for the original study on which the present article is based.

*Give information separately for cases and controls in case-control studies and, if applicable, for exposed and unexposed groups in cohort and cross-sectional studies.

Analogous to the CONSORT guidelines[29] for randomised controlled trials, the STROBE guidelines specify the requisite reporting elements for such studies (see Panel 4.2). The checklist is best used in conjunction with a 28-page article explaining the rationale for each of the 22 items in the checklist.[30] An example from the literature is given for each item on the checklist. The STROBE guidelines provide a roadmap for the reporting of cohort studies.

A decade after promulgation of the STROBE guidelines, reporting of cohort studies remains suboptimal. This is the assessment of both cross-sectional and before-after studies of report quality. In general-medical journals with a high-impact-factor, cohort studies published in 2010 adhered to about 70% of the items in the STROBE checklist.[31] Cohort studies in specialty journals fell further short of the mark. Assessments in hand surgery,[32] plastic surgery,[33] nephrology,[34] and dermatology[35] reveal even lower compliance with the checklist. We suspect that many researchers are simply unaware of the STROBE guidelines. Journal endorsement of the guidelines[34] and submission of a completed STROBE checklist as a prerequisite for manuscript review[33] may improve this chronic deficiency.

Variations on the Cohort Theme
BEFORE-AFTER STUDIES

Before-after studies (time series) have important limitations. Here, an investigator takes a measurement, exposes participants to an intervention (often a drug), repeats the measurements, and then compares them. First, regression to the mean is often ignored. If admission to the cohort includes extreme measurements, such as high laboratory values, then lower mean values will arise at follow-up, irrespective of treatment.[36] Second, secular trends, such as seasonal changes in the frequency of pneumonia, can affect results. Third, washout periods are often needed to avoid a carryover effect of drugs given during the initial observation period.

NESTED CASE-CONTROL STUDIES

Cohort studies sometimes spawn other studies. One of the most frequent is the nested case-control study. Why would an investigator carve out a case-control study in the midst of a cohort study? The answer often involves body fluids and a freezer. Some exposure or predictor variables are simply too expensive to determine on everyone in a study. A sophisticated blood test is the prototype. A clever way to skirt this financial obstacle is to do a cohort study that will yield a sufficient number of cases. All participants entering the cohort study have a tube of blood drawn at enrolment; serum is frozen until the study's conclusion. All those in the cohort study who develop the outcome of interest now become the cases for the nested study. The investigator then chooses a random sample of all participants who did not develop the outcome (controls). Next, the blood test is done on serum from only the cases and controls, not the whole group of exposed and unexposed. In this way, the laboratory cost is minimised while assuring that the exposure (e.g., a positive laboratory test) was present before development of the outcome. Controls are generally matched to cases by important characteristics such as age and sex.[9]

A nested case-control study within a large screening trial examined the potential relationship between mitochondrial DNA copy number and the risk of prostate cancer. Cases with prostate cancer (800) and an equal number of controls had DNA extracted from peripheral blood leucocytes. Thus only a fraction of those enrolled in the trial had to have this genetic testing done on their stored blood samples.[37] In view of the availability of banked blood specimens around the world, this type of research design is likely to become popular. Moreover, nested case-control studies might be useful for other studies that do not require blood tests but in which determination of the exposure is expensive (measuring the internal dimensions of the uterus by ultrasound)[38] or inconvenient (measurement of airway obstruction by spirometry).[39]

Conclusion

Cohort studies are common in medical research. Like other research designs, they entail important trade-offs. Readers should make sure that investigators provide clear, specific, and measurable definitions of exposures and outcomes. The unexposed group should resemble the exposed group in all important respects, and determination of outcomes should be objective and, whenever possible, blinded. Results for dichotomous outcomes should be provided as rates, relative risks, and confidence intervals, which offer more information than do p values. Reports of cohort studies should identify and describe the potential effect of biases. Importantly, investigators should measure and control for potential confounding.

References

1. Song, J.W., Chung, K.C., 2010. Observational studies: cohort and case-control studies. Plast. Reconstr. Surg. 126, 2234–2242.
2. Porta, M., 2014. A Dictionary of Epidemiology. Oxford University Press, New York.
3. Luke, B., 2017. Pregnancy and birth outcomes in couples with infertility with and without assisted reproductive technology: with an emphasis on US population-based studies. Am. J. Obstet. Gynecol. 217, 270–281.
4. Sessler, D.I., Imrey, P.B., 2015. Clinical research methodology 2: observational clinical research. Anesth. Analg. 121, 1043–1051.
5. Sergentanis, T.N., Diamantaras, A.A., Perlepe, C., Kanavidis, P., Skalkidou, A., Petridou, E.T., 2014. IVF and breast cancer: a systematic review and meta-analysis. Hum. Reprod. Update 20, 106–123.
6. Thadhani, R., Tonelli, M., 2006. Cohort studies: marching forward. Clin. J. Am. Soc. Nephrol. 1, 1117–1123.
7. Buonanotte, F., Burrone, M.S., Abeldano, R.A., et al., 2015. Prevalence of mental health disorders among patients who attended a service of neurology for chronic pain. Rev. Fac. Cien. Med. Univ. Nac. Cordoba 72, 304–308.
8. Euser, A.M., Zoccali, C., Jager, K.J., Dekker, F.W., 2009. Cohort studies: prospective versus retrospective. Nephron Clin. Pract. 113, c214–c217.
9. Bin Abd Razak, H.R., Ang, J.E., Attal, H., Howe, T.S., Allen, J.C., 2016. P-hacking in orthopaedic literature: a twist to the tail. J. Bone Joint Surg. Am. 98, e91
10. Pocock, S.J., Collier, T.J., Dandreo, K.J., et al., 2004. Issues in the reporting of epidemiological studies: a survey of recent practice. BMJ 329, 883.
11. Setia, M.S., 2016. Methodology series module 1: cohort studies. Indian J. Dermatol. 61, 21–25.
12. Hill, G., Connelly, J., Hebert, R., Lindsay, J., Millar, W., 2003. Neyman's bias re-visited. J. Clin. Epidemiol. 56, 293–296.
13. von Elm, E., Altman, D.G., Egger, M., Pocock, S.J., Gøtzsche, P.C., Vandenbroucke, J.P., 2007. The Strengthening the Reporting of Observational Studies in Epidemiology (STROBE) statement: guidelines for reporting observational studies. Lancet 370, 1453–1457.
14. Lang, T.A., Secic, M., 2006. How to Report Statistics in Medicine: Annotated Guidelines for Authors, Editors, and Reviewers, Second ed. American College of Physicians, Philadelphia.
15. Grimes, D.A., Schulz, K.F., 2008. Making sense of odds and odds ratios. Obstet. Gynecol. 111, 423–426.
16. Iversen, L., Sivasubramaniam, S., Lee, A.J., Fielding, S., Hannaford, P.C., 2017. Lifetime cancer risk and combined oral contraceptives: the Royal College of General Practitioners' Oral Contraception Study. Am. J. Obstet. Gynecol. 216, 580.e1–580.e9.
17. Barbhaiya, M., Lu, B., Sparks, J.A., et al., 2017. Influence of alcohol consumption on the risk of systemic lupus erythematosus among women in the Nurses' Health Study Cohorts. Arthritis Care Res. 69, 384–392.
18. Doll, R., Peto, R., Boreham, J., Sutherland, I., 2000. Smoking and dementia in male British doctors: prospective study. BMJ 320, 1097–1102.

19. Dinger, J., Bardenheuer, K., Heinemann, K., 2014. Cardiovascular and general safety of a 24-day regimen of drospirenone-containing combined oral contraceptives: final results from the International Active Surveillance Study of Women Taking Oral Contraceptives. Contraception 89, 253–263.

20. Dinger, J.C., Heinemann, L.A., Kuhl-Habich, D., 2007. The safety of a drospirenone-containing oral contraceptive: final results from the European Active Surveillance Study on oral contraceptives based on 142,475 women-years of observation. Contraception 75, 344–354.

21. Levgur, M., Duvivier, R., 2000. Pelvic inflammatory disease after tubal sterilization: a review. Obstet. Gynecol. Surv. 55, 41–50.

22. Lin, J.H., Jiang, C.Q., Ho, S.Y., et al., 2015. Smoking and nasopharyngeal carcinoma mortality: a cohort study of 101,823 adults in Guangzhou. China. BMC Cancer 15, 906.

23. Sullivan, E.A., Dickinson, J.E., Vaughan, G.A., et al., 2015. Maternal super-obesity and perinatal outcomes in Australia: a national population-based cohort study. BMC Pregnancy Childbirth 15, 322.

24. Mc Menamin, U.C., Murray, L.J., Hughes, C.M., Cardwell, C.R., 2016. Statin use and breast cancer survival: a nationwide cohort study in Scotland. BMC Cancer 16, 600.

25. Gronseth, G.S., 2005. Gulf war syndrome: a toxic exposure? A systematic review. Neurol. Clin. 23, 523–540.

26. Unger, E.R., Lin, J.M., Tian, H., Gurbaxani, B.M., Boneva, R.S., Jones, J.F., 2016. Methods of applying the 1994 case definition of chronic fatigue syndrome—impact on classification and observed illness characteristics. Popul. Health Metrics 14, 5.

27. Ghosh, A., 2011. The metabolic syndrome: a definition dilemma. Cardiovasc. J. Afr. 22, 295–296.

28. Dinger, J.C., Bardenheuer, K., Assmann, A., 2009. International Active Surveillance Study of Women Taking Oral Contraceptives (INAS-OC Study). BMC Med. Res. Methodol. 9, 77.

29. Schulz, K.F., Altman, D.G., Moher, D., CONSORT Group, 2010. CONSORT Group 2010 statement: updated guidelines for reporting parallel group randomised trials. BMJ 340, c332.

30. Vandenbroucke, J.P., von Elm, E., Altman, D.G., et al., 2007. Strengthening the Reporting of Observational Studies in Epidemiology (STROBE): explanation and elaboration. Ann. Intern. Med. 147, W163–W94.

31. Poorolajal, J., Cheraghi, Z., Irani, A.D., Rezaeian, S., 2011. Quality of cohort studies reporting post the Strengthening the Reporting of Observational Studies in Epidemiology (STROBE) Statement. Epidemiol. Health 33, e2011005.

32. Sorensen, A.A., Wojahn, R.D., Manske, M.C., Calfee, R.P., 2013. Using the Strengthening the Reporting of Observational Studies in Epidemiology (STROBE) Statement to assess reporting of observational trials in hand surgery. J. Hand Surg. 38, 1584-1589.e2.

33. Agha, R.A., Lee, S.Y., Jeong, K.J., Fowler, A.J., Orgill, D.P., 2016. Reporting quality of observational studies in plastic surgery needs improvement: a systematic review. Ann. Plast. Surg. 76, 585–589.

34. Rao, A., Bruck, K., Methven, S., et al., 2016. Quality of reporting and study design of CKD cohort studies assessing mortality in the elderly before and after STROBE: a systematic review. PLoS One 11, e0155078.

35. Bastuji-Garin, S., Sbidian, E., Gaudy-Marqueste, C., et al., 2013. Impact of STROBE statement publication on quality of observational study reporting: interrupted time series versus before-after analysis. PLoS One 8, e64733.

36. Cockrell Skinner, A., Goldsby, T.U., Allison, D.B., 2016. Regression to the mean: a commonly overlooked and misunderstood factor leading to unjustified conclusions in pediatric obesity research. Child. Obes. 12, 155–158.

37. Moore, A., Lan, Q., Hofmann, J.N., et al., 2017. A prospective study of mitochondrial DNA copy number and the risk of prostate cancer. Cancer Causes Control 28, 529–538.

38. Liang, H., Li, L., Yuan, W., et al., 2014. Dimensions of the endometrial cavity and intrauterine device expulsion or removal for displacement: a nested case-control study. BJOG 121, 997–1004.

39. Maldonado, F., Bartholmai, B.J., Swensen, S.J., Midthun, D.E., Decker, P.A., Jett, J.R., 2010. Are airflow obstruction and radiographic evidence of emphysema risk factors for lung cancer? A nested case-control study using quantitative emphysema analysis. Chest 138, 1295–1302.

Case-Control Studies: Research in Reverse

Epidemiologists benefit greatly from having case-control study designs in their research armamentarium. Case-control studies can yield important scientific findings with relatively little time, money, and effort compared with other study designs. This seemingly quick road to research results entices many newly trained epidemiologists. Indeed, investigators implement case-control studies more frequently than any other analytical epidemiological study. Unfortunately, case-control designs also tend to be more susceptible to biases than other comparative studies. Although easier to do, they are also easier to do wrong. Five main notions guide investigators who do, or readers who assess, case-control studies. First, investigators must explicitly define the criteria for diagnosis of a case and any eligibility criteria used for selection. Second, controls should come from the same population as the cases, and their selection should be independent of the exposures of interest. Third, investigators should blind the data gatherers to the case or control status of participants or, if impossible, at least blind them to the main hypothesis of the study. Fourth, data gatherers need to be thoroughly trained to elicit exposure in a similar manner from cases and controls; they should use memory aids to facilitate and balance recall between cases and controls. Finally, investigators should address confounding in case-control studies, either in the design stage or with analytical techniques. Devotion of meticulous attention to these points enhances the validity of the results and bolsters the reader's confidence in the findings.

Case-control studies contribute greatly to the research toolbox of an epidemiologist. They embody the strengths and weaknesses of observational epidemiology. Moreover, epidemiologists use them to study a huge variety of associations. To show this variety, we searched PubMed for topics investigated with case-control studies (Panel 5.1).[1-24] We identified diverse diseases and exposures, with outcomes ranging from hip fracture to premature ejaculation, and exposures ranging from hair dyes to vitamin D.

The strength of case-control studies can be appreciated in early research done by investigators hoping to understand the cause of AIDS. Case-control studies identified risk groups (e.g., homosexual men, intravenous drug users, and blood-transfusion recipients) and risk factors (e.g., multiple sex partners, receptive anal intercourse in homosexual men, and not using condoms) for AIDS. Based on such studies, blood banks restricted high-risk individuals from donating blood, and educational programmes began to promote safer behaviours. As a result of these precautions, the speed of transmission of HIV-1 was greatly reduced, even before the virus had been identified.

By comparison with other study types, case-control studies can yield important findings in a relatively short time, and with relatively little money and effort. This apparently quick road to research results entices many newly trained epidemiologists. However, case-control studies tend to be more susceptible to biases than other analytical, epidemiological designs.[25] A notable friend of ours (the late David L. Sackett, personal communication, 2001) told us that he would trust only six people in the world to do a proper case-control study. And Ken Rothman comments in his book that 'because it need not be extremely expensive nor time-consuming to conduct a case-control study, many studies have been conducted by would-be investigators who lack even a rudimentary appreciation for epidemiological principles. Occasionally such haphazard research can produce fruitful or even extremely important results, but often the results are wrong because basic research principles have been violated'.[26]

Basic Case-Control Study Design

Case-control designs might seem easy to understand, but many clinicians stumble over them. Because this type of study runs backwards by comparison with most other studies, it often confuses researchers and readers alike. Indeed, it so confuses researchers that they frequently do not know what type of study they have done (and readers do not know the difference). For example, in a review of 124 published articles in four US obstetrics and gynaecology journals labelled as 'case-control' studies, clearly 30% were not case-control studies.[27] Most of the mislabelled case-control

---

PANEL 5.1 ■ Examples of Topics in the Literature Investigated With Case-Control Studies

Exposure	*Outcome*
Uterine fibromas	Postpartum haemorrhage[1]
Breastfeeding	Pertussis[2]
Shiftwork	Violence against nurses[3]
Periodontitis	Breast cancer[4]
History of migraine	Concussion[5]
Hypothyroidism	Unruptured cerebral aneurysms [6]
Statins	Polyneuropathy[7]
Vitamin D	Early childhood fracture[8]
HPV	Invasive cervical cancer[9]
Vitamin B_{12}	Premature ejaculation[10]
Human Papillomavirus	Colorectal cancer[11]
Untreated psoriasis	Male fertility[12]
Atopy	Melanoma[13]
Body mass index, hormone therapy	Cutaneous melanoma[14]
Micronutrients	Hip fracture[15]
Antidepressants	Colorectal cancer[16]
Agricultural occupation	Testicular cancer[17]
Childhood obesity	Hypertriglyceridaemia[18]
Hair dyes	Connective tissue disorders[19]
Digital rectal examination	Metastatic prostate cancer[20]
Statins	Dementia[21]
Paracetamol use	Ovarian cancer[22]
Physical activity	Breast cancer[23]
Influenza vaccination	Recurrent myocardial infarction[24]

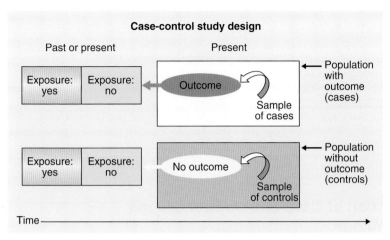

Fig. 5.1   Schematic diagram of a case-control study design.

studies were actually retrospective cohort studies. This mislabelling of studies as 'case-contol' extends to other specialties as well. In a review of studies in diabetes labelled as 'case-control', 43.8% were mislabelled and thereby misleading.[28] Certainly, researchers, reviewers, editors, and readers need better training in methods and terminology.[27]

In cohort studies, study groups are defined by exposure. In case-control studies, however, study groups are defined by outcome (Fig. 5.1). To study the association between smoking and lung cancer, therefore, people with lung cancer are enrolled to form the case group, and people without lung cancer are identified as controls. Researchers then look back in time to ascertain each person's exposure status (smoking history), hence the retrospective nature of this study design. Investigators compare the frequency of smoking exposure in the case group with that in the control group, and calculate a measure of association.[25,26,29]

Unlike cohort studies, case-control studies cannot yield incidence rates.[30] Instead, they provide an odds ratio, derived from the proportion of individuals exposed in each of the case and control groups. When the cumulative incidence rate of an outcome in the population of interest is low (usually under 5% suffices in both the exposed and unexposed),[25] the odds ratio from a case-control study is a good estimate of relative risk.[25,29] Epidemiologists refer to this condition as the rare disease assumption, which pertains to a type of case-control study that ascertains cases after the end of the risk period of interest, with controls being selected from among those who did not become cases.[31] This represents the type of case-control study that we address in this chapter, usually labelled a cumulative case-control study. Of note, although beyond the scope of this chapter, this rare disease assumption is not needed for other case-control study designs in which researchers estimate the incidence density ratio.[31]

Advantages and Disadvantages

Researchers often tout case-control studies as the most efficient epidemiological study design.[32] Indeed, they tend to take less time, less money, and less effort. That makes sense when the incidence rate of an outcome is low, because in a cohort design the researchers would have to follow up many individuals to identify one with the outcome. Case-control studies are also efficient in the investigation of diseases that have a long latency period (e.g., cancer), in which instance a cohort study would involve many years of follow-up before the outcome became evident.

However, cohort studies can be more efficient than case-control studies. If the frequency of exposure is low, for example, case-control studies quickly become inefficient. Researchers would have to examine many cases and controls to find one who had been exposed. For instance, a case-control study of oral contraceptive use and transmission of HIV-1 would be impractical in parts of Africa because of the rarity of use of oral contraceptives. As a rule of thumb, cohort designs are more efficient in settings in which the incidence of outcome is higher than the prevalence of exposure.

Finally, many methodological issues affect the validity of the results of case-control studies, and two factors (i.e., choosing a control group and obtaining exposure history) can greatly affect a study's vulnerability to bias.

Selection of Case and Control Groups
CASE GROUP

All the cases from a population could, theoretically, be included as participants in a case-control study. For practical reasons, however, only a sample is frequently studied.[26] Investigators should, therefore, state how the sample was selected, providing a clear definition of the outcome being studied, including, for example, clinical symptoms, laboratory results, and diagnostic methods used. Furthermore, researchers should detail eligibility criteria used for selection, such as age range and location (e.g., clinic, hospital, population-based). Finally, they should gather data, preferably from incident (new) rather than prevalent (both old and new) cases;[33] because diagnostic patterns change over time, recent diagnoses are likely to be more consistent than those obtained from different periods.

CONTROL GROUP

The control group provides the background proportion of exposure expected in the case group. Controls should, therefore, be free of the disease (outcome) being studied but should be representative of those individuals who would have been selected as cases had they developed the disease. In other words, controls should represent the population at risk of becoming cases.

Selection of controls must be independent of the exposure being investigated. Subjective investigator judgement enters the study design at this point, sometimes for the better and, unfortunately, sometimes for the worse. When investigators consider potential control groups, they must anticipate all the potential biases that could arise, making this task one of the hardest in epidemiology.

Suppose investigators selected individuals with myocardial infarction from the cardiology ward of a large, city hospital as cases, but identified people without infarction from the emergency department of the same hospital as controls. Bias might result. The cardiology ward is used as a referral centre for the entire state, whereas the emergency department primarily serves only the city. Unfortunately, the exposure history for patients from the city would not usually accurately reflect that of patients statewide. For example, the exposure of interest (e.g., a new blood-pressure drug) might not be available to patients in outlying areas of the state but be commonly prescribed in the city. In this example, therefore, either the controls should be chosen from the entire state, like the cases, or the investigators should exclude all individuals (cases and controls) who live outside the local community served by the emergency department. Moreover, controls should be selected independent of exposure. Assume that this new antihypertensive drug causes drowsiness and slows reaction time.

Such side effects might lead to automobile accidents, with injured drivers entering the emergency department. Thus the investigator's control group would include an abnormally high proportion of individuals exposed to the new antihypertensive, a biased comparison with the case group.

Another hypothetical example could be a case-control study of whether nonsteroidal antiinflammatory drugs (NSAIDs) prevent colorectal cancer. The study measures previous NSAID use by patients admitted to hospital with (cases) and without (controls) colorectal cancer. If the control group came from the rheumatology service, then the study would be biased, because individuals with arthritis use NSAIDs more often than do the general population from which the cases were chosen. Such a high level of NSAID use in controls would result in a spuriously low risk (odds ratio) calculation. Alternatively, if the control group came from the gastroenterology service, where many ulcer patients had been advised by their doctors to avoid NSAIDs, then that control group might yield a low level of NSAID use and a spuriously high-risk (odds ratio) calculation. In other words, if investigators do not select control groups independent of exposure, biases in either direction might result (Panel 5.2).

An early case-control study in AIDS serves as a good example of how inappropriate controls can result in biased findings.[34] In this instance, the researchers compared cases of AIDS diagnosed in San Francisco, CA, USA, between 1983 and 1984 with two HIV-uninfected control groups. One control group included individuals who attended a clinic for sexually transmitted diseases (STDs), and the other included people identified from the neighbourhoods of the cases. The investigators compared the risk of AIDS in individuals with more than 100 sexual partners with that in people with zero to five sexual partners. The resulting odds ratios were 2.9 with STD clinic controls, but 52.0 with neighbourhood controls. The magnitude of this difference shows the potential for huge biases due to selection of improper control groups. In this study, controls from the STD clinic proved inappropriate, because their selection was not independent of exposure (more than 100 sexual partners). Acquisition of STDs is associated with number of sexual partners; thus these controls generated a highly biased odds ratio estimate.

Investigators can reduce selection bias by minimising judgement in the selection process. For example, if the case group included all affected individuals in a specified geographical region, then the control group could be chosen at random from the general population of the same area. This approach was used in a case-control study of breast cancer and oral contraceptive use.[35] All women aged 20 to 54 years who had newly diagnosed breast cancer and who lived in one of eight geographical areas in the United States formed the case group. Women of the same ages and from the same areas, selected by random digital telephone dialling, formed the control group. Although this study represents an excellent example, such designs are not always feasible.

Readers of case-control studies should not accept results of studies without checking the appropriateness of the control group, as described in the methods section. If the researchers provide little insight into the choice of their control group, become sceptical. Examine whatever information the researcher has provided for indications about how well the control group represents the cases, independent of the exposure being studied.[33] This assessment takes time and energy, but it represents

---

PANEL 5.2 ■ Introduction of Bias Through Poor Choice of Controls

Cases	Control Selection	Nonrepresentativeness	Selection Bias
Colorectal cancer patients admitted to hospital	Patients admitted to hospital with arthritis	Controls probably have high degrees of exposure to NSAIDs	Would spuriously **reduce** the estimate of effect (odds ratio)
Colorectal cancer patients admitted to hospital	Patients admitted to hospital with peptic ulcers	Controls probably have low degrees of exposure to NSAIDs	Would spuriously **increase** the estimate of effect (odds ratio)

the crux of a case-control study. Indeed, many control groups are not appropriate. For example, in a review of case-control studies in periodontitis, the scheme to choose the control participants was appropriate in only 8.9% of the studies.[36]

Measurement of Exposure Information

Another difficulty in case-control studies involves the measurement of exposure information. Participants, both cases and controls, might inaccurately remember past exposures, especially those that happened a long time ago. Furthermore, cases often remember exposures to putative risk factors differently than controls. This differential recall (recall bias) causes information bias.[33]

In the study of breast cancer and oral contraceptive use,[35] for example, investigators asked participants about previous exposure to oral contraceptives. Women with breast cancer might have searched their minds for what could have caused their cancers, identifying oral contraceptives as a risk because of stories in the media about the postulated relation between contraceptives and breast cancer. Thus although some women in each group might have used a particular oral contraceptive 20 years ago, the case might remember taking it whereas the control might not. Such recall bias would generate an exaggerated relation between oral contraceptives and breast cancer. Information bias is especially pernicious because analytical techniques, irrespective of their sophistication, cannot moderate or eliminate it.

In a Swedish study,[37] investigators examined the potential link between induced abortion and later development of breast cancer. They gathered information about exposure (previous abortion) from cases and controls by means of personal interviews and by looking through national medical records. When interviewed, fewer controls admitted to having had an abortion than was evident in vital statistics. This discrepancy did not arise among cases. Differential recall between cases and controls led to a biased estimate of risk.

Bias from data gatherers presents further difficulties. If the individuals gathering information know the case or control status of the participants, they can elicit information differently, again leading to potential information bias. A data gatherer might delve more deeply into a case's background than a control's to obtain a hypothesised exposure. When possible, data gatherers (e.g., interviewers) should be unaware of the case or control status of the respondents. When blinding is not possible, investigators should keep the main hypothesis from the data gatherers.

Furthermore, researchers should train data gatherers to elicit information similarly for cases and controls. Obtaining exposure information from records as a solution to information bias rarely suffices, because such information does not always exist, and, if it does, it is usually insufficient to control adequately for confounding factors in the analysis.[26] Investigators who do case-control studies must be aware of the potential for information bias. They should address it in their study design and describe in their report approaches used to avoid such bias. Memory aids, such as photographs, diaries, and calendars, can help participants remember exposures. For example, in the case-control study of oral contraceptives,[35] the investigators used an album with colour photographs of every oral contraceptive marketed over the preceding decades and a blank calendar grid to help recall major life events and contraceptive use. Those colour photographs stimulated memories, both in cases and controls, to past exposure, and thus reduced recall bias. Reports of case-control studies that do not detail use of memory aids should make readers sceptical.

Control for Confounding

Case-control studies need to address confounding bias (Chapter 3).[25,26,38] This type of bias can be dealt with in the design phase by restriction or matching, but researchers generally prefer to handle it in the analysis phase with analytical techniques such as logistic regression or stratification with Mantel–Haenszel approaches.[25,26,33] If this second approach is used, investigators should plan carefully in advance what potentially confounding variables to obtain data for; irrespective of the analytical approach used, researchers cannot control for a variable for which they have no data. Moreover, invalid measurement of potential confounding factors leads to residual confounding, even after adjustment.[26]

Conclusion

Case-control studies that are well designed and carefully done can provide useful and valid results. Investigators must, however, devote meticulous attention to the selection of control groups and to measurement of exposure information. Awareness of these key elements should help readers to identify the strengths and weaknesses of a properly reported study. Accurate and thorough description of methods by investigators will enhance credibility.

References

1. Nyflot, L.T., Sandven, I., Stray-Pedersen, B., et al., 2017. Risk factors for severe postpartum hemorrhage: a case-control study. BMC Pregnancy Childbirth 17, 17.
2. Pandolfi, E., Gesualdo, F., Carloni, E., et al., 2017. Does breastfeeding protect young infants from pertussis? case-control study and immunologic evaluation. Pediatr. Infect. Dis. J. 36, e48–e53.
3. Sun, S., Gerberich, S.G., Ryan, A.D., 2017. The relationship between shiftwork and violence against nurses: a case control study. Workplace Health Saf. 65, 603–611.
4. Sfreddo, C.S., Maier, J., De David, S.C., Susin, C., Moreira, C.H.C., 2017. Periodontitis and breast cancer: a case-control study. Community Dent. Oral Epidemiol. 45, 545–551.
5. Eckner, J.T., Seifert, T., Pescovitz, A., Zeiger, M., Kutcher, J.S., 2017. Is migraine headache associated with concussion in athletes? A case-control study. Clin. J. Sport Med. 27, 266–270.
6. Atchaneeyasakul, K., Tipirneni, A., Zhang, T., et al., 2018. Association of hypothyroidism with unruptured cerebral aneurysms: a case-control study. J. Neurosurg. 128, 511–514.
7. Svendsen, T.K., Norregaard Hansen, P., Garcia Rodriguez, L.A., et al., 2017. Statins and polyneuropathy revisited: case-control study in Denmark, 1999-2013. Br. J. Clin. Pharmacol. 83, 2087–2095.
8. Anderson, L.N., Heong, S.W., Chen, Y., et al., 2017. Vitamin D and fracture risk in early childhood: a case-control study. Am. J. Epidemiol. 185, 1255–1262.
9. Berraho, M., Amarti-Riffi, A., El-Mzibri, M., et al., 2017. HPV and cofactors for invasive cervical cancer in Morocco: a multicentre case-control study. BMC Cancer 17, 435.
10. Kadihasanoglu, M., Kilciler, M., Kilciler, G., et al., 2017. Relation between blood vitamin B12 levels with premature ejaculation: case-control study. Andrologia 49. https://doi.org/10.1111/and.12657.
11. Vuitton, L., Jaillet, C., Jacquin, E., et al., 2017. Human papillomaviruses in colorectal cancers: a case-control study in western patients. Dig. Liver Dis. 49, 446–450.
12. Caldarola, G., Milardi, D., Grande, G., et al., 2017. Untreated psoriasis impairs male fertility: a case-control study. Dermatology, 233, 170–174.
13. Marasigan, V., Morren, M.A., Lambert, J., et al., 2017. Inverse association between atopy and melanoma: a case-control study. Acta Derm. Venereol. 97, 54–57.
14. De Giorgi, V., Gori, A., Savarese, I., et al., 2017. Role of BMI and hormone therapy in melanoma risk: a case-control study. J. Cancer Res. Clin. Oncol. 143, 1191–1197.
15. Torbergsen, A.C., Watne, L.O., Wyller, T.B., et al., 2017. Micronutrients and the risk of hip fracture: case-control study. Clin. Nutr. 36, 438–443.
16. Lee, H.C., Chiu, W.C., Wang, T.N., et al., 2017. Antidepressants and colorectal cancer: a population-based nested case-control study. J. Affect. Disord. 207, 353–358.
17. Moirano, G., Zugna, D., Grasso, C., et al., 2017. Postnatal risk factors for testicular cancer: the EPSAM case-control study. Int. J. Cancer 141, 1803–1810.
18. Hanh, N.T.H., Tuyet, L.T., Dao, D.T.A., Tao, Y., Chu, D.T., 2017. Childhood obesity is a high-risk factor for hypertriglyceridemia: a case-control study in Vietnam. Osong Public Health Res. Perspect. 8, 138–146.

19. Freni-Titulaer, L.W., Kelley, D.B., Grow, A.G., McKinley, T.W., Arnett, F.C., Hochberg, M.C., 1989. Connective tissue disease in southeastern Georgia: a case-control study of etiologic factors. Am. J. Epidemiol. 130, 404–409.

20. Friedman, G.D., Hiatt, R.A., Quesenberry, C.P., Selby, J.V., 1991. Case-control study of screening for prostatic cancer by digital rectal examinations. Lancet 337, 1526–1529.

21. Jick, H., Zornberg, G.L., Jick, S.S., Seshadri, S., Drachman, D.A., 2000. Statins and the risk of dementia. Lancet 356, 1627–1631.

22. Cramer, D.W., Harlow, B.L., Titus-Ernstoff, L., Bohlke, K., Welch, W.R., Greenberg, E.R., 1998. Over-the-counter analgesics and risk of ovarian cancer. Lancet 351, 104–107.

23. Verloop, J., Rookus, M.A., van der Kooy, K., van Leeuwen, F.E., 2000. Physical activity and breast cancer risk in women aged 20-54 years. J. Natl. Cancer Inst. 92, 128–135.

24. Naghavi, M., Barlas, Z., Siadaty, S., Naguib, S., Madjid, M., Casscells, W., 2000. Association of influenza vaccination and reduced risk of recurrent myocardial infarction. Circulation 102, 3039–3045.

25. Kelsey, J.L., Whittemore, A.S., Evans, A.S., Thompson, W.D., 1996. Methods in Observational Epidemiology. Oxford University Press, New York.

26. Rothman, K.J., 1986. Modern Epidemiology. Little, Brown and Company, Boston.

27. Grimes, D.A., 2009. "Case-control" confusion: mislabeled reports in obstetrics and gynecology journals. Obstet. Gynecol. 114, 1284–1286.

28. Ramos, A., Mendoza, L.C., Rabasa, F., Bolibar, I., Puig, T., Corcoy, R., 2017. Case-control studies in diabetes. Do they really use a case-control design? Acta Diabetol. 54, 631–634.

29. Grimes, D.A., Schulz, K.F., 2002. An overview of clinical research: the lay of the land. Lancet 359, 57–61.

30. Grimes, D.A., Schulz, K.F., 2002. Cohort studies: marching towards outcomes. Lancet 359, 341–345.

31. Rothman, K.J., 2017. Invited commentary: when case-control studies came of age. Am. J. Epidemiol. 185, 1012–1014.

32. van Stralen, K.J., Dekker, F.W., Zoccali, C., Jager, K.J., 2010. Case-control studies—an efficient observational study design. Nephron Clin. Pract. 114, c1–4.

33. Schlesselman, J., 1982. Case-control Studies: Design, Conduct, Analysis. Oxford University Press, New York.

34. Moss, A.R., Osmond, D., Bacchetti, P., Chermann, J.C., Barre-Sinoussi, F., Carlson, J., 1987. Risk factors for AIDS and HIV seropositivity in homosexual men. Am. J. Epidemiol. 125, 1035–1047.

35. Stadel, B.V., Rubin, G.L., Webster, L.A., Schlesselman, J.J., Wingo, P.A., 1985. Oral contraceptives and breast cancer in young women. Lancet 2, 970–973.

36. Lopez, R., Scheutz, F., Errboe, M., Baelum, V., 2007. Selection bias in case-control studies on periodontitis: a systematic review. Eur. J. Oral Sci. 115, 339–343.

37. Lindefors-Harris, B.M., Eklund, G., Adami, H.O., Meirik, O., 1991. Response bias in a case-control study: analysis utilizing comparative data concerning legal abortions from two independent Swedish studies. Am. J. Epidemiol. 134, 1003–1008.

38. Grimes, D.A., Schulz, K.F., 2002. Bias and causal associations in observational research. Lancet 359, 248–252.

CHAPTER 6

Compared to What? Finding Controls for Case-Control Studies

Use of control (comparison) groups is a powerful research tool. In case-control studies, controls estimate the frequency of an exposure in the population under study. Controls can be taken from known or unknown study populations. A known group consists of a defined population observed over a period, such as passengers on a cruise ship. When the study group is known, a sample of the population can be used as controls. If no population roster exists, then techniques such as random-digit dialling can be used. Sometimes, however, the study group is unknown (e.g., motor-vehicle crash victims brought to an emergency department, who may come from far away). In this situation, hospital controls, neighbourhood controls, and friend, associate, or relative controls can be used. In general, one well-selected control group is better than two or more. When the number of cases is small, the ratio of controls to cases can be raised to improve the ability to find important differences. Although no ideal control group exists, readers need to think carefully about how representative the controls are. Poor choice of controls can lead to both wrong results and possible medical harm.

When asked 'How's your wife?', comedian Henny Youngman would quip, 'Compared to what?' Although sexist by contemporary standards, this old vaudeville line frames the question relating to the results of case-control studies: compared to what? Valid conclusions hinge on finding an appropriate comparison group. Stated alternatively, use of suboptimal control groups has undermined much research.

Use of control groups is a powerful scientific tool—and an old one. The first documentation of a comparison group appears in *The Holy Bible* in the Book of Daniel.[1] Daniel (Fig. 6.1) and his three colleagues, captured by King Nebuchadnezzar of Babylon, carried out a 10-day trial of healthy food versus the royal diet of the court. At the end, Daniel and his buddies appeared healthier than did the Babylonian youth who enjoyed the usual fare. This trial has been criticised over the years for an inadequate duration of exposure to note any change in appearance and, thus, probable divine confounding. The experiment took place around 600 BC and was finally published four centuries later.

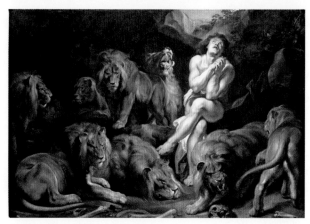

Fig. 6.1 Daniel, world's first recorded clinical trialist,[1] visiting with lions.

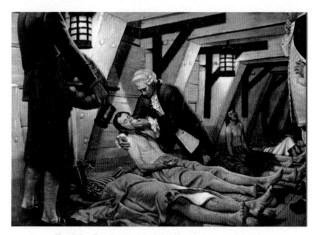

Fig. 6.2 Dr. James Lind treating scurvy on board.

Delay in publishing is not a new problem: Daniel perished, then published. Perhaps as a result, control groups disappeared from published work for millennia.

James Lind's (Fig. 6.2) 1747 trial of scurvy treatments rekindled interest in contemporaneous controls.[2] Despite its small size (six treatment groups with two sailors assigned to each), the trial showed the benefit of citrus-fruit supplementation. In studies without randomisation, finding an appropriate control group can sometimes be challenging. We will explain the role of control groups in case-control studies, describe special difficulties in choosing them, and discuss some implications of these choices.

Aim of Controls

Controls in a case-control study (Chapter 5), which progresses backwards in time from outcome to exposure, indicate the background frequency of an exposure in individuals who are free of the disease in question. Controls do not need to be healthy; inclusion of sick people is sometimes

> **PANEL 6.1 ■ Attributes of Controls in a Case-Control Study**
>
> ■ Free of the outcome of interest
> ■ Representative of the population at risk of the outcome
> ■ Selected independent of the exposure of interest

appropriate. Indeed, exclusion of ill people as controls can distort the results.[3] (Like healthy individuals, ill people can develop a different condition of interest.) The final point is key: controls in a case-control study should represent those at risk of becoming a case.[4] Stated another way, controls should have the same risk of exposure as the cases, if the exposure and disease are unrelated (Panel 6.1).[5]

If cases (with the disease) have a higher frequency of the exposure than do the controls, then a positive association emerges (e.g., multiple sexual partners are more common among cases of cervical cancer than among controls without cervical cancer). If the exposure prevalence among cases is lower than among controls, a protective association exists (e.g., oral contraceptive use is less common among ovarian cancer cases than among controls without this cancer).

Avoidance of bias is important when choosing controls for a case-control study. Selection bias arises if controls are not representative of those at risk of the disease in question. An early case-control study of cigarette smoking and lung cancer[6] underestimated the effect of smoking. Controls in this hospital-based case-control study included 709 hospitalised patients without lung cancer. In that era, myocardial infarction patients routinely spent 3 weeks in hospital recuperating and would have been readily available controls. Thus the controls chosen likely had a higher proportion of smokers than in the general population, which would overestimate the background smoking rate and underestimate the association between smoking and lung cancer.[7]

Case-control studies of potential protection against colorectal cancer associated with nonsteroidal antiinflammatory drugs (NSAIDs)[8,9] provide another example (Fig. 6.3). Assume that colorectal cancer cases are identified at the time of their operations in hospital. Controls are hospital patients without colorectal cancer. If the researcher identified controls from the rheumatology service, this selection would bias the results: patients with arthritis would be more likely than most people in the community to be exposed to NSAIDs, thereby reducing the estimate of the association between these drugs and colorectal cancer. By contrast, if controls were selected from the gastroenterology service, this choice would bias the results in the opposite direction. Patients with ulcers would be less likely than the general population at risk of colorectal cancer to be exposed to NSAIDs, because of warnings from their clinicians. This bias would increase the estimate of the effect.

Research in endometriosis provides another example of challenges in selection of a control group. Because endometriosis needs an operation for diagnosis, investigators frequently use as controls women having laparoscopy or laparotomy without this diagnosis being made. However, women having operations are unlikely to be representative of all those at risk of developing endometriosis, because operations do not occur at random.[10]

Control selection	Flaw in control group	Effect on estimate of NSAID effect
Patients with arthritis	Probable atypically high exposure to NSAIDs	↓
Patients with peptic ulcers	Probable atypically low exposure to NSAIDs	↑

Fig. 6.3 Introduction of bias in a case-control study of nonsteroidal antiinflammatory drugs (NSAIDs) and colorectal cancer.

Where to Find Controls?

The investigator (and, ultimately, the reader) need to determine the group of individuals from which cases and controls will be drawn. A known group[11] consists of a defined population observed over a period (Fig. 6.4). This group might consist of passengers and crew on a week-long cruise of the Caribbean or all individuals living in Sweden over a decade. Cases are those who develop the disorder of interest, and controls are those in the same group without the condition. Thus case-control studies can be thought of as occurring in the midst of a larger cohort study (nested case-control studies[12] being a nice example). The task here is to find the cases in the group in question; choosing controls is easier in a defined population.

Usually the group from which cases come is unknown.[11] For example, victims of motor-vehicle crashes in a hospital emergency department pose this sort of challenge. Some might live nearby, others could be passing through on a highway, and others may arrive from rural areas by helicopter. Here, the cases are chosen before the study group is deduced. Finding cases is the simple part; the challenge now is to define the group from which controls should come. They should come from the same group. (One approach would be to limit both cases and controls to people who live within the city limits.)

Poor control groups can lead to big mistakes. The case-control study of AIDS in homosexual men in San Francisco described in Chapter 5 is illustrative.[13] Use of sexually transmitted disease clinic controls grossly underestimated the true risk, because the likelihood of using a clinic was strongly related to the exposure of interest (i.e., it was not independent of the number of partners). Controls in a public clinic at which sexually transmitted diseases are treated were much more likely to have multiple partners than were other homosexual men in San Francisco. Neighbourhood controls were the better control group.

Controls From a Known Group

When possible, random samples of people without the disease can serve as controls; this approach helps avoid selection bias. Investigation of an outbreak of food-borne illness on a cruise ship generally uses a case-control approach. Cases are those who develop gastroenteritis; controls are those on board who do not. The study seeks to identify food exposures that are more common among the cases than the controls. Moreover, no one who had not eaten the suspect food should have become ill. On the ship, probability sampling among those unaffected could be done.[14] Thus controls could be a random sample of everyone on board without food poisoning.

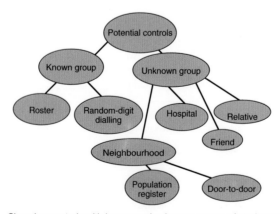

Fig. 6.4 Choosing controls with known and unknown groups of study participants.

Population controls have both advantages and disadvantages. Random sampling should provide representative controls, and extrapolation of results to the study group is easily justified. On the other hand, population controls can be inappropriate when cases have not been completely identified in the population or when substantial numbers of potential controls cannot be reached (e.g., those on holiday). Moreover, population controls could be less motivated to take part in research than individuals in a healthcare setting, such as hospitalised patients.[15]

RANDOM-DIGIT DIALLING

When no roster of the population exists, random-digit dialling of telephone numbers has been used to sample potential controls. A random sample of incomplete telephone numbers (e.g., eight digits) is taken from working telephone exchanges; random two-digit numbers then complete the number to be called (Fig. 6.5). This approach has strengths and weaknesses. It attempts to sample residential telephone numbers equally while keeping calls to commercial numbers to a minimum. The strategy reaches both new numbers and unlisted numbers not available through directories.

However, the heyday of random-digit dialling has passed. First, response rates have been steadily declining from over 90% in the 1980s to less than 70% by 2007.[16] More recently, an overall response rate for telephone landlines as low as 11% has been reported.[17] Declining response rates both reduce the efficiency of finding controls and undermine how representative respondents may be of the population at risk.[18] Changing communications technology over the past few decades has revolutionised telephone use. Answering devices and caller-identification features likely reduce response rates.

Second, more and more people have no landline. At least 30% of US residents live in a home with only wireless connectivity.[18] Thus researchers are now suggesting that cell phones be added to the random-digit dialling approach to reach those without landlines.[19,20] The portability of cellphone numbers since 1996 has compounded this problem; area codes are no longer tethered to a locale. This further drives down the efficiency of selecting controls in a geographical area. For example, many Atlanta residents in area code 404 have cells phones from other area codes and will be missed by random-digit dialling in 404.

Third, respondents to random-digit dialling may not be representative of those at risk of becoming a case. Evaluations of the technique have found that respondents differ from the broader population in education,[21] socioeconomic status,[22] and other demographic characteristics.[20] Selection bias is a growing concern. This has led to exploration of other sources for potential controls, including birth certificates[23] and commercial vendors of marketing databases.[18]

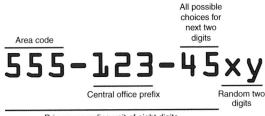

Fig. 6.5 Random-digit dialling for controls. Primary sampling unit included eight-digit central-office prefixes in the county, plus all combinations of next two digits. For all these eight-digit numbers randomly chosen, a computer generated the two final digits, creating a 10-digit number to be called.

Controls From an Unknown Group

NEIGHBOURHOOD CONTROLS

Neighbourhood controls generally are drawn in a specified pattern from the block in which the case lives. As always, selection of controls should be independent of the exposure of interest. To avoid selection bias, interviewers are given a specific pattern of houses to approach. Researchers have used several approaches to identify houses of controls: a population register or door-to-door canvassing.[24,25] A useful aid for the former is the cross-reference (also termed 'criss-cross' or 'reverse-street') directory that lists addresses and corresponding telephone numbers.

We participated in a case-control study of oral contraceptives and hepatocellular adenomas that used door-to-door canvassing; researchers interviewed every case in her home and then attempted to find three controls on the same street (Fig. 6.6).[26] A recent case-control study of leptospirosis in India chose the three houses nearest to the case for controls.[27]

Advantages of neighbourhood controls include no need for a roster, and many confounding factors are accounted for (e.g., socioeconomic status, climate). On the other hand, canvassing neighbourhoods is expensive, and using homes rather than people as the sampling unit is a problem shared with random-digit dialling. Nonresponse can pose challenges. In one report, an average of nine household contacts was needed for one successful control,[24] although in our experience, this ratio can be as much as 150:1. Multiunit buildings require identification of all units and then gain of access. This challenge is not unique to urban settings; in a case-control study in which we participated, interviewers dealt with German Shepherd dogs, barbed wire fences, and arrest by suspicious local police.[26]

A modern alternative to 'walking the neighbourhood' involves using a commercial marketing database to identify dwellings within a given distance from the case residence. For example, proximity to the case was deemed important in a case-control study of Lyme disease because of its transmission by tick vector.[18]

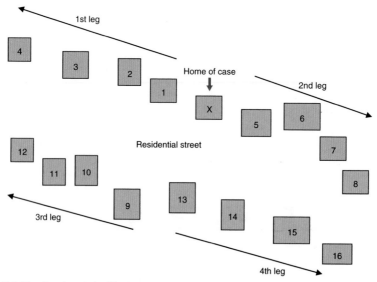

Fig. 6.6 Neighbourhood controls. After interviewing the case in her home, the investigator canvasses up to 16 homes in a predetermined H-shaped pattern until three controls are identified and interviewed. Every rectangle represents a home along the same street.

HOSPITAL CONTROLS

Hospital controls have been widely used—and criticised—in case-control studies. They have several appealing features: convenience, low cost to identify and interview, comparable information quality as cases, motivation to participate, and comparable healthcare-seeking behaviour.[15,28] However, the disadvantages are notable. Use of hospital controls assumes that they are representative of the background rate of exposure among people in the study group that produced the cases, meaning that the exposure is unrelated to the disease leading to hospitalisation of the control.

The best way to avoid this pitfall is to exclude as controls those whose admission diagnosis is likely to be related to the exposure of interest. For example, in a hospital-based case-control study of contraception and systemic lupus erythematosus, controls admitted to the obstetrics and gynaecology service were excluded.[29] The rationale for this exclusion was that women having reproductive care at tertiary-care hospitals might have had obstetrical and gynaecological histories different than most women in the community. Different diseases can have different catchment areas for a hospital; control diagnoses should have the same catchment area as the cases.

Admission rate bias (Berkson's bias, discussed in Chapter 3) can also cause difficulties. For example, if women wearing an intrauterine device (IUD) are more likely to be admitted for treatment of salpingitis than are women with salpingitis but no device, this difference would exaggerate the apparent odds ratio of salpingitis associated with IUD use.[30] Knowledge of the exposure of interest (an IUD) leads to an increased likelihood of becoming a case in a hospital-based study, resulting in an abnormally high proportion of IUD-using cases.

Several reports suggest that hospital controls might not be representative of the population at risk. Hospital controls can resemble cases more than do population controls, biasing odds ratios towards the null.[31,32] Others have noted differences between hospital and population controls in weight, smoking patterns, and burden of illness.[33]

FRIEND OR ASSOCIATE CONTROLS

Friends or work associates of cases sometimes serve as controls. This approach has both critics and supporters. An advantage is generation of a control group similar to the cases in several important respects, such as socioeconomic status and education. However, asking cases to name potential controls is the antithesis of random selection. Those named might be more gregarious and sociable than other potential controls, leading to the controls not being representative.[15] Introvert cases might not be able to nominate potential controls as easily as extrovert cases.[34] Cases with cancer may be unwilling to nominate possible controls because they do not want the nature of their disease known.[28]

Another concern about friend or family controls is potential overmatching.[35] Matching too closely or on too many characteristics can mask real associations between exposure and outcome.[36] On the other hand, cases tend to nominate as potential controls those who are better off than they in terms of education and socioeconomic status.[37]

In hidden populations for which socially unacceptable behaviours are being studied (e.g., drug abuse), friend controls have been suggested to be convenient and unlikely to introduce selection bias. In one study, drug misusers were asked to nominate a friend who was a drug misuser (a new case) and another friend who had never been involved with drugs (a control). This chain referral or snowball technique concluded that cases and controls came from the same population.[38] Although not ideal, friend controls appear to provide a representative comparison group with a sufficiently high response rate.[34,36]

RELATIVE CONTROLS

Relatives share many traits with cases. When genetic factors are deemed to be confounding, relatives have been used to control for this bias.[34] Many other exposures will be similar (e.g., siblings are likely to have diet, environment, lifestyle, and socioeconomic status in common as well). For example, when siblings serve as controls, the potential effect of family size cannot be examined.[15] Some researchers have concluded that as long as the exposure-specific risks remain stable over time, use of relatives as controls does not distort the results.[39] A study of stroke found that only 65% of surviving stroke cases had a living spouse, limiting the usefulness of this approach.[40]

How Many Control Groups?

Some authors have argued for using two separate control groups; if results are consistent, then findings are deemed more credible.[14,41] For example, a case-control study of oestrogen therapy and endometrial cancer used both hospital and community controls.[42] In the unhappy circumstance of disparate results, however, which result should be ignored?[15] Another immediate disadvantage is the added cost in time and resources. For example, in the case-control study of endometrial cancer cited previously,[42] adding a community control group increased the number of study participants to be interviewed from 480 to 801, a 67% rise.

Alternatively, in a case-control study of cancer, community controls without cancer might underestimate relevant exposures (recall bias), because they have no motivation to search their memories. Choosing a second comparison group of patients with cancers other than the cancer being studied might reduce this problem, because they would be similarly concerned about their health.[43] In general, we suggest selecting the one best control group possible.[44]

How Many Controls Per Case?

Readers are sometimes surprised to discover large disparities between the numbers of cases and controls in a case-control report; clinicians intuitively expect similar group sizes (a problem not limited to views of randomised trials). This inequality reflects attempts by investigators to boost the power (i.e., the ability of the study to find differences of importance, should they exist). In unmatched case-control studies, having roughly equal numbers of cases and controls is most efficient if costs are similar for cases and controls. However, sometimes the number of cases is small and cannot be increased. For example, in the early days of toxic shock syndrome (TSS) in the United States, the Centers for Disease Control and Prevention surveillance identified 28 cases of nonmenstrual TSS. Investigators chose four age-matched controls per case to increase the power of the study.[45] Increasing the number of controls up to a ratio of about 4:1 improves the power of the study.[46,47] This rise is not linear, however. Beyond a ratio of about 4:1, little power improvement results from increasing the number of controls. Boosting the ratio of controls to cases narrows the width of the confidence interval (the precision of the results) around the odds ratios but does not address the more critical issue of bias.

Stevens-Johnson syndrome, another rare condition, easily satisfies the rare disease assumption for a case-control study. An investigation from Taiwan had 35 cases and chose three controls per case, matched on age, sex, and admission date.[48] Even when substantial numbers of cases are available, researchers sometimes choose more controls than cases, especially when readily available on a computerised database. A UK study of prior antibiotic use and primary liver cancer collected 1195 cases from a large database. These were matched to 4640 controls in the same database. No danger signal emerged.[49]

What to Look for in Controls

The validity of case-control studies depends on selection of appropriate control groups. Choosing controls might seem deceptively simple, but it can be treacherous. Controls should reflect the background frequency of the exposure in the population. Hence, they should be similar in all important respects to cases, except that they do not have the disorder in question. Indeed, a person could be a control and then develop the disease in question during the study and be admitted as a case.[43] Their selection must be independent of exposure.

When the study group of potential controls is known, a good approach is to take all, or, if not feasible, a random sample of them. When the group of potential controls is unknown, choosing controls gets tough. Generally, we suggest using individuals chosen from the same time and place as cases. Look for one good control group; if the appropriateness of a control group is uncertain, sometimes a second control group is added. If the number of cases is small, having up to four times as many controls improves study power. However, this strategy does not improve validity.

Use of inappropriate control groups generally leads to both wrong conclusions and potential medical harm.[50] Readers of case-control reports need to think carefully about the characteristics of the controls. The results hang in the balance.

Conclusion

Controls in a case-control study estimate the frequency of an exposure in the population under study. When the study group is known, a random sample of controls without the outcome can be taken. If the study group is unknown, controls should be chosen from the same time and place as cases. Controls should be representative of those at risk of the outcome of interest. Choosing appropriate controls is the Achilles heel of case-control studies.

References

1. Grimes, D.A., 1995. Clinical research in ancient Babylon: methodologic insights from the book of Daniel. Obstet. Gynecol. 86, 1031–1034.
2. Feinstein, A.R., 1985. Clinical Epidemiology: The Architecture of Clinical Research. W. B. Saunders Company, Philadelphia.
3. Marbach, J.J., Schwartz, S., Link, B.G., 1992. The control group conundrum in chronic pain case/control studies. Clin. J. Pain 8, 39–43.
4. Rothman, K.J., Greenland, S., Lash, T.L., 2012. Modern Epidemiology. Lippincott Williams & Wilkins, Philadelphia.
5. Schlesselman, J.J., 1982. Case-Control Studies. Design, Conduct, Analysis. Oxford University Press, New York.
6. Doll, R., Hill, A.B., 1950. Smoking and carcinoma of the lung; preliminary report. Br. Med. J. 2, 739–748.
7. Sessler, D.I., Imrey, P.B., 2015. Clinical research methodology 2: observational clinical research. Anesth. Analg. 121, 1043–1051.
8. Chan, A.T., Giovannucci, E.L., 2010. Primary prevention of colorectal cancer. Gastroenterology 138, 2029-2043.e10.
9. Cao, Y., Nishihara, R., Qian, Z.R., et al., 2016. Regular aspirin use associates with lower risk of colorectal cancers with low numbers of tumor-infiltrating lymphocytes. Gastroenterology 151, 879-892.e4.
10. Zondervan, K.T., Cardon, L.R., Kennedy, S.H., 2002. What makes a good case-control study? Design issues for complex traits such as endometriosis. Hum. Reprod. 17, 1415–1423.
11. Wacholder, S., McLaughlin, J.K., Silverman, D.T., Mandel, J.S., 1992. Selection of controls in case-control studies. I. Principles. Am. J. Epidemiol. 135, 1019–1028.
12. Franchi, M., Asciutto, R., Nicotra, F., et al., 2017. Metformin, other antidiabetic drugs, and endometrial cancer risk: a nested case-control study within Italian healthcare utilization databases. Eur. J. Cancer Prev. 26, 225–231.

13. Moss, A.R., Osmond, D., Bacchetti, P., Chermann, J.C., Barre-Sinoussi, F., Carlson, J., 1987. Risk factors for AIDS and HIV seropositivity in homosexual men. Am. J. Epidemiol. 125, 1035–1047.

14. Perillo, M.G., 1993. Choice of controls in case-control studies. J. Manip. Physiol. Ther. 16, 578–585.

15. Wacholder, S., Silverman, D.T., McLaughlin, J.K., Mandel, J.S., 1992. Selection of controls in case-control studies. II. Types of controls. Am. J. Epidemiol. 135, 1029–1041.

16. Bunin, G.R., Spector, L.G., Olshan, A.F., et al., 2007. Secular trends in response rates for controls selected by random digit dialing in childhood cancer studies: a report from the Children's Oncology Group. Am. J. Epidemiol. 166, 109–116.

17. Clagett, B., Nathanson, K.L., Ciosek, S.L., et al., 2013. Comparison of address-based sampling and random-digit dialing methods for recruiting young men as controls in a case-control study of testicular cancer susceptibility. Am. J. Epidemiol. 178, 1638–1647.

18. Connally, N.P., Yousey-Hindes, K., Meek, J., 2013. Selection of neighborhood controls for a population-based Lyme disease case-control study by using a commercial marketing database. Am. J. Epidemiol. 178, 276–279.

19. Badcock, P.B., Patrick, K., Smith, A.M., et al., 2017. Differences between landline and mobile phone users in sexual behavior research. Arch. Sex. Behav. 46, 1711–1721.

20. Voigt, L.F., Schwartz, S.M., Doody, D.R., Lee, S.C., Li, C.I., 2011. Feasibility of including cellular telephone numbers in random digit dialing for epidemiologic case-control studies. Am. J. Epidemiol. 173, 118–126.

21. Wang, P.P., Dicks, E., Gong, X., et al., 2009. Validity of random-digit-dialing in recruiting controls in a case-control study. Am. J. Health Behav. 33, 513–520.

22. Bailey, H.D., Milne, E., de Klerk, N., et al., 2010. Representativeness of child controls recruited by random digit dialling. Paediatr. Perinat. Epidemiol. 24, 293–302.

23. Puumala, S.E., Spector, L.G., Robison, L.L., et al., 2009. Comparability and representativeness of control groups in a case-control study of infant leukemia: a report from the Children's Oncology Group. Am. J. Epidemiol. 170, 379–387.

24. Vernick, L.J., Vernick, S.L., Kuller, L.H., 1984. Selection of neighborhood controls: logistics and fieldwork. J. Chronic Dis. 37, 177–182.

25. Ryu, J.E., Thompson, C.J., Crouse, J.R. 3rd., 1989. Selection of neighborhood controls for a study of coronary artery disease. Am. J. Epidemiol. 129, 407–414.

26. Rooks, J.B., Ory, H.W., Ishak, K.G., et al., 1979. Epidemiology of hepatocellular adenoma. The role of oral contraceptive use. JAMA 242, 644–648.

27. Desai, K.T., Patel, F., Patel, P.B., Nayak, S., Patel, N.B., Bansal, R.K., 2016. A case-control study of epidemiological factors associated with leptospirosis in South Gujarat region. J. Postgrad. Med. 62, 223–227.

28. Lasky, T., Stolley, P.D., 1994. Selection of cases and controls. Epidemiol. Rev. 16, 6–17.

29. Grimes, D.A., LeBolt, S.A., Grimes, K.R., Wingo, P.A., 1985. Systemic lupus erythematosus and reproductive function: a case-control study. Am. J. Obstet. Gynecol. 153, 179–186.

30. Grimes, D.A., 1987. Intrauterine devices and pelvic inflammatory disease: recent developments. Contraception 36, 97–109.

31. West, D.W., Schuman, K.L., Lyon, J.L., Robison, L.M., Allred, R., 1984. Differences in risk estimations from a hospital and a population-based case-control study. Int. J. Epidemiol. 13, 235–239.

32. Infante-Rivard, C., 2003. Hospital or population controls for case-control studies of severe childhood diseases? Am. J. Epidemiol. 157, 176–182.

33. Olson, S.H., Kelsey, J.L., Pearson, T.A., Levin, B., 1994. Characteristics of a hypothetical group of hospital controls for a case-control study. Am. J. Epidemiol. 139, 302–311.

34. Zhong, C., Cockburn, M., Cozen, W., et al., 2017. Evaluating the use of friend or family controls in epidemiologic case-control studies. Cancer Epidemiol. 46, 9–13.

35. Porta, M., 2014. A Dictionary of Epidemiology. Oxford University Press, New York.

36. Bunin, G.R., Vardhanabhuti, S., Lin, A., Anschuetz, G.L., Mitra, N., 2011. Practical and analytical aspects of using friend controls in case-control studies: experience from a case-control study of childhood cancer. Paediatr. Perinat. Epidemiol. 25, 402–412.

37. Kaplan, S., Novikov, I., Modan, B., 1998. A methodological note on the selection of friends as controls. Int. J. Epidemiol. 27, 727–729.

38. Lopes, C.S., Rodrigues, L.C., Sichieri, R., 1996. The lack of selection bias in a snowball sampled case-control study on drug abuse. Int. J. Epidemiol. 25, 1267–1270.
39. Goldstein, A.M., Hodge, S.E., Haile, R.W., 1989. Selection bias in case-control studies using relatives as the controls. Int. J. Epidemiol. 18, 985–989.
40. Worrall, B.B., Brown, D.L., Brott, T.G., Brown, R.D., Silliman, S.L., Meschia, J.F., 2003. Spouses and unrelated friends of probands as controls for stroke genetics studies. Neuroepidemiology 22, 239–244.
41. Ibrahim, M.A., Spitzer, W.O., 1979. The case control study: the problem and the prospect. J. Chronic Dis. 32, 139–144.
42. Hulka, B.S., Fowler, W.C.J., Kaufman, D.G., et al., 1980. Estrogen and endometrial cancer: cases and two control groups from North Carolina. Am. J. Obstet. Gynecol. 137, 92–101.
43. Checkoway, H., Pearce, N., Kriebel, D., 2007. Selecting appropriate study designs to address specific research questions in occupational epidemiology. Occup. Environ. Med. 64, 633–638.
44. Moritz, D.J., Kelsey, J.L., Grisso, J.A., 1997. Hospital controls versus community controls: differences in inferences regarding risk factors for hip fracture. Am. J. Epidemiol. 145, 653–660.
45. Schwartz, B., Gaventa, S., Broome, C.V., et al., 1989. Nonmenstrual toxic shock syndrome associated with barrier contraceptives: report of a case-control study. Rev. Infect. Dis. 11 (Suppl 1), S43–S48; discussion S8–S89.
46. Song, J.W., Chung, K.C., 2010. Observational studies: cohort and case-control studies. Plast. Reconstr. Surg. 126, 2234–2242.
47. Gamble, J.M., 2014. An introduction to the fundamentals of cohort and case-control studies. Can. J. Hosp. Pharm. 67, 366–372.
48. Lin, M.S., Dai, Y.S., Pwu, R.F., Chen, Y.H., Chang, N.C., 2005. Risk estimates for drugs suspected of being associated with Stevens-Johnson syndrome and toxic epidermal necrolysis: a case-control study. Intern. Med. J. 35, 188–190.
49. Yang, B., Hagberg, K.W., Chen, J., et al., 2016. Associations of antibiotic use with risk of primary liver cancer in the Clinical Practice Research Datalink. Br. J. Cancer 115, 85–89.
50. Grimes, D.A., Lobo, R.A., 2002. Perspectives on the Women's Health Initiative trial of hormone replacement therapy. Obstet. Gynecol. 100, 1344–1353.

CHAPTER 7

The Limitations of Observational Epidemiology

Observational research dominates the biomedical literature. However, few readers of that literature appreciate its tenuous scientific foundation. Most published findings of observational research are false. Of those findings that are true, most are exaggerated. Reporting is generally poor, and the inability to reproduce results is a generic problem in both the biomedical and behavioural sciences. Research with large administrative databases often produces precisely wrong results. Weak associations, below the discrimination limits of observational research, are routinely reported without caveats. Biomedical researchers are usually amateurs; most have no formal training in research methods, and the peer-review process at journals has little evidence of value. Retractions due to fraud are increasing dramatically. Observational studies have caused great harm and wasted precious resources. Indeed, an estimated 85% of the annual research investment is wasted. This chapter outlines some of the limitations of observational research and suggests some ways to address these problems.

False Claims

'There is now enough evidence to say what many have long thought: that any claim coming from an observational study is most likely to be wrong – wrong in the sense that it will not replicate if tested rigorously'.[1]

In 2005 Ioannidis shocked the medical world with his mathematical models showing that most reported research findings are wrong.[2] He extended this observation by noting that of those associations that are true, most are exaggerated.[3] The problem of false-positive claims is more acute with small studies, weak associations, more teams in pursuit of significant findings, and greater methodological bias or investigator prejudice. Indeed, large statistical associations may reflect large net bias, not any causality. At the other extreme, with massive study sizes, trivial effects (due to built-in bias) become statistically significant.[4] Unsuspected or unmeasured residual confounding and confounding by indication handicap observational studies, and no easy remedies are available.[5]

Others have confirmed that most observational study findings cannot be replicated. For example, 12 randomised trials tested claims from observational studies (including large ones) about diet,

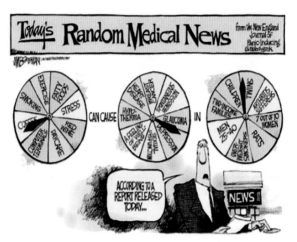

Fig. 7.1 Today's random medical news. Borgman ©1977 The Cincinnati Inquirer. (Reproduced with permission from Andrews McMeel Syndication.)

vitamins, and minerals. A total of 52 observational report claims were examined, and not one could be confirmed. Ironically, randomised trials found an effect in the opposite direction for 10% of the observational claims.[1] Researchers and the lay public must grapple daily with an epidemic of false claims[6] based on poor-quality research (Fig. 7.1). Although observational studies and randomised trials in pulmonary and critical care sometimes concur, numerous interventions found beneficial in observational studies have been refuted by randomised controlled trials. Basing therapy on observational studies instead of randomised trials may be more costly in the long run and more dangerous to patients.[7]

The medical literature is replete with bogus findings (Panel 7.1). Cigarette smoking was falsely linked with suicide due to inadequate control of confounding. Betacarotene was shown to have no benefit in reducing lung-cancer risk. Selection bias led to a consistent, but incorrect, conclusion that oestrogen in menopause was associated with a reduced risk of heart disease. Poor-quality case-control studies falsely linked reserpine (an antihypertensive drug) with breast cancer and coffee drinking with pancreatic cancer. Social desirability bias (healthy controls not reporting sensitive information) linked abortion with breast cancer. Junk science[8] led to the disappearance of a safe and effective antiemetic widely used in pregnancy. Inappropriate control groups, information bias, and failure to control for the confounding effect of sexually transmitted diseases led to the near disappearance of the intrauterine device (IUD) in the United States in the 1980s. Lack of control of confounding led researchers to believe that oral contraceptives were linked with pituitary tumours. A recent news report linking wearing high heel shoes and cancer[9] has led both authors to abandon our stilettos for good. Better safe than sorry!

Amateurs at Work

For millennia, medicine was learned through apprenticeship. By the early 1900s the deficiencies in this approach were evident. Abraham Flexner's review of American medical schools[10] led to the closure of many for-profit schools. Thereafter, medical schools joined forces with teaching hospitals. For the past century, medical education has featured clear objectives, formal curricula, postgraduate training, and national testing for competence.

In contrast, biomedical research continues to be learned through apprenticeship. As a result, few researchers today have any advanced training in research methods.[11] Most young researchers learn

PANEL 7.1 ■ Examples of Spurious Associations in Observational Epidemiology Studies

Exposure	Outcome	Explanation
Cigarette smoking	Increased risk of suicide	Smoking associated with factors predisposing to mental state that increases suicide risk[49,70]
Beta-carotene	Reduced risk of lung cancer	Information bias and residual confounding[71]
Menopausal oestrogen therapy	Reduced risk of coronary artery disease	Selection bias: women who chose to use oestrogen were at lower risk of coronary artery disease[72]
Reserpine therapy	Increased risk of breast cancer	Flawed case-control studies; findings not replicated by later, larger studies[73]
Coffee drinking	Increased risk of pancreatic cancer	Gravely flawed case-control study; finding refuted by later studies[43,73]
Induced abortion	Increased risk of breast cancer	Information bias; underreporting of abortion among healthy controls[43,74]
Bendectin (pyridox-ine/doxylamine) exposure	Increased risk of birth defects	Junk science[27]
IUD use	Increased risk of salpingitis and infertility	Wrong comparison groups, information bias (systematic overdiagnosis in IUD users), failure to control for confounding by sexually transmitted diseases[75]
Oral contraceptive use	Increased risk of pituitary adenoma	Confounding by indication[76]

Reproduced with permission from Grimes, D.A., Schulz, K.F., 2012. False alarms and pseudoepidemics. The limitations of observational epidemiology. Obstet. Gynecol. 120, 920–927.

on the job under the guidance of an older colleague, who generally has no formal research training either. As a result of the lower standards for medical research than for medical practice, most research today is suboptimal, as is its reporting. The desire to be a surgeon is insufficient to gain operating-room privileges. Not so in research. No formal training or certification is required before doing research and submitting a manuscript for publication.

The poor quality of biomedical research and its reporting is well documented. Many reports make no mention of limitations of the study.[12,13] Even in high-profile general medical journals, description of control for confounding bias remains poor.[14,15] Statistical errors include multiple unplanned comparisons to find something statistically significant ('p-value hacking'), single imputation of missing data, ignoring regression to the mean, and inferring causation from statistical associations in observational studies.[16] Discussion sections of manuscripts, where limitations and caveats should be discussed, are often chaotic and loosely tethered to the results.[17] Structured discussion sections, akin to structured abstracts, might promote transparency regarding the limitations of observational reports.[18]

Many clinical practice recommendations cannot be supported by the published literature.[19] Because of these deficiencies, international guidelines now exist for reporting observational studies. The Strengthening the Reporting of Observational Studies in Epidemiology (STROBE) guidelines[20] are available on the Internet (http://www.strobe-statement.org/index.php?id = strobe-home, accessed 9 March 2017) and on the Equator Network website (www.equator-network.org, accessed 9 March 2017). Compliance with the checklist for various types of observational studies will promote transparency concerning methods.

Moreover, over the past decade, formal approaches to grading the quality of evidence and strength of recommendations have gained popularity. The Grading of Recommendations Assessment, Development and Evaluation (GRADE) system evaluates the quality of evidence, including susceptibility to bias, then makes either strong or weak recommendations based on that evidence.[21,22]

Administrative Databases

Big data invite big problems. The term 'big data' denotes large, complex, and linkable information.[23] Poring over databases built for insurance or other purposes has become a burgeoning industry in medical research. Although such databases can monitor trends over time or provide crude measures of frequency, most databases are simply inadequate for credible epidemiological research. Eager researchers often start data dredging without a specified hypothesis and written plan of analysis. The process may degenerate into a scavenger hunt, derisively termed 'risk factorology'.[24] As Ioannidis has lamented, 'Risk factor epidemiology has excelled in salami-sliced data-dredged articles'.[25] The resultant spurious associations and false alarms needlessly frighten the public[26] and fill courtrooms with bogus, but remunerative, litigation.[27]

The advantages of administrative databases are readily apparent: the data are already gathered, computerised, and often vast in scope. The advantages of speed, previous data entry, and precision from large numbers are offset by two insurmountable problems: lack of validation of diagnosis and lack of information about potentially confounding factors.[28,29]

Accurate coding of patient outcomes is mandatory for study validity. Indeed, the US Food and Drug Administration cautions that for drug epidemiology studies using electronic databases, confirmation of the diagnosis requires going to the patient's medical record: 'Although validation can be performed using different techniques, the determination of the positive predictive value of a code-based (e.g., ICD) operational outcome definition often involves selecting all or a sample of cases with the codes of interest from the data source and conducting a review of their primary medical data (generally medical charts) to determine whether or not each patient actually experienced the coded event'.[30]

Diagnoses in many administrative databases are invalid, which precludes their use in epidemiological research. For example, an analysis of the Danish Patient Registry suggested differing risk of venous thromboembolism by type of progestin in oral contraceptives.[4] In contrast, large, rigorous, targeted cohort studies have consistently found the risk comparable with all progestins.[31,32] One explanation is that the diagnosis of venous thromboembolism in that database is often wrong.[33] Indeed, the positive predictive value for diseases and treatments in this database ranges from <15% to 100%.[34] The problem of invalid diagnoses in administrative databases is widespread. It includes insurance,[35] healthcare,[36] and vital statistics databases.[37]

The second deficiency of administrative databases is the usual lack of information about important potential confounding factors. For example, database studies of venous thrombosis commonly lack information on body mass index, family history of thrombosis, and socioeconomic status.[38,39] Missing data pose other irremediable challenges. Insurance claims data are often incomplete and error ridden.[40] Diet may play a role in the aetiology of many diseases, including cancer.[41] What information on fruit and vegetable consumption is found on insurance databases or national registries? Missing data are the norm in electronic health records, and these missing data are not missing at random.

Another danger of administrative database studies is 'mass significance'. Because of large sample sizes, almost any weak association, real or bogus, has a narrow confidence interval and an impressive statistical significance level with lots of zeroes after the decimal point. Big data can find significant differences of no consequence.[40] Trivial, often spurious, associations have achieved statistical significance but have no clinical relevance. Because of inaccurate diagnoses and lack of control for potential confounding, these studies may have precision but not validity. Stated another way, they may be precisely wrong.[4] Administrative databases have a role to play, but the notion that bigger is better in clinical research is demonstrably false.[40]

Weak Associations: Size Matters

Many researchers are unaware of the limitations of their craft. All observational research (and poorly done randomised controlled trials)[42] are susceptible to bias. Even after attempts to minimise selection and information biases and after control for known potential confounding factors, bias often remains. These biases can easily account for small associations. As a result, weak associations (which dominate in published studies) must be viewed with circumspection and humility.[43] Weak associations, defined as relative risks between 0.5 and 2.0, in a cohort study can readily be accounted for by residual bias (Fig. 7.2). Because case-control studies are more susceptible to bias than are cohort studies, the bar must be set higher. In case-control studies, weak associations can be viewed as odds ratios between 0.33 and 3.0 (Fig. 7.3). Results that fall within these zones may be due to bias. Results that fall outside these bounds in either direction may deserve attention.

Strength of association is one of the most important considerations in judging causality. In Austin Bradford Hill's classic essay, the relative risks for smoking and death from lung cancer ranged from 8 to 32, depending on smoking exposure. In his other example, the risk of cholera from drinking contaminated water was 14 compared with drinking water from another supplier.[44] Large relative risks are less likely to be due to bias than are small ones. This guideline is not absolute: large bias can produce large relative risks. For example, a British cohort study found a risk of pelvic inflammatory disease associated with IUDs of 11.[45] When a later reanalysis of the same cohort corrected for several biases, the risk associated with medicated IUDs was no longer statistically significant.[46] Unsuspected bias had accounted for a spurious 11-fold increase.

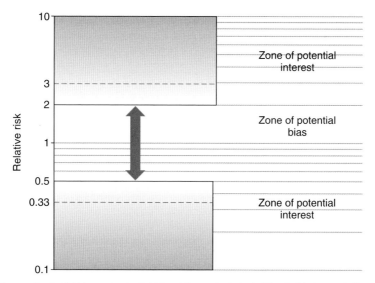

Fig. 7.2 Zones of potential bias and potential interest in a cohort study. Threshold of potential interest starts at 2 to 3 (dashed line) for increased risk and 0.5 to 0.33 (dashed line) for decreased risk. (Reproduced with permission from Grimes, D.A., Schulz, K.F., 2012. False alarms and pseudoepidemics. The limitations of observational epidemiology. Obstet. Gynecol. 120, 920–927.)

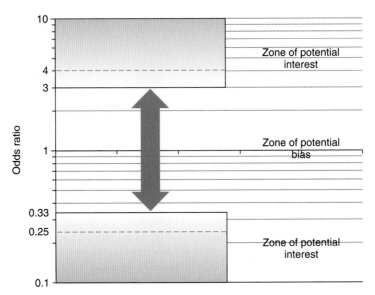

Fig. 7.3 Zones of potential bias and potential interest in a case-control study. Threshold of potential interest starts at 3 or 4 (dashed line) for increased risk and 0.33 to 0.25 (dashed line) for decreased risk. (Reproduced with permission from Grimes, D.A., Schulz, K.F., 2012. False alarms and pseudoepidemics. The limitations of observational epidemiology. Obstet. Gynecol. 120, 920–927.)

The medical literature is strewn with false alarms and pseudoepidemics due to flawed research (see Panel 7.1). The literature is replete with,[47] if not dominated by,[48] reports of weak associations. In observational studies, one cannot differentiate between bias and causation. This is simply beyond the discriminatory ability of observational research with its inherent biases. Even the most elegant statistical machinations cannot eliminate bias, especially unsuspected confounding. Meta-analysis of flawed observational studies offers no remedy; it provides more precision without addressing the more critical problem with validity.[49,50] Stated alternatively, most observational studies cannot separate noise from signal.[51]

Porous Peer Review

Scholarly critique of submitted manuscripts is a cornerstone of biomedical publishing and has been so for decades. As with institutional review boards (IRBs, or ethical review boards),[52] little evidence supports the value of this hoary tradition.[53] In contrast, the limited evidence is generally negative. As one editor noted, peer review is 'slow, expensive, ineffective, something of a lottery, prone to bias and abuse, and hopeless at spotting errors and fraud'.[54]

'Unfortunately, many medical editors who oversee their journal are largely untrained and certainly uncertified'.[55] Peer reviewers generally have even less training in research methods than editors, many are overburdened with other responsibilities, and the time invested in reviews goes unrewarded. One jaded male colleague told us that performing peer reviews for journals was akin to wetting his pants in a dark suit: it gave him a warm feeling, but nobody noticed. Some journals bestow continuing medical education credits for peer reviews done; although this may help ensure state licensure, it does little to advance one's career. Stated alternatively, doing peer reviews may be a poor investment of one's time.

The quality of peer reviews varies greatly. Our experience on editorial boards suggests that the quality of peer reviews is often inversely related to the age of the reviewer. Fellows and young academicians may devote more time and effort to this thankless task than more senior faculty who are inundated with such requests or just burned out.

Designed to provide objective assessments of the quality of submitted manuscripts, the peer-review system is easily corrupted. Some authors have steered reviews away from hostile reviewers by thanking them (without permission) for their (nonexistent) contributions to the manuscript. Some journals request the names and contact information for three potential reviewers when manuscripts are submitted; filling the list with friends (or those who owe the author money) is an obvious response. Other authors have fabricated names and e-mail addresses of potential reviewers; review invitations are then diverted back to the authors' own accounts.[56] This tactic is not novel: Walt Whitman wrote favourable anonymous reviews of his *Leaves of Grass* in New York newspapers.[57]

The peer-review process is a coarse net. Almost any manuscript can and will get published somewhere,[58] especially in light of the explosion of online journals. A follow-up of rejected manuscripts by one journal found that 42% were published in open-access journals within 10 months after rejection.[56] Open-access journals are especially problematic. To demonstrate the fallibility of their review process, the journal *Science* wrote a flagrantly flawed bogus paper and submitted it to more than 300 open-access journals; most accepted it. This sting operation revealed that academic publishing today is the 'Wild West'.[59]

'Regardless of the reason for doing peer review, most reviewers do it without training or reward'.[55] To expect referees to identify methodological flaws in submitted manuscripts without training in research methods or appropriate rewards for their efforts seems unrealistic.[56] Training in core competencies should be a prerequisite for serving as a peer reviewer. Some have suggested mandatory university full- or half-semester courses as part of degree requirements for graduate students to learn these skills.[55] These skills would, of course, transfer to the role of author. Skilled and motivated reviewers might help the peer-review process reach its intended goals.

Fraud

Fraud, which includes fabrication, falsification, and plagiarism,[60] poses a growing threat to medical research. In addition to 'dry labbing' false data, misconduct includes purging outliers ('trimming') and selectively using data ('cooking').[61] Since 1975 the proportion of published articles that has subsequently been retracted because of fraud or suspected fraud has increased 10-fold.[62] This worrisome trend may reflect increased attention to the problem,[61] an absolute increase in its frequency, or both. Retractions due to plagiarism and duplicate publication are a newer trend and may also account for some of the increase.[61]

Estimates of the prevalence of fraud vary. In a recent survey of Belgian researchers concerning fraud, the response rate was low (12% completed two questionnaires). Nevertheless, 15% of respondents admitted to scientific misconduct in the past three years. An earlier meta-analysis of 18 published surveys on the prevalence of fraud revealed that 2% of scientists admitted to scientific misconduct. A higher percentage reported other dubious research practices that could influence research validity. When asked if they knew of a colleague committing fraud, 14% of respondents replied affirmatively. Again, the frequency of suspect research practices by colleagues was higher than that of fraud.[63] Given the sensitivity of these issues,[64] these results should be considered conservative estimates of the frequency.

Retractions are more often due to dishonesty than to error. A review of more than 2000 retracted articles identified in PubMed found that 43% were retracted for confirmed or suspected fraud, 14% because of duplicate publication, and 10% for plagiarism. Only 21% were retracted because of error.[62] In general, fraudulent publications came from industrialised nations and high-profile journals; in contrast, plagiarism was associated with developing countries and lower-profile journals.

Improper incentives for researchers encourage fraud. In academic medicine, the quantity of publications counts more than quality.[65] Campbell's Law suggests that if researchers have incentives to produce more papers, then they will adjust their methods to maximise productivity, not quality.[66] In an evolutionary sense, the current reward system in biomedical research selects for poor methods that yield large numbers of publications (i.e., chaff, not wheat). Surveys confirm that young investigators in university hospitals, in particular, feel pressured to publish.[60] A simple remedy would be to change the incentives: have candidates for promotion and tenure provide their five best papers, not a list of all publications.

Conclusion

Learning medicine by apprenticeship was abandoned a century ago because of its deficiencies, yet a double standard in medical research continues to be tolerated. Researchers should have formal training and certification. Promotion and tenure should be based on the quality and not the quantity of publications. Peer review might function usefully with editors, authors, and peer reviewers having had some training in research methods.[54,55] Similarly, if peer reviews are a prerequisite to publication, then reviewer competence should be documented and the efforts rewarded. Researchers need more circumspection regarding the results of observational research. Reports with weak associations must provide caveats that the associations are likely wrong and of no clinical relevance. Editors need to raise the bar for acceptance of such manuscripts. Data mining of large administrative databases should be discouraged.[67] Such research is both quick and dirty, with the emphasis on the second adjective. As noted by Altman in a seminal essay,[68] what is needed today is 'less research, better research, and research done for the right reasons'.[69] That advice holds true today.

References

1. Young, S.S., Karr, A., 2011. Deming, data and observational studies. A process out of control and needing fixing. Significance 8, 116–120. https://doi.org/10.1111/j.1740-9713.2011.00506.x.
2. Ioannidis, J.P., 2005. Why most published research findings are false. PLoS Med 2, e124.
3. Ioannidis, J.P., 2008. Why most discovered true associations are inflated. Epidemiology 19, 640–648.
4. Lidegaard, O., Nielsen, L.H., Skovlund, C.W., Skjeldestad, F.E., Lokkegaard, E., 2011. Risk of venous thromboembolism from use of oral contraceptives containing different progestogens and oestrogen doses: Danish cohort study, 2001–9. BMJ 343, d6423.
5. Boyko, E.J., 2013. Observational research—opportunities and limitations. J. Diabetes Complicat. 27, 642–648.
6. Ioannidis, J.P., 2011. An epidemic of false claims. Competition and conflicts of interest distort too many medical findings. Sci. Am. 304, 16.
7. Albert, R.K., 2013. "Lies, damned lies …" and observational studies in comparative effectiveness research. Am. J. Respir. Crit. Care Med. 187, 1173–1177.
8. Crane, M., 1996. Is "junk science" finally on the way out? Med. Econ. 73, 59–61, 5–6.
9. Liviakis, V. Study: wearing high heels could lead to cancer. http://kron4.com/2017/03/06/study-wearing-high-heels-could-lead-to-cancer/.
10. Markel, H., 2010. Abraham Flexner and his remarkable report on medical education: a century later. JAMA 303, 888–890.
11. Luepker, R.V., 2005. Observational studies in clinical research. J. Lab. Clin. Med. 146, 9–12.
12. Ioannidis, J.P., 2007. Limitations are not properly acknowledged in the scientific literature. J. Clin. Epidemiol. 60, 324–329.
13. Ter Riet, G., Chesley, P., Gross, A.G., et al., 2013. All that glitters isn't gold: a survey on acknowledgment of limitations in biomedical studies. PLoS One 8, e73623.

14. Groenwold, R.H., Van Deursen, A.M., Hoes, A.W., Hak, E., 2008. Poor quality of reporting confounding bias in observational intervention studies: a systematic review. Ann. Epidemiol. 18, 746–751.
15. Groenwold, R.H., Hak, E., Hoes, A.W., 2009. Quantitative assessment of unobserved confounding is mandatory in nonrandomized intervention studies. J. Clin. Epidemiol. 62, 22–28.
16. George, B.J., Beasley, T.M., Brown, A.W., et al., 2016. Common scientific and statistical errors in obesity research. Obesity (Silver Spring, Md) 24, 781–790.
17. Horton, R., 2002. The hidden research paper. JAMA 287, 2775–2778.
18. Puhan, M.A., Akl, E.A., Bryant, D., Xie, F., Apolone, G., ter Riet, G., 2012. Discussing study limitations in reports of biomedical studies—the need for more transparency. Health Qual. Life Outcomes 10, 23.
19. Chauhan, S.P., Hammad, I.A., Weyer, K.L., Ananth, C.V., 2016. False alarms, pseudoepidemics, and reality: a case study with American College of Obstetricians and Gynecologists Practice Bulletins. Am. J. Perinatol. 33, 442–448.
20. von Elm, E., Altman, D.G., Egger, M., Pocock, S.J., Gøtzsche, P.C., Vandenbroucke, J.P., 2007. The Strengthening the Reporting of Observational Studies in Epidemiology (STROBE) statement: guidelines for reporting observational studies. Lancet 370, 1453–1457.
21. Guyatt, G.H., Oxman, A.D., Vist, G.E., et al., 2008. GRADE: an emerging consensus on rating quality of evidence and strength of recommendations. BMJ 336, 924–926.
22. Guyatt, G., Oxman, A.D., Akl, E.A., et al., 2011. GRADE guidelines: 1. Introduction-GRADE evidence profiles and summary of findings tables. J. Clin. Epidemiol. 64, 383–394.
23. Khoury, M.J., Ioannidis, J.P., 2014. Medicine. Big data meets public health. Science 346, 1054–1055.
24. Smith, G.D., 2001. Reflections on the limitations to epidemiology. J. Clin. Epidemiol. 54, 325–331.
25. Ioannidis, J.P., 2016. Evidence-based medicine has been hijacked: a report to David Sackett. J. Clin. Epidemiol. 73, 82–86.
26. Furedi, A., 1999. The public health implications of the 1995 'pill scare'. Hum. Reprod. Update 5, 621–626.
27. Brent, R.L., 1995. Bendectin: review of the medical literature of a comprehensively studied human non-teratogen and the most prevalent tortogen-litigen. Reprod. Toxicol. 9, 337–349.
28. Suissa, S., Garbe, E., 2007. Primer: administrative health databases in observational studies of drug effects—advantages and disadvantages. Nat. Clin. Pract. Rheumatol. 3, 725–732.
29. Grimes, D.A., 2010. Epidemiologic research using administrative databases: garbage in, garbage out. Obstet. Gynecol. 116, 1018–1019.
30. Food and Drug Administration, 2013. Best Practices for Conducting and Reporting Pharmacoepidemiologic Safety Studies Using Electronic Healthcare Data. Food and Drug Administration, Rockville, MD.
31. Dinger, J., Bardenheuer, K., Heinemann, K., 2014. Cardiovascular and general safety of a 24-day regimen of drospirenone-containing combined oral contraceptives: final results from the International Active Surveillance Study of Women Taking Oral Contraceptives. Contraception 89, 253–263.
32. Dinger, J.C., Heinemann, L.A., Kuhl-Habich, D., 2007. The safety of a drospirenone-containing oral contraceptive: final results from the European Active Surveillance Study on oral contraceptives based on 142,475 women-years of observation. Contraception 75, 344–354.
33. Severinsen, M.T., Kristensen, S.R., Overvad, K., Dethlefsen, C., Tjonneland, A., Johnsen, S.P., 2010. Venous thromboembolism discharge diagnoses in the Danish National Patient Registry should be used with caution. J. Clin. Epidemiol. 63, 223–228.
34. Schmidt, M., Schmidt, S.A., Sandegaard, J.L., Ehrenstein, V., Pedersen, L., Sorensen, H.T., 2015. The Danish National Patient Registry: a review of content, data quality, and research potential. Clin. Epidemiol. 7, 449–490.
35. Kern, D.M., Davis, J., Williams, S.A., et al., 2015. Validation of an administrative claims-based diagnostic code for pneumonia in a US-based commercially insured COPD population. Int. J. Chron. Obstruct. Pulmon. Dis. 10, 1417–1425.
36. Molnar, A.O., van Walraven, C., McArthur, E., Fergusson, D., Garg, A.X., Knoll, G., 2016. Validation of administrative database codes for acute kidney injury in kidney transplant recipients. Can. J. Kidney Health Dis. 3, 18.
37. Northam, S., Knapp, T.R., 2006. The reliability and validity of birth certificates. J. Obstet. Gynecol. Neonatal. Nurs. 35, 3–12.
38. Shapiro, S., Dinger, J., 2010. Risk of venous thromboembolism among users of oral contraceptives: a review of two recently published studies. J. Fam. Plann. Reprod. Health Care 36, 33–38.

39. Dinger, J., Shapiro, S., 2012. Combined oral contraceptives, venous thromboembolism, and the problem of interpreting large but incomplete datasets. J. Fam. Plann. Reprod. Health Care 38, 2–6.
40. Kaplan, R.M., Chambers, D.A., Glasgow, R.E., 2014. Big data and large sample size: a cautionary note on the potential for bias. Clin. Transl. Sci. 7, 342–346.
41. Martinez, M.E., Marshall, J.R., Giovannucci, E., 2008. Diet and cancer prevention: the roles of observation and experimentation. Nat. Rev. Cancer 8, 694–703.
42. Wood, L., Egger, M., Gluud, L.L., et al., 2008. Empirical evidence of bias in treatment effect estimates in controlled trials with different interventions and outcomes: meta-epidemiological study. BMJ 336, 601–605.
43. Boffetta, P., McLaughlin, J.K., La Vecchia, C., Tarone, R.E., Lipworth, L., Blot, W.J., 2008. False-positive results in cancer epidemiology: a plea for epistemological modesty. J. Natl. Cancer Inst. 100, 988–995.
44. Hill, A.B., 1965. The environment and disease association or causation. Proc. R. Soc. Med. 58, 295–300.
45. Vessey, M.P., Yeates, D., Flavel, R., McPherson, K., 1981. Pelvic inflammatory disease and the intrauterine device: findings in a large cohort study. Br. Med. J. (Clin. Res. Ed.) 282, 855–857.
46. Buchan, H., Villard-Mackintosh, L., Vessey, M., Yeates, D., McPherson, K., 1990. Epidemiology of pelvic inflammatory disease in parous women with special reference to intrauterine device use. Br. J. Obstet. Gynaecol. 97, 780–788.
47. Shapiro, S., 2008. Causation, bias and confounding: a hitchhiker's guide to the epidemiological galaxy Part 2. Principles of causality in epidemiological research: confounding, effect modification and strength of association. J. Fam. Plann. Reprod. Health Care 34, 185–190.
48. Khoury, M.J., Little, J., Gwinn, M., Ioannidis, J.P., 2007. On the synthesis and interpretation of consistent but weak gene-disease associations in the era of genome-wide association studies. Int. J. Epidemiol. 36, 439–445.
49. Egger, M., Schneider, M., Davey Smith, G., 1998. Spurious precision? Meta-analysis of observational studies. BMJ 316, 140–144.
50. Shapiro, S., 1997. Is meta-analysis a valid approach to the evaluation of small effects in observational studies? J. Clin. Epidemiol. 50, 223–229.
51. Silver, N., 2012. The Signal and the Noise. The Penguin Press, New York.
52. Silberman, G., Kahn, K.L., 2011. Burdens on research imposed by institutional review boards: the state of the evidence and its implications for regulatory reform. Milbank Q. 89, 599–627.
53. Jefferson, T., Rudin, M., Brodney Folse, S., Davidoff, F., 2007. Editorial peer review for improving the quality of reports of biomedical studies. Cochrane Database Syst. Rev. MR000016.
54. Smith, R., 2006. The trouble with medical journals. J. R. Soc. Med. 99, 115–119.
55. Moher, D., Altman, D.G., 2015. Four proposals to help improve the medical research literature. PLoS Med. 12, e1001864.
56. Stahel, P.F., Moore, E.E., 2014. Peer review for biomedical publications: we can improve the system. BMC Med. 12, 179.
57. Library of Congress, Revising himself: Walt Whitman and Leaves of Grass. https://www.loc.gov/exhibits/whitman/leavesofgrass.html.
58. Ioannidis, J.P., Tatsioni, A., Karassa, F.B., 2010. Who is afraid of reviewers' comments? Or, why anything can be published and anything can be cited. Eur. J. Clin. Investig. 40, 285–287.
59. Bohannon, J., 2013. Who's afraid of peer review? Science 342, 60–65.
60. Tijdink, J.K., Verbeke, R., Smulders, Y.M., 2014. Publication pressure and scientific misconduct in medical scientists. J. Empir. Res. Hum. Res. Ethics. 9 (5), 64–71. https://doi.org/10.1177/1556264614552421. Epub 2014 Oct 2.
61. Gross, C., 2016. Scientific misconduct. Annu. Rev. Psychol. 67, 693–711.
62. Fang, F.C., Steen, R.G., Casadevall, A., 2012. Misconduct accounts for the majority of retracted scientific publications. Proc. Natl. Acad. Sci. U. S. A. 109, 17028–17033.
63. Fanelli, D., 2009. How many scientists fabricate and falsify research? A systematic review and meta-analysis of survey data. PLoS ONE 4, e5738.
64. Stuart, G.S., Grimes, D.A., 2009. Social desirability bias in family planning studies: a neglected problem. Contraception 80, 108–112.
65. Ioannidis, J.P., 2014. How to make more published research true. PLoS Med 11, e1001747.

66. Smaldino, P.E., McElreath, R., 2016. The natural selection of bad science. R. Soc. Open Sci. 3, 160384.
67. Hauben, M., Reich, L., Van Puijenbroek, E.P., Gerrits, C.M., Patadia, V.K., 2006. Data mining in pharmacovigilance: lessons from phantom ships. Eur. J. Clin. Pharmacol. 62, 967–970.
68. Altman, D.G., 1994. The scandal of poor medical research. BMJ 308, 283–284.
69. von Elm, E., Egger, M., 2004. The scandal of poor epidemiological research. BMJ 329, 868–869.
70. Smith, G.D., Phillips, A.N., Neaton, J.D., 1992. Smoking as "independent" risk factor for suicide: illustration of an artifact from observational epidemiology? Lancet 340, 709–712.
71. Marshall, J.R., 1999. Beta-carotene: a miss for epidemiology. J. Natl. Cancer Inst. 91, 2068–2069.
72. Grimes, D.A., Lobo, R.A., 2002. Perspectives on the Women's Health Initiative trial of hormone replacement therapy. Obstet. Gynecol. 100, 1344–1353.
73. Spector, R., Vesell, E.S., 2000. The pursuit of clinical truth: role of epidemiology/observation studies. J. Clin. Pharmacol. 40, 1205–1210.
74. Bartholomew, L.L., Grimes, D.A., 1998. The alleged association between induced abortion and risk of breast cancer: biology or bias? Obstet. Gynecol. Surv. 53, 708–714.
75. Grimes, D.A., 1987. Intrauterine devices and pelvic inflammatory disease: recent developments. Contraception 36, 97–109.
76. Shy, K.K., McTiernan, A.M., Daling, J.R., Weiss, N.S., 1983. Oral contraceptive use and the occurrence of pituitary prolactinoma. JAMA 249, 2204–2207.

Uses and Abuses of Screening Tests

Despite extensive use of screening tests in contemporary practice, the underlying principles of screening are poorly understood by clinicians and the lay public alike. Screening is the testing of apparently well people to find those at increased risk of having a disease or disorder. Although an earlier diagnosis generally has intuitive appeal, earlier might not always be better or worth the cost. Four terms describe the validity of a screening test: sensitivity, specificity, predictive value positive, and predictive value negative. For tests with continuous variables (e.g., blood glucose), sensitivity and specificity are inversely related; where the cut-off for abnormal is placed should indicate the clinical effect of wrong results. The prevalence of disease in a population affects screening test performance: in low-prevalence settings, even very good tests have poor predictive value positives. Hence, knowledge of the approximate prevalence of disease is a prerequisite to interpreting screening test results. Tests are often done in sequence, as is true for syphilis and HIV-1 infection. Lead time, length, and other biases distort the apparent value of screening programmes; randomised controlled trials are the only way to avoid these biases. The STARD guidelines specify the steps needed to assess tests. Screening can improve health; for example, strong indirect evidence links cervical cytology programmes to declines in cervical cancer mortality. However, inappropriate application or interpretation of screening tests can rob people of their perceived health, initiate harmful diagnostic testing, and squander healthcare resources. Screening for ovarian cancer is a notable example.

Screening is a 'double-edged sword', sometimes wielded clumsily by the well-intended. Although ubiquitous in contemporary medical practice, screening remains widely misunderstood and misused. Indeed, most clinicians are unaware of the pitfalls of screening. Screening is defined as 'The presumptive identification of unrecognised disease or defect by the application of tests, examinations, or other procedures which can be applied rapidly. Screening tests sort out apparently well persons who probably have a disease from those who probably do not'.[1] Looking for additional

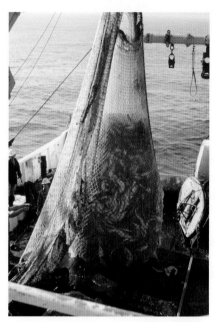

Fig. 8.1   Cod in commercial trawler net. Analogous to screening, as the prevalence of cod decreases, the cost of finding one increases. (Source: https://commons.wikimedia.org/wiki/File:Fish_on_Trawler.jpg, accessed July 3, 2017.)

illnesses in those with medical problems is termed case finding[1]; screening is limited to those apparently well.

One screening fallacy is that if we simply do enough testing, then we can eradicate a disease such as cervical cancer.[2] Fishing for cod explains why this optimism is naïve. Cod were so abundant in the Georges Bank on the continental shelf of North America that the Basques of Spain had established trade routes by AD 1000.[3] The fish were so plentiful that transoceanic expeditions were profitable centuries before Columbus wandered across. The cost of catching cod was negligible. As the Bank was aggressively overfished by traditional hand lines, then commercial trawlers, the fish population diminished greatly over the centuries. By the 1990s the Bank had few cod left (Fig. 8.1) Correspondingly the cost of catching a fish escalated dramatically. As the frequency of cod (or a disease) decreases, the cost of finding one increases. To catch the last cod in the Atlantic Ocean (or the last case of cervical cancer worldwide) would take extraordinary resources.

The number needed to screen (NNS) reflects this aspect of screening effectiveness. For cancer, this is the number of persons who would have to be screened to prevent one premature death from cancer (usually in the range of 500–1110 persons).[4] For mammography among women older than 50 years, an estimate is 543. For faecal occult blood testing for colorectal cancer, the corresponding number ranges from 600 to 1000 persons. For uncommon cancers, such as oral malignancies in developed countries, the NNS becomes prohibitively large. In the UK, the estimated NNS to prevent one death is >53,000, and to decrease oral cancer mortality rates by 1% is >1,125,000.[5] As the disease becomes more rare, the false-positive results dwarf the true positives, often wreaking harm by chasing false positives and wasting money.[6] Stated alternatively, finding the last case of any cancer (or fish in the sea) becomes impossibly expensive.

Screening can improve health. For example, strong indirect evidence supports cytology screening for cervical cancer. Insufficient use of this screening method accounts for a large proportion of invasive cervical cancers in industrialised nations.[7] Other beneficial examples include screening for hypertension in adults; screening for hepatitis B and C virus antigen, HIV, chlamydia infection, and syphilis in pregnant women; routine urine culture in pregnant women at 12 to 16 weeks' gestation; and phenylketonuria screening in newborns.[8] However, inappropriate screening harms healthy individuals and squanders precious resources. Here, we review the purposes of screening, the selection of tests, measurement of validity, the effect of prevalence on test outcome, and some biases that can distort interpretation of tests.

Ethical Implications
WHAT ARE THE POTENTIAL HARMS OF SCREENING?

Screening differs from the traditional clinical use of tests in several important ways. Ordinarily, patients consult with clinicians about complaints or problems; this prompts testing to confirm or exclude a diagnosis. Because the patient feels unwell and requests our help, the risk and expense of tests are usually deemed acceptable by the patient. By contrast, screening engages apparently healthy individuals who are not seeking medical help (and who might prefer to be left alone). Alternatively, consumer-generated demand for screening, such as for osteoporosis and ovarian cancer, might lead to expensive programmes of no clear value.[9] Hence the cost, injury, and stigmatisation related to screening are especially important (though often ignored in our zeal for earlier diagnosis); the medical and ethical standards of screening should be, correspondingly, higher than with diagnostic tests.[10] Bluntly put: every adverse outcome of screening is iatrogenic and inconsistent with the ethical principle of nonmaleficence.

Screening has a darker side that is often overlooked. It can be nauseating (oral glucose tolerance test for gestational diabetes), unpleasant (bowel preparation before colonoscopy), and both expensive and uncomfortable (mammography). Ovarian cancer screening is a prototype. The deadliest gynaecological cancer is usually detected when metastatic, and 5-year survival rates are grim. Hence some enthusiasts urged mounting screening programmes with vaginal ultrasound rather than waiting for empirical evidence of benefit.[11] Fortunately, large randomised trials of ovarian cancer screening with ultrasound and CA-125 were subsequently done. In the UK trial, no significant survival benefit was found with screening.[12] In the US trial among 78,216 women aged 55 to 74 years studied, no benefit in cancer mortality was found; this was confirmed by follow-up at a median of 15 years.[13] Screening enthusiasts[11] usually ignore the harms occasioned by screening. In the US trial, 3285 women had false-positive results; of these, 1080 had an operation as a result. Among these surgical patients, 163 had one or more serious complications, with a surgical morbidity rate of 21%. Stated alternatively, screening for ovarian cancer in this age group caused net harm to women and wasted resources. That is unethical.[14]

Cervical cancer screening, although likely useful, has important harms as well. In the late 1990s liquid-based cytology was developed as an alternative to the venerable Pap smear.[15] Based on unsubstantiated claims of better sensitivity than a Pap smear, the new and more expensive screening test soon dominated the US market. Claims of superiority over the traditional Pap smear subsequently were refuted,[16] by which time the liquid-based cytology had become firmly entrenched in practice. This change to liquid-based cytology drove up the cost of finding cervical cancer, a clear setback in public health.[17] Other harms of cervical cancer screening include the stigma of labelling, anxiety about cancer and loss of childbearing, extended and frequent future surveillance, and operations on the cervix. Excisional procedures on the cervix are linked with adverse pregnancy outcomes.[7] One report estimated that in the United States in 2007, more than 4 million women had health problems related to cervical cancer screening, 800,000 experienced anxiety, and more than 3 million had adverse events related to biopsy or treatment. Moreover, cervical cancer screening practices may have led to an estimated 5300 preterm births.[18]

The appropriate role of mammography screening remains in flux, despite its wide use and aggressive promotion.[19] An evaluation of three decades of mammography in the United States was discouraging. The rate of early-stage cancers detected doubled, while that of late-stage disease decreased only 8%.[20] A by-product of screening was substantial overdiagnosis of cancer. Because the natural history of ductal carcinoma in situ of the breast remains unclear, a recommendation has been made to delete the anxiety-provoking word 'carcinoma' from the term.[21] Until it metastasises, it is not cancer. The same holds true for in situ lesions of the prostate. More men die *with* prostate cancer than *of* prostate cancer. About half of all diagnosed cases of prostate cancer do not benefit from treatment.[22]

Prenatal testing for foetal chromosomal abnormalities poses another emerging crisis in screening practice. Noninvasive testing uses cell-free foetal DNA found in the pregnant woman's plasma. These tests first became commercially available in 2011 and have been aggressively promoted to the lay public.[23] Direct-to-consumer advertising has touted 'near-perfect accuracy', and uptake sky-rocketed in the absence of adequate evaluation and genetic counselling regarding interpretation of results. What consumers do not understand is that predictive-value-positive results, even if the test is accurate, are poor for rare disease such as genetic abnormalities.[24] Frightened women are now bypassing the requisite confirmatory tests and proceeding directly to abortion based on a screening test. One report found that 6% of women who were informed of a foetus at high risk aborted their pregnancies without a confirmatory amniocentesis and karyotype.[25] The use of diagnostic testing plummeted after introduction of noninvasive screening, raising concerns about clinicians' skill with amniocentesis and chorionic villus sampling dwindling as a result.[26]

A second wave of injury can arise after the initial screening insult. Although the stigma associated with correct labelling of people as ill might be acceptable, those incorrectly labelled as sick suffer as well. For example, labelling productive steelworkers as being hypertensive led to increased absenteeism and adoption of a sick role, independent of treatment or disease severity.[27] Women labelled as having gestational diabetes reported deterioration in their health and that of their children over the 5 years after diagnosis.[28] Awareness, as opposed to ignorance of hypothyroidism, diabetes, and hypertension, is associated with worse self-reported health status.[29] For some diseases, 'ignorance may be bliss'.

Treatment of hyperlipidaemia with clofibrate several decades ago provides another sobering example. Treatment of the cholesterol count (a surrogate endpoint, rather than an illness itself) inadvertently led to a 17% increase in mortality among middle-aged men given the drug (Chapter 18). This screening misadventure cost the lives of more than 5000 men in the United States alone. Because of these mishaps, screening practices should be more selective.

Criteria for Screening
IF A TEST IS AVAILABLE, SHOULD IT BE USED?

The availability of a screening test does not imply that it should be used. Indeed, before screening is done, the strategy must meet stringent criteria. Many of these were included in early guidance from the World Health Organization.[30] The disease should be medically important and clearly defined, and its prevalence reasonably well known. The natural history should be known, and an effective intervention must exist. The screening programme must be cost-effective, facilities for diagnosis and treatment must be readily available, and the course of action after a positive result must be generally agreed on and acceptable to those screened.

Finally, the test must do its job. It should be safe, have a reasonable cut-off level defined, and be both valid and reliable. The latter two terms, often used interchangeably, are distinct. Validity is the ability of a test to measure what it sets out to measure, usually differentiating between those with and without the disease. By contrast, reliability indicates repeatability. For example, a bathroom scale that consistently measures 2 kg heavier than a hospital scale ('the gold standard') provides an invalid but highly reliable result.

Although an early diagnosis generally has intuitive appeal, earlier might not always be better. For example, what benefit would accrue (and at what cost) from early diagnosis of Alzheimer disease, which to date has no effective treatment? What merit has earlier diagnosis of cervical cancer in developing countries if no treatment is available? The net effect of screening would be deprivation of one's sense of well-being. Sackett and colleagues[31] proposed a pragmatic checklist to help decide when (or if) seeking a diagnosis earlier than usual is worth the expense and bother. Does early diagnosis really benefit those screened, for example, in survival or quality of life? Can the clinician manage the additional time required to confirm the diagnosis and deal with those diagnosed before symptoms developed? Will those diagnosed earlier comply with the proposed treatment? Has the effectiveness of the screening strategy been established empirically rather than theoretically? Finally, are the cost and accuracy of the test clinically acceptable?

Assessment of Test Effectiveness

IS THE TEST VALID?

For over half a century,[32] four indices of test validity have been widely used: sensitivity, specificity, predictive value positive, and predictive value negative. Although clinically useful (and far improved over clinical hunches), these terms are predicated on an assumption that is often clinically unrealistic (i.e., that all people can be dichotomised as ill or well). Indeed, one definition of an epidemiologist is a person who sees the entire world in a 2×2 table. Often, those tested simply do not fit neatly into these designations: they might be possibly ill, early ill, probably well, or some other variant. Likelihood ratios, which incorporate varying (not just dichotomous) degrees of test results, can be used to refine clinicians' judgements about the probability of disease in a particular person (Chapter 9).

For simplicity, however, assume a population has been tested and assigned to the four mutually exclusive cells shown in Fig. 8.2. Sensitivity, sometimes termed the detection rate, is the ability of a test to find those with the disease. All those with disease are in the left column. Hence, the sensitivity is simply those correctly identified by the test (**a**) divided by all those sick (**a** + **c**). Specificity denotes the ability of a test to identify those without the condition. Calculation of this proportion is trickier, however. By analogy to sensitivity, some assume (incorrectly) that the formula here is **b/(b + d)**. However, the numerator for specificity is cell **d** (the true negatives), which is divided by all those healthy (**b + d**).

Sensitivity and specificity were traditionally thought not to vary with disease prevalence.[33] Empirical evidence has now disproved that concept.[34] This belies the simple arithmetic depicted previously. The variability of sensitivity and specificity with disease prevalence may reflect the patients' spectrum of disease, the filter of referral to studies, verification bias, and problems with the reference standard, discussed later.[35] Evidence from meta-analyses suggests that with high-prevalence diseases, the specificity tends to be lower; no clear effect was seen for sensitivity.[35] For clinicians, this means that validity of tests should be drawn from studies in populations with similar disease prevalence as their own. Although sensitivity and specificity are of interest to public-health policymakers, they are of little interest to the clinician. Stated alternatively, sensitivity and specificity (population measures) look backward (at results gathered over time).

Clinicians have to interpret test results to those tested. Thus what clinicians need to know are the predictive values of the test (individual measures, which look forward). To consider predictive values, one needs to rotate the orientation in Fig. 8.2 by 90°: predictive values work horizontally (rows), not vertically (columns). In the top row are all those with a positive test, but only those

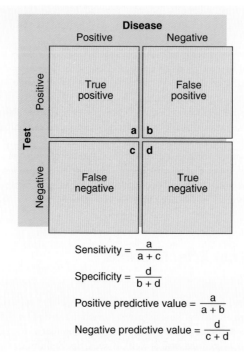

Fig. 8.2   Template for calculation of test validity.

in cell **a** are sick. Thus the predictive value positive is **a**/(**a** + **b**). The 'odds of being affected given a positive result' (OAPR) is the ratio of true positives to false positives, or **a** to **b**. Advocates of use of the OAPR note that these odds better describe test effectiveness than do probabilities (predictive values). On the other hand, most clinicians are more familiar with percentages than odds.[36]

In the bottom row of Fig. 8.2 are those with negative tests, but only those in cell **d** are free of disease. Hence the predictive value negative is **d**/(**c** + **d**). Memorising (and promptly forgetting) these formulas was an annual ritual for many of us in our clinical training. If readers understand the previous definitions and can recall the 2 × 2 table shell, then they can quickly derive these formulas when needed. As a mnemonic, disease goes at the top of the table shell, because it is our top priority. By default, test goes on the left border.

Through the years, researchers have tried to simplify these four indices of test validity by condensing them into a single term. However, none adequately depicts the important trade-offs between sensitivity and specificity that generally arise. An example is diagnostic accuracy, which is the proportion of correct results. It is the sum of the correctly identified ill and well divided by all those tested, or (**a** + **d**)/(**a** + **b** + **c** + **d**). Cells **b** and **c** are noise in the system. Another early attempt, Youden's *J*, is simply the sensitivity plus specificity minus one.[37] The range of values extends from zero to 1.0, when tests are perfect.

Benchmarks are helpful when considering screening tests. One rule of thumb is that a good test should have sensitivity plus specificity that add to ≥1.5 (or ≥150%). A very good test should have sensitivity plus specificity that add to ≥1.8 (or ≥180%). Modern polymerase chain reaction (PCR) tests for chlamydial infection have values that add to nearly 2.0,[38] while electronic foetal monitoring has a sum of about 1.3, indicating a mediocre test.[39]

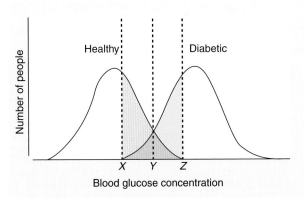

Fig. 8.3   Hypothetical distribution of blood glucose concentrations in people with and without diabetes. Setting cut-off for abnormal at *X* yields perfect sensitivity at the expense of specificity. Setting cut-off at *Z* results in perfect specificity at the cost of lower sensitivity. Cut-off *Y* is a compromise.

Trade-Offs Between Sensitivity and Specificity

WHERE SHOULD THE CUT-OFF FOR ABNORMAL BE?

The ideal test would perfectly discriminate between those with and without the disorder. The distributions of test results for the two groups would not overlap. More commonly in human biology, test values for those with and without a disease overlap, sometimes widely. The placement of the cut-off defining normal versus abnormal determines the sensitivity and specificity. For any continuous outcome measurement (e.g., blood pressure, intraocular pressure, or blood glucose), the sensitivity and specificity of a test will be inversely related. Fig. 8.3 shows that placing the cut-off for abnormal blood glucose at point *X* produces nearly perfect sensitivity; this low cut-off identifies all those with diabetes. However, the trade-off is poor specificity: those in the part of the healthy distribution in pink and purple are incorrectly identified as having abnormal values. Placing the cut-off higher at point *Z* yields the opposite result: all those healthy are correctly identified (nearly perfect specificity), but the cost here is missing a proportion of ill individuals (portion of the diabetic distribution in purple and blue). Placing the cut-off at point *Y* is a compromise, mislabelling some healthy people and some people with diabetes.

Where the cut-off should be depends on the implications of the test, and receiver operator characteristic curves, described further in Chapter 9, are useful in making this decision. For example, screening for phenylketonuria in newborns places a premium on sensitivity rather than on specificity; the cost of missing a case is high, and effective treatment exists. The downside is a large number of false-positive tests, which cause anguish and further testing. By contrast, screening for breast cancer should favour specificity over sensitivity, because further assessment of those tested positive entails costly and invasive biopsies. Moreover, false-positive results are associated with delayed subsequent screening and a later stage at diagnosis.[40]

Prevalence and Predictive Values

CAN TEST RESULTS BE TRUSTED?

A badly understood feature of screening is the dramatic effect of disease prevalence on predictive values. Clinicians must know the approximate prevalence of the condition of interest in the

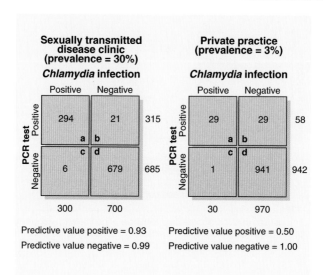

Fig. 8.4 Predictive values of a polymerase chain reaction (PCR) test for *Chlamydia trachomatis* in high-prevalence and low-prevalence settings.

population being tested; if not, reasonable interpretation is impossible. Consider a new PCR test for *Chlamydia trachomatis*, with a sensitivity of 0.98 and specificity of 0.97 (a superb test). As shown in the left panel of Fig. 8.4, a doctor uses the test in a municipal sexually transmitted disease clinic, where the prevalence of *C. trachomatis* is 30%. In this high-prevalence setting, the predictive value of a positive test is high, 93% (i.e., 93% of those with a positive test actually have the infection).

Impressed with the new test, the doctor now takes it to her private practice in the suburbs, which has a clientele that is mostly older than age 35 years (see Fig. 8.4, right panel). Here, the prevalence of chlamydial infection is only 3%. Now the same excellent test has a predictive positive value of only 0.50. When the results of the test are positive, what should the doctor tell the patient, and what, in turn, should the patient tell her husband? Here, flipping a coin has the same predictive positive value (cheaper, simpler, and no need for a speculum examination). This message is important, yet not widely understood: when used in low-prevalence settings, even excellent tests have poor predictive positive value. This is why routine electronic foetal monitoring and newer variants[39] are doomed to fail: the diseases they seek (foetal death in labour or later cerebral palsy) are too rare to enable screening. The reverse is true for negative predictive values, which are nearly perfect in Fig. 8.4. Although failing to diagnose sexually transmitted diseases can have important health implications, incorrectly labelling people as infected can wreck marriages and damage lives.

Tests in Combination
SHOULD A FOLLOW-UP TEST BE DONE?

Clinicians rarely use tests in isolation. Few tests have sufficiently high sensitivity and specificity, so a common approach is to do tests in sequence. With syphilis, a sensitive (but not specific) reagin test is the initial screen. Those who test positive then get a second, more specific test, a diagnostic treponemal test. Only those who test positive on both receive the diagnosis. This strategy generally increases the specificity compared with a single test and limits the use of the more expensive treponemal test. Traditional testing for HIV used an analogous two-step procedure with repeatedly reactive immunoassay followed by a supplemental test, such as western blot or indirect immunofluorescence assay. Other HIV diagnostic algorithms are under investigation.[41]

Alternatively, tests can be done in tandem (parallel or simultaneous testing). For example, two different tests might both have poor sensitivity, but one might be better at picking up early disease, whereas the other is better at identifying late disease. A positive result from either test would then lead to diagnostic assessment. This approach results in higher sensitivity than would arise with either test used alone.

Benefit or Bias?

DOES A SCREENING PROGRAMME REALLY IMPROVE HEALTH?

Even worthless screening tests often seem to have benefit. This cruel irony underlies many inappropriate screening programmes used today. Two common pitfalls lead to the conclusion that screening improves health: one is an artefact and the other a reflection of biology.

LEAD-TIME BIAS

Lead-time bias refers to a spurious increase in longevity associated with screening. For example, assume that mammography screening leads to cancer detection two years earlier than would have ordinarily occurred, yet the screening does not prolong life. On average, women with breast cancer detected through screening live two years longer than those with cancers diagnosed through traditional means. This gain in longevity is apparent and not real: the screening allows women to live two years longer with the knowledge that they have cancer, but it does not prolong survival, an example of zero-time shift.

The cartoon character tied to the railroad tracks awaiting the oncoming train (the fatal disease) illustrates this bias. Use of binoculars (the screening test) would enable an earlier diagnosis of the impending lethal event. However, unless this knowledge enables escape, death will occur when the train arrives on schedule. The screening allows the character to live longer with the knowledge of his impending death.[42] This probably adds to the discomfort of being tied to the tracks.

LENGTH BIAS

Length bias is more subtle than lead-time bias: the longevity association is real, but indirect. Assume that community-based mammography screening is done at 10-year intervals. Further assume that women whose breast cancers were detected through screening live 5 years longer on average from cancer initiation to death than those whose cancers were detected through usual means. That screening is associated with longer survival implies clear benefit. However, in this hypothetical example, this benefit reflects the inherent variability in cancer growth rates and not a benefit of screening. Women with indolent, slow-growing cancers are more likely to live long enough to be identified in decennial screening. Conversely, those with rapidly progressing tumours are less likely to survive until screening.[42]

The only way to avoid these pervasive biases is to do randomised controlled trials and then to assess age-specific mortality rates for those screened versus those not screened. Moreover, the trials must be done well. The quality of published trials of mammography screening has raised serious questions about the utility of this massive and expensive enterprise; the net effect on women's health appears smaller than anticipated.[20,43]

Still other biases can impair test accuracy.[44] 'Incorporation bias' occurs when the index test in question plays a role in whether the reference standard test is done. If the reference test is only done on persons with a positive index test, this circularity biases the sensitivity upward. Similarly, if an expert panel serves as the reference standard and the panel is not blinded as to the index test result, the same bias occurs. If a physician's final diagnosis provides the reference standard, knowledge of the index test likely played a role in the physician's final diagnosis; the reference standard was not independent of the index test result.

'Differential verification bias' happens when those with a positive index test are more likely to get the reference test, and only those with a positive reference test are included in the study. An example would be a sign or symptom being the index test, and a positive result (e.g., right lower quadrant pain) prompts further evaluation. Again, the decision to perform the reference test is not independent of the index test.

'Imperfect gold-standard bias' reflects the fallibility of the reference test. Assume that PCR is the index test for *Bordetella pertussis* infection, and bacterial culture is the reference standard. False-negative cultures are a problem; false-positive cultures are rare. Evaluating the index PCR against the imperfect bacterial culture will exaggerate its sensitivity.

'Spectrum bias' reflects the variation in disease and health in the population sampled.[45] Sensitivity is influenced by the spectrum of disease, and specificity by the spectrum of nondisease. If only severe cases of illness are included in a study, the sensitivity of the test will be exaggerated. Similarly, if only the healthiest of the well are included, the specificity will be overestimated.

GUIDELINES FOR TEST EVALUATIONS

In 2015, the **St**andards for **R**eporting **D**iagnostic Accuracy Studies (STARD) guidelines were updated[34] from the original version.[46] The revised checklist includes 30 items deemed essential for evaluating tests. The checklist and STARD statement are also available on the EQUATOR network website (http://www.equator-network.org, accessed 8 May 2017). These guidelines aim to improve the transparency and rigour of test evaluations. For researchers performing systematic reviews of diagnostic accuracy, the **Qu**ality **A**ssessment of **D**iagnostic **A**ccuracy **S**tudies (QUADAS) tool features a 14-item checklist.[47] A second version of QUADAS breaks down the items into four areas: selection of patients, the index test, the reference (gold) standard, and flow and timing of the study.[48]

Conclusion

Screening can promote or impair health, depending on its application. Unlike a diagnostic test, a screening test is done in apparently healthy people, which raises unique ethical concerns. Sensitivity and specificity tend to be inversely related, and choice of the cut-off point for abnormal should indicate the implications of incorrect results. Even excellent tests have poor predictive value positive when applied to low-prevalence populations. Lead time, length, and other biases distort the apparent benefit of screening programmes, underscoring the need for rigorous assessment in randomised controlled trials before use of screening programmes or their promotion to the lay public.

References

1. Porta, M., 2014. A Dictionary of Epidemiology. Oxford University Press, New York.
2. Ness, A.B., 2015. How We Can Eliminate Cervical Cancer Worldwide. http://www.gereports.com/post/123031815163/alicia-bonner-ness-how-we-can-eliminate-cervical-cancer/. Accessed 4 January 2016.
3. The sorry story of Georges Bank. http://www.amnh.org/explore/science-bulletins/bio/documentaries/will-the-fish-return/the-sorry-story-of-georges-bank. Accessed 4 January 2016.
4. Fields, M.M., Chevlen, E., 2006. Screening for disease: making evidence-based choices. Clin. J. Oncol. Nurs. 10, 73–76.
5. Petti, S., Scully, C., 2015. How many individuals must be screened to reduce oral cancer mortality rate in the Western context? A challenge. Oral Dis. 21, 949–954.

6. Petti, S., 2016. Oral cancer screening usefulness: between true and perceived effectiveness. Oral Dis. 22, 104–108.
7. Sawaya, G.F., 2009. Cervical-cancer screening—new guidelines and the balance between benefits and harms. N. Engl. J. Med. 361, 2503–2505.
8. US Preventive Services Task Force Guides to Clinical Preventive Services, 2014. The Guide to Clinical Preventive Services 2014: Recommendations of the US Preventive Services Task Force. Agency for Healthcare Research and Quality (US), Rockville (MD).
9. Andersen, M.R., Peacock, S., Nelson, J., et al., 2002. Worry about ovarian cancer risk and use of ovarian cancer screening by women at risk for ovarian cancer. Gynecol. Oncol. 85, 3–8.
10. Chiolero, A., Paccaud, F., Aujesky, D., Santschi, V., Rodondi, N., 2015. How to prevent overdiagnosis. Swiss Med. Wkly. 145, w14060.
11. Gosink, B.B., 1992. Ovarian cancer screening. Am. J. Obstet. Gynecol. 166, 1591–1593.
12. Jacobs, I.J., Menon, U., Ryan, A., et al., 2016. Ovarian cancer screening and mortality in the UK Collaborative Trial of Ovarian Cancer Screening (UKCTOCS): a randomised controlled trial. Lancet 387, 945–956.
13. Pinsky, P.F., Yu, K., Kramer, B.S., et al., 2016. Extended mortality results for ovarian cancer screening in the PLCO trial with median 15 years follow-up. Gynecol. Oncol. 143, 270–275.
14. American College of Obstetricians and Gynecologists, 2004. Ethics in Obstetrics and Gynecology, second ed. American College of Obstetricians and Gynecologists, Washington, D.C.
15. Sawaya, G.F., Grimes, D.A., 1999. New technologies in cervical cytology screening: a word of caution. Obstet. Gynecol. 94, 307–310.
16. Arbyn, M., Bergeron, C., Klinkhamer, P., Martin-Hirsch, P., Siebers, A.G., Bulten, J., 2008. Liquid compared with conventional cervical cytology: a systematic review and meta-analysis. Obstet. Gynecol. 111, 167–177.
17. Relman, A.S., 1980. The new medical-industrial complex. N. Engl. J. Med. 303, 963–970.
18. Habbema, D., Weinmann, S., Arbyn, M., et al., 2017. Harms of cervical cancer screening in the United States and the Netherlands. Int. J. Cancer 140, 1215–1222.
19. Myers, E.R., Moorman, P., Gierisch, J.M., et al., 2015. Benefits and harms of breast cancer screening: a systematic review. JAMA 314, 1615–1634.
20. Bleyer, A., Welch, H.G., 2012. Effect of three decades of screening mammography on breast-cancer incidence. N. Engl. J. Med. 367, 1998–2005.
21. Allegra, C.J., Aberle, D.R., Ganschow, P., et al., 2010. National Institutes of Health State-of-the-Science Conference statement: diagnosis and management of ductal carcinoma in situ September 22–24, 2009. J. Natl. Cancer Inst. 102, 161–169.
22. Jahn, J.L., Giovannucci, E.L., Stampfer, M.J., 2015. The high prevalence of undiagnosed prostate cancer at autopsy: implications for epidemiology and treatment of prostate cancer in the Prostate-specific Antigen-era. Int. J. Cancer 137, 2795–2802.
23. Meredith, S., Kaposy, C., Miller, V.J., Allyse, M., Chandrasekharan, S., Michie, M., 2016. Impact of the increased adoption of prenatal cfDNA screening on non-profit patient advocacy organizations in the United States. Prenat. Diagn. 36, 714–719.
24. Gekas, J., Langlois, S., Ravitsky, V., et al., 2016. Non-invasive prenatal testing for fetal chromosome abnormalities: review of clinical and ethical issues. Appl. Clin. Genet. 9, 15–26.
25. Daley, B., 2014. Oversold and misunderstood. Prenatal screening tests prompt abortions. https://eye.necir.org/2014/12/13/prenatal-testing/. Accessed 3 January 2017.
26. Warsof, S.L., Larion, S., Abuhamad, A.Z., 2015. Overview of the impact of noninvasive prenatal testing on diagnostic procedures. Prenat. Diagn. 35, 972–979.
27. Haynes, R.B., Sackett, D.L., Taylor, D.W., Gibson, E.S., Johnson, A.L., 1978. Increased absenteeism from work after detection and labeling of hypertensive patients. N. Engl. J. Med. 299, 741–744.
28. Feig, D.S., Chen, E., Naylor, C.D., 1998. Self-perceived health status of women three to five years after the diagnosis of gestational diabetes: a survey of cases and matched controls. Am. J. Obstet. Gynecol. 178, 386–393.
29. Jorgensen, P., Langhammer, A., Krokstad, S., Forsmo, S., 2015. Diagnostic labelling influences self-rated health. A prospective cohort study: the HUNT Study, Norway. Fam. Pract. 32, 492–499.
30. Wilson, J.M.G., Jungner, G., 1968. Principles and Practice of Screening for Disease. World Health Organization, Geneva.

31. Sackett, D., Haynes, R., Guyatt, G., Tugwell, P., 1991. Clinical Epidemiology. A Basic Science for Clinical Medicine, second ed. Little, Brown and Company, Boston.
32. Yerushalmy, J., 1947. Statistical problems in assessing methods of medical diagnosis, with special reference to X-ray techniques. Public Health Rep. 62, 1432–1449.
33. Streiner, D.L., 2003. Diagnosing tests: using and misusing diagnostic and screening tests. J. Pers. Assess. 81, 209–219.
34. Bossuyt, P.M., Reitsma, J.B., Bruns, D.E., et al., 2015. STARD 2015: an updated list of essential items for reporting diagnostic accuracy studies. Clin. Chem. 61, 1446–1452.
35. Leeflang, M.M., Rutjes, A.W., Reitsma, J.B., Hooft, L., Bossuyt, P.M., 2013. Variation of a test's sensitivity and specificity with disease prevalence. CMAJ 185, E537–44.
36. Grimes, D.A., Schulz, K.F., 2008. Making sense of odds and odds ratios. Obstet. Gynecol. 111, 423–426.
37. Youden, W.J., 1950. Index for rating diagnostic tests. Cancer 3, 32–35.
38. Dos Santos, C.G., Sabido, M., Leturiondo, A.L., Ferreira, C.O., da Cruz, T.P., Benzaken, A.S., 2017. Development, validation and testing costs of an in-house real-time polymerase chain reaction assay for the detection of *Chlamydia trachomatis*. J. Med. Microbiol. 66, 312–317.
39. Grimes, D.A., Peipert, J.F., 2010. Electronic fetal monitoring as a public health screening program: the arithmetic of failure. Obstet. Gynecol. 116, 1397–1400.
40. Dabbous, F.M., Dolecek, T.A., Berbaum, M.L., et al., 2017. Impact of a false-positive screening mammogram on subsequent screening behavior and stage at breast cancer diagnosis. Cancer Epidemiol. Biomark. Prev. 26, 397–403.
41. Detection of acute HIV infection in two evaluations of a new HIV diagnostic testing algorithm—United States, 2011-2013, 2013. MMWR Morb. Mortal. Wkly. Rep. 62, 489–494.
42. Hsu, J.L., Banerjee, D., Kuschner, W.G., 2008. Understanding and identifying bias and confounding in the medical literature. South. Med. J. 101, 1240–1245.
43. Gøtzsche, P.C., Jorgensen, K.J., 2013. Screening for breast cancer with mammography. Cochrane Database Syst. Rev., CD001877.
44. Kohn, M.A., Carpenter, C.R., Newman, T.B., 2013. Understanding the direction of bias in studies of diagnostic test accuracy. Acad. Emerg. Med. 20, 1194–1206.
45. Sica, G.T., 2006. Bias in research studies. Radiology 238, 780–789.
46. Bossuyt, P.M., Reitsma, J.B., Bruns, D.E., et al., 2003. Towards complete and accurate reporting of studies of diagnostic accuracy: the STARD initiative. Standards for Reporting of Diagnostic Accuracy. Clin. Chem. 49, 1–6.
47. Whiting, P., Rutjes, A.W., Reitsma, J.B., Bossuyt, P.M., Kleijnen, J., 2003. The development of QUADAS: a tool for the quality assessment of studies of diagnostic accuracy included in systematic reviews. BMC Med. Res. Methodol. 3, 25.
48. Whiting, P.F., Rutjes, A.W., Westwood, M.E., et al., 2011. QUADAS-2: a revised tool for the quality assessment of diagnostic accuracy studies. Ann. Intern. Med. 155, 529–536.

CHAPTER 9

Refining Clinical Diagnosis With Likelihood Ratios

Likelihood ratios can refine clinical diagnosis on the basis of signs and symptoms; however, they are grossly underused for patient care. A likelihood ratio is the percentage of ill people with a given test result divided by the percentage of well individuals with the same result. Ideally, abnormal test results should be much more frequent in ill individuals than in those who are well (high likelihood ratio), and normal test results should be more frequent in well people than in sick people (low likelihood ratio). Likelihood ratios near unity have little effect on decision making; by contrast, high or low ratios can shift (sometimes dramatically) the clinician's estimate of the probability of disease. Likelihood ratios can be calculated not only for dichotomous (positive or negative) tests but also for tests with multiple levels of results, such as helical computerised tomography (CT) scans. When combined with an accurate clinical diagnosis, likelihood ratios from ancillary tests improve diagnostic accuracy in a synergistic manner.

Despite their usefulness in interpretation of clinical findings, laboratory tests, and imaging studies, likelihood ratios remain little used. Most doctors are unfamiliar with likelihood ratios,[1,2] and few use them in practice. In a survey of 300 doctors in different specialties, only two (both internists) reported using likelihood ratios for test results.[3] The underuse of likelihood ratios may reflect the dominance of therapeutic studies in the medical literature, as opposed to diagnostic studies.[2] Because simple descriptions help clinicians to understand such ideas,[4] we will try to make likelihood ratios both simple and clinically relevant. Our aim is to enhance clinicians' familiarity with and use of likelihood ratios.

If everyone could be categorised as diseased or healthy, and if a dichotomous test for that disease were universally administered, then all seven billion of us will fit (albeit crowded) into one such table (Fig. 9.1). Regrettably, neither life nor tests are so simple; grey zones abound. Likelihood ratios help clinicians to navigate these seas of uncertainty.

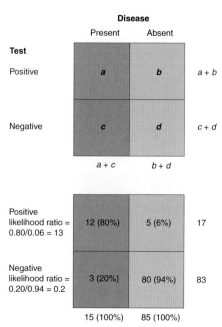

Fig. 9.1   2 × 2 tables. Top: distribution of population by disease status and dichotomous test result. Bottom: hypothetical distribution of 100 people by disease status and dichotomous test result.

A likelihood ratio, as its name implies, is the likelihood of a given test result in a person with a disease compared with the likelihood of this result in a person without the disease. Stated alternatively, a likelihood ratio is simply the percentage of sick people with a given test result divided by the percentage of well individuals with the same result. Percentage and likelihood are used interchangeably here. The implications are clear: ill people should be much more likely to have an abnormal test result than healthy individuals, and vice versa. The size of this discrepancy has clinical importance.

Likelihood Ratios for Tests With Two Outcomes

The simple 2 × 2 table in the bottom of Fig. 9.1 shows the calculation for the likelihood ratio. In this example, 15 people are sick and 12 (80%) have a true-positive test for the disease. By contrast, 85 are well but five (6%) have a false-positive test. Thus the likelihood ratio for a positive test is simply the ratio of these two percentages (80%/6%), which is 13. Stated in another way, people with the disease are 13 times more likely to have a positive test than are those who are well. For a dichotomous test (positive or negative), this is called the positive likelihood ratio (abbreviated LR+). The flip side, the negative likelihood ratio (LR–), is calculated similarly. Three of 15 sick people (20%) have a false-negative test, whereas 80 of 85 healthy individuals (94%) have a true-negative test. So LR– is the ratio of these percentages (20%/94%), which is 0.2. Thus a negative test is one-fifth as likely in someone who is sick than in a well person. Panel 9.1 outlines three approaches to calculate likelihood ratios for dichotomous data.

The Prospective Investigation of Pulmonary Embolism Diagnosis III (PIOPED III) study examined the usefulness of gadolinium-enhanced magnetic resonance angiography in diagnosing this disease.[5] A total of 371 patients were included. This imaging technique proved technically inadequate in a quarter of patients, which limits its clinical usefulness (Panel 9.2). The reference standard incorporated clinical assessment, D-dimer tests, and other imaging studies.

PANEL 9.1 ■ Calculation of Likelihood Ratios for Dichotomous Results

If sensitivity and specificity have already been determined, then:
    LR+ is sensitivity/(1 – specificity)
    LR– is (1 – sensitivity)/specificity
If raw numbers for the 2 × 2 table are available, then:
    LR+ is (a/[a + c])/(b/[b + d])
    LR– is (c/[a + c])/(d/[b + d])
If mathematical formulas are unappealing, then:
    LR+ is the true-positive percentage divided by the false-positive percentage
    LR– is the false-negative percentage divided by the true-negative percentage

---

PANEL 9.2 ■ Magnetic Resonance Angiography Compared With Reference Standard[5]

Angiography Result	Reference Standard		Total
Positive	59	2	61
Negative	17	201	218
Technically inadequate	28	64	92
Total	104	267	371

PANEL 9.3 ■ Magnetic Resonance Angiography Compared With Reference Standard in Those With Adequate Studies[5]

Angiography Result	Reference Standard		Total	Likelihood Ratio
Positive	59 (0.776)	2 (0.001)	61	78.8
Negative	17 (0.224)	201 (0.990)	218	0.226
Total	76 (1.000)	203 (1.000)	279	

For patients with adequate imaging studies (Panel 9.3), the sensitivity was 0.78 and the specificity was 0.99. The distribution of results is presented, and the likelihood ratios are calculated in the right column. A positive test had a high LR+, useful for establishing the diagnosis. The LR– approached the threshold of 0.1.

Why Bother?

As most doctors are generally familiar with terms such as 'sensitivity' and 'specificity',[1,6] is learning to use likelihood ratios worth the additional effort? Likelihood ratios have several attractive features that the traditional indices of test validity (Chapter 8) do not share.

First, not all tests have dichotomous results. Formulae for test validity do not work when results are anything other than just positive or negative. Many tests in clinical medicine have continuous results (e.g., blood pressure) or multiple ordinal levels (fine-needle biopsy of breast masses).

Public-domain software will calculate indices of validity and likelihood ratios for 2 × 2 tables. For 2 × n tables, the software will calculate level-specific likelihood ratios, plot a receiver operating characteristic (ROC) curve, and determine the area under the curve (http://www.openepi.com/DiagnosticTest/DiagnosticTest.htm, accessed 2 April 2017). Another useful calculator can be found at http://ebm-tools.knowledgetranslation.net/calculator/diagnostic/ (accessed 21 April 2017).

Likelihood ratios express the richness of test results and can influence patient management. Collapsing multiple categories into positive and negative sacrifices information. Likelihood ratios enable clinicians to interpret and use the full range of diagnostic test results instead of arbitrarily dichotomizing results. Although predictive values relate test characteristics to populations, likelihood ratios can be applied to a specific patient. Moreover, likelihood ratios, unlike traditional indices of validity, incorporate all four cells of a 2 × 2 table (see Panel 9.1).

Reliance on sensitivity and specificity frequently leads to exaggeration of the benefits of tests.[7] In a comparison of two obstetrical tests (foetal fibronectin measurement to predict premature birth, and uterine artery Doppler wave-form analysis to predict pre-eclampsia), two-thirds of published reports overestimated the value of the tests. Use of likelihood ratios, rather than just sensitivity and specificity, might have prevented this misinterpretation.

Finally, and most important, likelihood ratios refine clinical judgement. Application of a likelihood ratio to a working diagnosis may change the diagnostic probability—sometimes radically.

When tests are done in sequence, the post-test odds of the first test become the pretest odds for the second test; one builds on the other. An example is sequential use of the D-dimer followed by a ventilation/perfusion scan or helical CT scan to diagnose pulmonary embolism.[8]

Shift Happens

Likelihood ratios were traditionally thought to be invariable (i.e., unaffected by the prevalence of a disease).[9] By their definitions, sensitivity, specificity, and likelihood ratios should not shift with different disease prevalences. However, numerous examples have now refuted this notion of invariability.[10] This variability may reflect the patient spectrum involved, distorted inclusion of patients, verification bias, faulty reference standards, or other clinical issues.

A likelihood ratio derives from sensitivity and specificity, which are known to vary by disease prevalence, as discussed in Chapter 8. Thus a likelihood ratio derived from a population with a low prevalence may not apply to one with a higher prevalence. Rather than being fixed values, sensitivity, specificity, and likelihood ratios reflect how a test performs in a specific population.[11] Accordingly, clinicians should seek likelihood ratios derived from populations similar to their own.

Choosing Cut Points

ROC curves can help identify where cut points should be for continuous variables, like blood glucose, intraocular pressure, and blood pressure. An ROC curve (Fig. 9.2) plots the true-positive rate (TPR) on the vertical axis and the false-positive rate (FPR) on the horizontal axis. For a worthless test, the plot is a diagonal line, and the area under the curve is 0.5. The closer the curve approaches

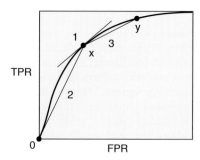

Fig. 9.2 Receiver operating characteristic curve and slopes relevant to likelihood ratios. (Redrawn, with permission, from Choi.[14])

the upper left-hand corner, the better is the test (and the greater is the area under the curve). In general, the best cut point is the point on the curve closest to the upper left-hand corner of the box.[12]

ROC curve slopes have several useful features concerning their relationship to likelihood ratios. First, the slope (#1 in Fig. 9.2) of the tangent to any point on the curve is equal to the likelihood ratio of the test result for that point.[13] Second, the slope (#2 in Fig. 9.2) between the origin (lower left-hand corner) and any point on the curve is the positive likelihood ratio when using that point as the threshold for test 'positive'. Third, the slope (#3 in Fig. 9.2) between any two points on the curve (*x* and *y*) corresponds to the likelihood ratio for a test result using those two points to define an interval when multiple intervals are used.[14]

Fagan Nomogram

Tests are not undertaken in a vacuum; a clinician always has an estimate (although usually not quantified) of the probability of a given disease before doing any test. According to Bayesian principles, the pretest odds of disease multiplied by the likelihood ratio gives the post-test odds of disease. For example, a pretest odds of 3/1 multiplied by a likelihood ratio of 2 would yield a post-test odds of 6/1. Unlike gamblers (or statisticians), most clinicians do not think in terms of odds; we usually use percentages. For example, a probability of 75% (75% yes/25% no) is the same as an odds of 3/1.[15]

Although the conversion back and forth between odds and probabilities involves simple arithmetic,[15] a widely used nomogram[16] (Fig. 9.3A) skirts this step altogether. A nomogram is a graphical calculator that solves a specific equation; given two known values, the nomogram calculates a third value.[17] A straight edge is placed on the pretest probability of disease (left column) and aligned with the likelihood ratio (middle column); the post-test probability (right column) can be read off this line. This procedure shows how much the test result has altered the pretest probability. For example, in the bottom of Fig. 9.1, the likelihood ratio for a positive test was 13 and for a

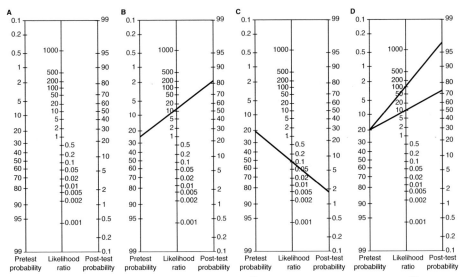

Fig. 9.3 Nomograms for probabilities and likelihood ratios.[16] (A) Nomogram reprinted from Fagan[16] with permission of the Massachusetts Medical Association. (B) Straight edge applied for pretest probability of 0.25 and likelihood ratio of 13. (C) Straight edge applied for pretest probability of 0.20 and likelihood ratio of 0.1. (D) Effect of likelihood ratios of 10 and 100 on pretest probability of 0.2.

negative test, 0.2. Assume that the pretest probability of the hypothetical disease is 0.25 and that the test is positive. Placing a straight edge on a pretest probability of 0.25 and intercepting the likelihood ratio column at 13 yields a post-test probability of about 0.80, a large shift in diagnostic probability (Fig. 9.3B). This value is close to the post-test probability of 0.81 calculated with the Bayesian formula.

A laminated copy of the Fagan nomogram is a useful tool in a white coat pocket. The Fagan nomogram can also be downloaded as a pdf for printing (http://www.cebm.net/wp-content/uploads/2014/02/likelihood-ratio.png, accessed 2 April 2017).

Two-Step Fagan Nomogram

Detractors of likelihood ratios rightfully complain that the chain of calculations involved can be tedious and off-putting to clinicians.[18] In addition, likelihood ratios for some tests can be difficult to find. Caraguel and Vanderstichel crafted an elegant workaround.[19] They added a linear scale for sensitivity and another for specificity adjacent to the likelihood ratio scale in the original Fagan nomogram. The new sensitivity and specificity scales are coloured red on the left for positive results and blue on the right for negative results. (Fig. 9.4). The revised two-step nomogram enables clinicians first to determine the likelihood ratio from the sensitivity and specificity of the test. In the next step, the post-test probability is calculated as in the original Fagan nomogram using the pretest probability and likelihood ratio scales. The two-step nomogram can be downloaded at http://www.adelaide.edu.au/vetsci/research/pub_pop/2step-nomogram (accessed 21 April 2017). Caraguel has even provided a colourful, free app for the iPhone (DocNomo) that will do the calculations painlessly (https://itunes.apple.com/us/app/docnomo/id901279945?mt=8, accessed 21 April 2017).

Nomogram Alternatives

Nomograms and computers are often not available at the bedside. Hence a mnemonic suggested by McGee for simplifying the use of likelihood ratios has appeal.[20] He notes that for pretest probabilities between 10% and 90% (the usual situation), the change in probability from a test or clinical finding is approximated by a constant. The clinician needs to remember only three benchmark likelihood ratios: 2, 5, and 10 (Panel 9.4). These correspond to the first three multiples of 15%: a likelihood ratio of 2 increases the probability by about 15%, 5 by 30%, and 10 by 45%. For example, with a pretest probability of 40% and a likelihood ratio of 2, the post-test probability is 40% + 15% = 55% (quite close to the 57% when calculated by formula). For likelihood ratios less than 1, the rule works in the opposite direction. The reciprocal of 2 is 0.5, that of 5 is 0.2, and that of 10 is 0.1. A likelihood ratio of 0.5 would reduce the pretest probability by about 15%, while a ratio of 0.1 would drop it by about 45 absolute percentage points. Another algorithm for likelihood ratios has been suggested, but it requires juggling six numbers in one's head (which we think is too cumbersome and have not included).[21]

Size Matters

Likelihood ratios of different sizes have different clinical implications. Clinicians intuitively understand that a likelihood ratio of 1.0 is unhelpful: the percentage of sick and well people with the test result is the same. The result does not discriminate between illness and health, and the pretest probability is unchanged despite the inconvenience and cost (and perhaps risk) of the test.

As with all ratios, likelihood ratios start at unity and extend down to zero and up to infinity. Hence the further the likelihood ratio is from 1.0, the greater its effect on the probability of disease. Likelihood ratios from 2 to 5 yield small increases in the post-test probability of disease, from 5 to

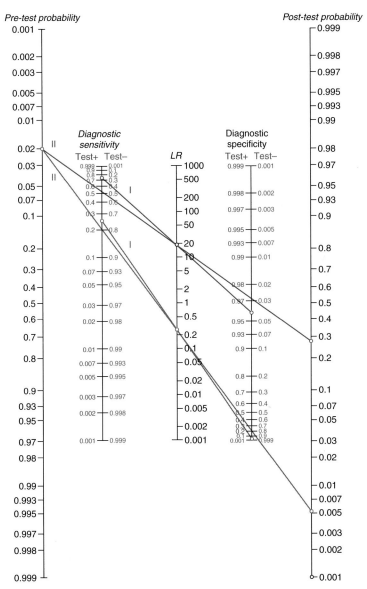

Fig. 9.4 Two-step Fagan nomogram, which calculates the likelihood ratio from sensitivity and specificity. (Redrawn, with permission, from Caraguel and Vanderstichel.[19])

10 yield moderate increases, and above 10 yield large increases. For ratios less than unity, the smaller the likelihood ratio, the greater the decrease in probability.

Only extreme values would shift the probability much. Consider a 28-year-old man with a 20% pretest probability of pulmonary embolism. He has a ventilation-perfusion scan interpreted as normal, which has a likelihood ratio positive of 0.1.[22] If we place a straight edge at 20% in the left scale of the nomogram and align it with 0.1 in the middle scale, the right scale indicates a post-test probability around 2% (Fig. 9.3C).

PANEL 9.4 ■ Likelihood Ratios and Bedside Estimates*

Approximate Change in Probability (%)

Likelihood Ratios Between 0 and 1 Reduce the Probability of Disease

0.1	−45
0.2	−30
0.3	−25
0.4	−20
0.5	−15
1.0	0

Likelihood Ratios Greater Than 1 Increase the Probability of Disease

2	+ 15
3	+ 20
4	+ 25
5	+ 30
6	+ 35
7	
8	+ 40
9	
10	+ 45

---

*Reproduced from McGee[20] with permission of Blackwell Publishing.

Some Large Likelihood Ratios

Large likelihood ratios are helpful. Diagnostic tests used to evaluate possible pulmonary embolism provide some examples. A ventilation-perfusion scan with a 'high probability' result has a likelihood ratio of about 18. For helical computed tomography, the corresponding 'high probability' likelihood ratio is about 24. Hence for patients with a moderate to high pretest probability based on clinical findings, a positive result with either of these tests yields a post-test probability of embolism greater than 85%.[23] When evaluating a potential myocardial infarction, any ST segment elevation on electrocardiogram has a likelihood ratio of about 11.[24]

For evaluating possible urinary tract infection, traditional dipstick tests for either leucocyte esterase or nitrite have a modest positive likelihood ratio of about 4[25] to 7.[26] In contrast, a dipslide with an agar-covered paddle that can be cultured features a positive likelihood ratio of 225.[26] Likelihood ratios of this magnitude can produce big shifts in diagnostic probability. Stated alternatively a high likelihood ratio indicates that a positive test is good at ruling in a diagnosis. Correspondingly a low likelihood ratio indicates that a negative test is useful in ruling out the condition.

Likelihood Ratios for Tests With Multiple Outcomes

A longitudinal study in Sweden examined the likelihood ratios for prostate-specific antigen (PSA) in predicting prostate cancer.[27] The researchers calculated sensitivity and specificity for a number of PSA cut-off values (Panel 9.5). As noted earlier in this chapter, LR+ was calculated as sensitivity/(1 − specificity), and LR− was calculated as (1 − sensitivity)/specificity.

As discussed in Chapter 8, sensitivity and specificity for this continuous variable are inversely related; as the PSA cut-off level increases, the sensitivity drops, and specificity rises. Likelihood ratios > 10 are useful for ruling in a diagnosis; in this study, PSA values higher than 10 ng/mL had positive likelihood values in this range. Conversely, negative likelihood values < 0.1 are useful

PANEL 9.5 ■ Likelihood Ratios for Prostate-Specific Antigen (PSA) and Subsequent Prostate Cancer[27]				
PSA Cut-Off (ng/mL)	*Sensitivity*	*Likelihood Ratio +*	*Specificity*	*Likelihood Ratio −*
0.5	0.99	1.2	0.13	0.04
1	0.96	1.7	0.44	0.08
2	0.78	3.2	0.75	0.30
3	0.59	4.5	0.87	0.47
4	0.44	5.5	0.92	0.61
5	0.33	6.4	0.95	0.70
10	0.13	12.3	0.99	0.88
20	0.05	28.1	1.00	0.95

for excluding a diagnosis. PSA levels of 1 ng/mL or lower had ratios this extreme. The commonly used cut-off of 4 ng/mL had sensitivity and specificity less than 1.5, which explains the ongoing controversy about the utility of PSA screening.[28]

The Importance of Accurate Pretest Probability

The medical history and physical examination remain fundamentally important. Indeed, a precise assessment of the chance of disease can be far more important than the likelihood ratios stemming from expensive, sometimes invasive tests.[29,30] For some diseases, such as Alzheimer dementia and sinusitis, clinical findings yield a highly accurate diagnosis. For other diseases, clinicians lack information about the predictive value of signs and symptoms; here they must rely on epidemiological data, education, and clinical acumen. For example, if additional patient history revised a pretest probability of coronary disease from 75% to less than 5%, this change would affect the post-test probability of disease more than would a stress test with positive and negative likelihood ratios of 3 and 0.5, respectively. Although the medical history and clinical diagnosis might not necessarily be more accurate than ancillary testing, their precision greatly influences the interpretation of any test results that follow.[31] The usefulness of likelihood ratios is less when pretest probabilities are unclear.[32] Methods are available for judging the effect of uncertainty in pretest probability of disease.[33] The bottom line: an accurate pretest probability and subsequent testing can greatly improve clinical diagnosis.

Diagnostic Thresholds

Tests should only be used when they will affect management. If a clinician's pretest probability of disease securely rules in or out a diagnosis, further testing is unwarranted. More testing should be considered only in the murky middle zone of clinical uncertainty (Fig. 9.5). The location of these

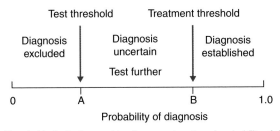

Fig. 9.5 Thresholds for testing and treating, as a function of probability of diagnosis.

decision thresholds[34] (A and B) along the continuum of diagnostic certainty needs to be determined before testing is done. Probabilities lower than point A effectively exclude the diagnosis in question. Hence point A becomes the testing threshold: pretest probabilities greater than A but lower than B could benefit from further testing. Point B is the treatment threshold: probabilities greater than this point justify beginning treatment without further delay.

The locations of these decision thresholds (A and B) should be tailored to the specific patient. Using the nomogram (see Fig. 9.3A) a clinician can estimate how high or low a likelihood ratio would have to be to shift the pretest probability below A (exclude the diagnosis) or above B (begin treatment). A clinician can consult published likelihood ratios for tests to find the corresponding test values (http://www.lrdatabase.com/, accessed 21 April 2017). If no test result would achieve this shift in probability, the test should not be done—a fundamentally important point. Moreover, when the clinician's pretest probability is very high, any negative test is likely wrong (a false negative). When the pretest probability is extremely low, any positive test is likely to be a false positive.[35]

Limitations of Likelihood Ratios

The effect of likelihood ratios on pretest probabilities is not linear. A likelihood ratio of 100 does not increase the pretest probability 10 times more than does a ratio of 10, as Fig. 9.3D shows.

For tests with several categories of results, extreme test values yield imprecise likelihood ratios because of sparse numbers. Few patients having values that are either very high or low result in little precision. Small changes in the numbers of patients in these cells can produce very different likelihood ratios. Stated alternatively, imprecision in likelihood ratios is greatest at the top and bottom of test-result distributions. Combining continuous categories at the extremes of the test-result distribution provides larger numbers and more precision (i.e., narrower confidence intervals).[36]

Conversely, many test results will fall towards the centre of the distribution. Here, likelihood ratios are closer to 1 and thus help little. The big payoffs stem from high or low likelihood ratios. An additional problem is that pretest probabilities developed in tertiary-care settings might not be applicable because of differences in patient populations. Panel 9.6 provides some guidelines for ordering tests on the basis of pretest probabilities.

Likelihood ratios have a broad array of clinical applications, including symptoms, physical examinations, laboratory tests, imaging procedures, and scoring systems. Building on an accurate pretest probability of disease, likelihood ratios from ancillary tests can refine clinical judgement–often in important ways. This can pay big dividends for patients and their clinicians.

PANEL 9.6 ■ Tips on Testing

- Clinicians should be wary of ordering tests when the pretest probability of disease is high or low. Tests are unlikely to alter disease probability and will only confuse the situation: unexpected results will usually be false positives or false negatives.
- Tests are most useful when the pretest probability is 50%.[37] Numerical changes in the post-test column of the nomogram (see Fig. 9.3) are greater when the starting point in the pretest column is at 50% than elsewhere.
- The higher the pretest probability of disease, the higher will be the post-test probability, no matter what the test result. For example, three times a high probability will be larger than three times a low one.[37]
- LR+ greater than 10 means that a positive test is good at ruling in a diagnosis.[35]
- A negative likelihood ratio less than 0.1 means that a negative test is good at ruling out a diagnosis.[35]
- When using tests in sequence, the post-test probability of the first test becomes the pretest probability for the next one. Tests can build on each other in sequence.

Conclusion

Likelihood ratios are a neglected clinical tool. Nomograms and other tools facilitate their use at the bedside. The further a likelihood ratio is from 1.0, the greater will be its impact on diagnostic probability. Careful clinical assessment followed by testing with use of likelihood ratios can improve a clinician's diagnostic accuracy.

References

1. Whiting, P.F., Davenport, C., Jameson, C., et al., 2015. How well do health professionals interpret diagnostic information? A systematic review. BMJ Open 5, e008155.
2. Estellat, C., Faisy, C., Colombet, I., Chatellier, G., Burnand, B., Durieux, P., 2006. French academic physicians had a poor knowledge of terms used in clinical epidemiology. J. Clin. Epidemiol. 59, 1009–1014.
3. Reid, M.C., Lane, D.A., Feinstein, A.R., 1998. Academic calculations versus clinical judgments: practicing physicians' use of quantitative measures of test accuracy. Am. J. Med. 104, 374–380.
4. Steurer, J., Fischer, J.E., Bachmann, L.M., Koller, M., ter Riet, G., 2002. Communicating accuracy of tests to general practitioners: a controlled study. BMJ 324, 824–826.
5. Stein, P.D., Chenevert, T.L., Fowler, S.E., et al., 2010. Gadolinium-enhanced magnetic resonance angiography for pulmonary embolism: a multicenter prospective study (PIOPED III). Ann. Intern. Med. 152, 434–443. w142-3.
6. Hubbard, T.W., 1999. The predictive value of symptoms in diagnosing childhood tinea capitis. Arch. Pediatr. Adolesc. Med. 153, 1150–1153.
7. Khan, K.S., Khan, S.F., Nwosu, C.R., Arnott, N., Chien, P.F., 1999. Misleading authors' inferences in obstetric diagnostic test literature. Am. J. Obstet. Gynecol. 181, 112–115.
8. Chu, K., Brown, A.F., 2005. Likelihood ratios increase diagnostic certainty in pulmonary embolism. Emerg. Med. Australas. 17, 322–329.
9. Scales Jr., C.D., Dahm, P., Sultan, S., Campbell-Scherer, D., Devereaux, P.J., 2008. How to use an article about a diagnostic test. J. Urol. 180, 469–476.
10. Leeflang, M.M., Bossuyt, P.M., Irwig, L., 2009. Diagnostic test accuracy may vary with prevalence: implications for evidence-based diagnosis. J. Clin. Epidemiol. 62, 5–12.
11. Bai, A.D., Showler, A., Burry, L., et al., 2017. Clinicians should use likelihood ratios when comparing tests. Eur. J. Clin. Microbiol. Infect. Dis. 36, 197–198.
12. Christensen, E., 2009. Methodology of diagnostic tests in hepatology. Ann. Hepatol. 8, 177–183.
13. Brown, M.D., Reeves, M.J., 2003. Evidence-based emergency medicine/skills for evidence-based emergency care. Interval likelihood ratios: another advantage for the evidence-based diagnostician. Ann. Emerg. Med. 42, 292–297.
14. Choi, B.C., 1998. Slopes of a receiver operating characteristic curve and likelihood ratios for a diagnostic test. Am. J. Epidemiol. 148, 1127–1132.
15. Grimes, D.A., Schulz, K.F., 2008. Making sense of odds and odds ratios. Obstet. Gynecol. 111, 423–426.
16. Fagan, T.J., 1975. Letter: Nomogram for Bayes theorem. N. Engl. J. Med. 293, 257.
17. Grimes, D.A., 2008. The nomogram epidemic: resurgence of a medical relic. Ann. Intern. Med. 149, 273–275.
18. Van den Ende, J., Moreira, J., Basinga, P., Bisoffi, Z., 2005. The trouble with likelihood ratios. Lancet 366, 548.
19. Caraguel, C.G., Vanderstichel, R., 2013. The two-step Fagan's nomogram: ad hoc interpretation of a diagnostic test result without calculation. Evid. Based Med. 18, 125–128.
20. McGee, S., 2002. Simplifying likelihood ratios. J. Gen. Intern. Med. 17, 646–649.
21. Sotos, J.G., 2007. Simplified calculations using likelihood ratios. ACP J. Club 146, A10.
22. Jaeschke, R., Guyatt, G.H., Sackett, D.L., 1994. Users' guides to the medical literature. III. How to use an article about a diagnostic test. B. What are the results and will they help me in caring for my patients? The Evidence-Based Medicine Working Group. JAMA 271, 703–707.
23. Roy, P.M., Colombet, I., Durieux, P., Chatellier, G., Sors, H., Meyer, G., 2005. Systematic review and meta-analysis of strategies for the diagnosis of suspected pulmonary embolism. BMJ 331, 259.

24. Soltani, A., Moayyeri, A., 2006. Towards evidence-based diagnosis in developing countries: the use of likelihood ratios for robust quick diagnosis. Ann. Saudi Med. 26, 211–215.

25. Moosapour, H., Raza, M., Rambod, M., Soltani, A., 2011. Conceptualization of category-oriented likelihood ratio: a useful tool for clinical diagnostic reasoning. BMC Med. Educ. 11, 94.

26. Mignini, L., Carroli, G., Abalos, E., et al., 2009. Accuracy of diagnostic tests to detect asymptomatic bacteriuria during pregnancy. Obstet. Gynecol. 113, 346–352.

27. Holmstrom, B., Johansson, M., Bergh, A., Stenman, U.H., Hallmans, G., Stattin, P., 2009. Prostate specific antigen for early detection of prostate cancer: longitudinal study. BMJ 339, b3537.

28. Eapen, R.S., Herlemann, A., Washington, S.L., 3rd, Cooperberg, M.R., 2017. Impact of the United States Preventive Services Task Force 'D' recommendation on prostate cancer screening and staging. Curr. Opin. Urol. 27, 205–209.

29. Phelps, J.R., Ghaemi, S.N., 2006. Improving the diagnosis of bipolar disorder: predictive value of screening tests. J. Affect. Disord. 92, 141–148.

30. Kent, P., Hancock, M.J., 2016. Interpretation of dichotomous outcomes: sensitivity, specificity, likelihood ratios, and pre-test and post-test probability. J. Physiother. 62, 231–233.

31. Summerton, N., 2008. The medical history as a diagnostic technology. Br. J. Gen. Pract. 58, 273–276.

32. Morgan, A.A., Chen, R., Butte, A.J., 2010. Likelihood ratios for genome medicine. Genome Med. 2, 30.

33. Srinivasan, P., Westover, M.B., Bianchi, M.T., 2012. Propagation of uncertainty in Bayesian diagnostic test interpretation. South. Med. J. 105, 452–459.

34. Pauker, S.G., Kassirer, J.P., 1980. The threshold approach to clinical decision making. N. Engl. J. Med. 302, 1109–1117.

35. Davidson, M., 2002. The interpretation of diagnostic test: a primer for physiotherapists. Aust. J. Physiother. 48, 227–232.

36. Sonis, J., 1999. How to use and interpret interval likelihood ratios. Fam. Med. 31, 432–437.

37. Sharma, S., 1997. The likelihood ratio and ophthalmology: a review of how to critically appraise diagnostic studies. Can. J. Ophthalmol. 32, 475–478.

CHAPTER 10

Boosting Recruitment to Randomised Controlled Trials

Recruitment to randomised controlled trials is a widespread problem. Poor recruitment can lead to inadequate power, nonrepresentative participants, abandonment of trials, and squandered resources. Most importantly, patients may suffer needlessly in the absence of trial results. Eligibility fractions and enrolment fractions describe the recruitment process. Several alternatives to traditional trials have been suggested to skirt recruitment challenges. These include single randomised consent (Zelen method), double randomised consent, partially randomised patient-preference trial, and cohort multiple randomised controlled trial (cmRCT). Special populations, such as the elderly or minorities, can be hard to reach; special efforts are often required. Cochrane systematic reviews indicate that four strategies improve recruitment: open-label designs (participants are not blinded to treatment), opt-out strategies (every potential participant is approached unless expressly declined), telephone contacts, and financial compensation. Use of social media, smartphone applications, and business models may facilitate recruitment in the future.

The greater the obstacle, the more glory in overcoming it.
—Molière

For researchers around the world, failing to accrue participants in a timely manner and in sufficient numbers remains a daunting challenge. As a result, a voluminous literature exists on strategies for overcoming this hurdle. This chapter describes the scope of the problem, identifies some of its adverse consequences, reviews several alternatives to traditional trials, summarises the evidence regarding what works to improve recruitment, and considers new approaches to the problem.

Scope of the Problem

Failure to reach the intended sample size frustrates many randomised controlled trials. Several surveys of registered trials have documented widespread difficulties. Among 114 trials funded by UK agencies, only 31% met their sample-size target, and 53% requested an extension to enable additional recruitment.[1] About one-third of these trials modified the sample size, usually downward (86%). Regrettably, these extensions rarely translated into substantial improvements in enrolment. Most trials (63%) experienced problems with recruitment early on. In 11% of trials, recruitment was halted before the intended close of recruitment, usually due to slow enrolment.

An update to this UK study[1] found modest improvement in recruitment.[2] Fifty-five percent of publicly funded trials met their planned sample size, but nearly half (45%) had to request an extension. A compilation of all randomised trials published over 6 months in six journals documented that 21% of 133 trials failed to attain intended sample sizes.[3]

A review of more than 6000 cardiovascular trials of all types confirmed that slow recruitment was the most common reason for premature termination of the study. This occurred in 11% of the trials.[4] Trials with US federal funding, studies of dietary or behavioural interventions, and those without a comparison group had a lower risk of premature stopping.

Consequences of Poor Recruitment

TRIAL ABANDONMENT

Some researchers simply 'throw in the towel' and quit. A follow-up survey of randomised controlled trials in Canada, Switzerland, and Germany from 2000 to 2003 found that 25% were discontinued.[5] Once again, poor recruitment was the most common reason. Among these, the median percentage of sample size achieved was only 41%. These discontinued trials were less likely to be published, which is itself unethical.[6] Industry-sponsored research was less likely to be discontinued than were investigator-sponsored trials. Only a minority of investigators (38%) reported the trial discontinuation to the relevant institutional review board (IRB). Surveys from other countries have reported trial discontinuation rates ranging from 11% to 45%.[5]

POWER

Poor recruitment has potential harms that are both methodological and ethical. Failure to reach the intended sample size often means less power than intended; the risk of a type II error (saying no difference exists when a difference exists) is increased. Stated alternatively, clinically important findings may be overlooked.

Although some allege that underpowered trials are unethical,[7] we disagree (Chapter 11). If trials are free of bias, then they can contribute important information, especially when the alternative is continuing ignorance about the safety and usefulness of therapy.[8] 'New' is not a synonym for 'improved'. For example, in a sample of publicly funded trials, only about half of new therapies proved better than existing treatments.[9]

EXTERNAL VALIDITY

Randomised controlled trials inevitably involve trade-offs. Because of methodological rigour, trials have the best internal validity (avoiding bias) in the hierarchy of research types. However, because they include only screened and consented volunteers, the generalisability of results (external validity) may be a concern. Recruitment of representative participants, especially in special populations such as the elderly or visually impaired, is often challenging.

Eligibility criteria vary by the purpose of a trial. 'Efficacy' (also termed 'explanatory') trials aim to find whether a treatment *can* work in the best of circumstances. In contrast, 'effectiveness trials' (also called 'pragmatic trials') hope to determine whether a treatment *will* work in usual conditions. Less restrictive eligibility criteria are used for the latter, which hope to have good external validity.

Some trials impose exacting eligibility criteria that deter recruitment and diminish external validity. Taken to its extreme, this approach to trials can yield such eclectic participants that although the trial results are internally valid, they may not be capable of extrapolation to the population of interest. This weakness is common in pharmaceutical industry trials, which may exclude participants who are elderly, obese, or complicated by comorbidities. Alternatively, in surgical trials, the skill levels of participating surgeons may be so high that the results cannot be generalised to community surgeons.[10]

In order to recruit participants, some trials have run-in periods before randomisation to identify those with poor compliance or poor retention, who are then excluded from the main study. Although this approach may improve the overall compliance or retention rate of the main study,[11] the results may not relate to the general population, which includes many who struggle with treatment adherence and follow-up. A variation on this theme is 'enrichment', in which those who have previously responded well to therapy are preferentially recruited.[10] This, too, undermines external validity because the participants no longer represent the general population.

Ethical Concerns

Slow recruitment frustrates everyone involved. Those recruiting potential participants may get discouraged; funding agencies may be disinclined to provide future funding to research teams that are struggling.

Requests for supplemental funding to achieve target sample size may divert money that could be invested in other trials. If these other trials are more important, then this diversion has a net negative effect on health.

Slow accrual of participants can delay identification of potentially life-saving treatments. For example, slow recruitment of participants to a trial of streptokinase may have led to the preventable deaths of 10,000 patients in the United States.[12]

GREAT EXPECTATIONS?

Researchers routinely underestimate the difficulties recruiting to randomised controlled trials. Louis Lasagna, a pioneering clinical pharmacologist, commented on the challenges he faced in recruiting surgical patients to a trial of a single dose of an analgesic.[13] More than 8000 surgical patients had operations on the surgery service during the recruitment phase; 100 were successfully enrolled. The unjustified optimism about recruitment rates over time subsequently became known informally as 'Lasagna's Law'. Other early trialists noted that recruitment takes much longer than anticipated. 'Muench's Third Law' states that the number of potential participants who can be recruited should be divided by 10 to provide a more accurate estimate.[14] In our experience (admittedly more favourable), we have used a rule of π: take the estimate of how long recruitment will require, then multiply by 3.14. For trials in developing countries, where logistical challenges are greater, the multiplier is 2π. These provide a ballpark estimate and help novice researchers with reality testing.

Recruitment Terminology

A randomised controlled trial involves only a tiny fraction of the target population. The sampled fraction of the target population gets progressively smaller during recruitment (Fig. 10.1). In this Venn diagram, a subset (A) of the target population is identified as potential participants and

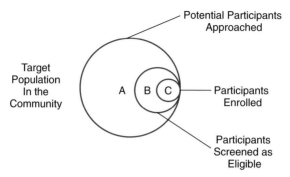

Fig. 10.1 Venn diagram of recruitment to randomised controlled trials.

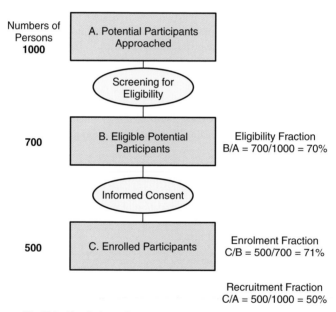

Fig. 10.2 Terminology of recruitment to randomised controlled trials.

approached about the study. A subset of these (B) is then screened and found to be eligible to take part. Yet another subset (C) agrees to participate.[15]

Several terms describe this selection process. The proportion of potential participants (A) who is screened as eligible for the study (B) is called the 'eligibility fraction' (Fig. 10.2). In Fig. 10.2, 700 of 1000 potential participants approached were found eligible, for an eligibility fraction of 70%. The proportion of potential eligible participants (B) who subsequently agrees to enroll (C) is termed the 'enrolment fraction'. In Fig. 10.2, 500 of 700 medically eligible potential participants enrolled, for an enrolment fraction of 71%. The 'recruitment fraction' is the proportion of potential participants (A) who subsequently enroll (C). In Fig. 10.2, 500 of 1000 potential participants enrolled, for an overall recruitment fraction of 50%.

A study of 172 randomised trial reports found that a minority provided sufficient detail to calculate these various fractions.[15] The median number of persons needed to screen to enroll one participant was 1.8, with a range of 1 to 68. Stated alternatively, one trial enrolled every person screened, while another had to approach 68 to admit one to the trial. The eligibility fraction in those reporting data had a median of 65% (interquartile range 41–82). The enrolment fraction had a median of 93% (interquartile range 79–100). The overall recruitment fraction had a median of 54% (interquartile range 32–77). These data should be viewed with caution, because 20 reports claimed that they enrolled *all* eligible patients; this suggests that some reports deemed those who declined participation as 'ineligible'. Better reporting of the recruitment process through use of the CONSORT flow diagram[16] will help readers judge the external validity of trial results.

KEEPING TABS

Recruitment progress should be monitored as the trial progresses. A graph of anticipated versus actual recruitment numbers over time alerts investigators to problems.[17] Should recruitment lag, researchers need to take corrective actions (e.g., adding new study sites or allocating more participants to sites with fast accrual). Other approaches include easing eligibility criteria, simplifying the trial for participants and clinicians, bolstering funds for recruitment, or extending the recruitment phase. Onerous data-collection forms and ponderous informed-consent documents (some running 20 pages) are common problems needing remedy. Many IRBs do not realise that trial participants often do not read or understand these documents.[18,19]

Alternatives to the Traditional Randomised Trial

Several alternative research designs have been advanced to skirt some of the challenges to recruitment; these vary widely in their ethical and scientific rigour.

SINGLE RANDOMISED CONSENT

Zelen ignited an ongoing controversy with his suggestion to obtain consent after, rather than before, randomisation to treatment.[20] For example, patients would be randomised to a new versus a standard treatment; only those randomised to the new treatment would be told of the experiment and consent requested. Should they decline participation, they would receive the standard therapy instead (Fig. 10.3, top). Zelen claimed that any loss in statistical inefficiency (unimportant except with gross disparities in treatment group sizes) would be offset by easier recruitment. He correctly observed that trial participants prefer to know their treatment.

This single randomised consent approach met with stiff resistance for several reasons. First, informed consent was denied to half of the participants. Second, considerable contamination (participants randomised to the new treatment crossing over and receiving the standard treatment) would dilute the experimental treatment effect in an intention-to-treat analysis. This would increase the likelihood of a type II error, unless a compensatory increase in sample size was made. Crossover (also called 'transfer') rates of 10% to 36% have been observed in cancer trials.[21] More recently, crossover rates of zero to 74% have been seen.[22] Moreover, neither allocation concealment nor treatment blinding would be possible for clinicians.[23]

DOUBLE RANDOMISED CONSENT

The ethical defects of the Zelen design are insurmountable. Withholding relevant information from participants[24] in research violates the ethical principles of autonomy and beneficence.[25] To avoid this problem, double randomised consent was suggested (Fig. 10.3, bottom). With this design, patients are randomised to treatment, after which both treatment groups learn of the trial and are asked to provide informed consent for their allocated treatment. Those who decline the assigned

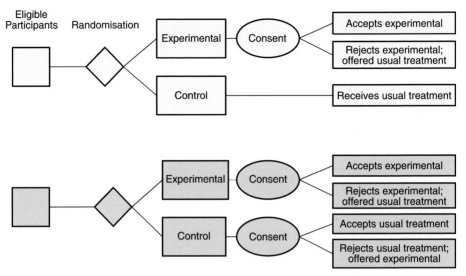

Fig. 10.3   Single- and double-consent randomised controlled trials.

treatment can cross over to the alternative, or perhaps, still other treatments. In the decades since its introduction, the Zelen approach has been used infrequently and generally inappropriately.[26] We find little to recommend it.

PARTIALLY RANDOMISED PATIENT-PREFERENCE TRIAL

In the mid-1980s, a hybrid approach was suggested to address both recruitment and external validity concerns. Initially termed 'comprehensive cohort study', [27] this design combines a cohort study and a randomised controlled trial in one study. After recruitment and informed consent, participants are asked if they are willing to be randomised to treatment (Fig. 10.4, top). If so, they are randomised in usual fashion. If not, they choose their treatment (cohort study). Participants in the cohort study and randomised trial receive the same follow-up observations. This allows a direct comparison of cohort and randomised trial results. For example, in German studies of breast cancer therapy, only 35% of women were willing to be randomised to loss of a breast; the remainder chose therapy in conjunction with their physicians.[28]

'Partially randomised patient-preference trial' is a more descriptive term for this design: patient preference plays a key role, and only some participants are randomised. This approach has both strengths and weaknesses. In an unblinded randomised trial (Fig. 10.4, bottom), some participants assigned to the standard or control treatment may have their hopes shattered. This may be especially true if the new treatment is available only through the trial. If comfort with the treatment is related to compliance or if a main outcome is satisfaction, then 'resentful demoralization' [22] may bias the results.[29] The cohort component of the study may provide better external validity.

Partially randomised patient-preference trials have drawbacks as well. The sample size will nearly double if the same power is desired in the randomised and nonrandomised comparisons. An overwhelming preference for one therapy over another could compromise the power of the cohort comparison. Unsuspected bias may remain in the cohort comparison.

This approach has been used to examine several questions in reproductive health. In the early 1990s, researchers in Aberdeen compared the acceptability of medical versus surgical abortion

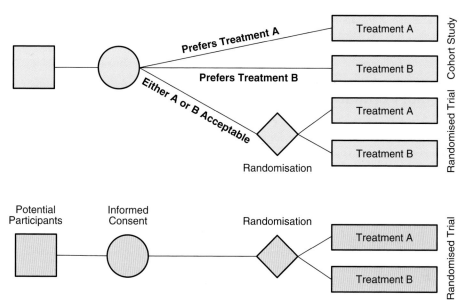

Fig. 10.4   Partially randomised patient-preference trial.

in early pregnancy.[30] Women who wanted a surgical procedure got their choice; those who requested a medical abortion received this regimen. The 'mushy middle' of women without a preference were approached and randomised to treatment. Overall, women liked their chosen method; among women indifferent to method, surgical abortion was better tolerated at later gestational ages.

Another trial compared treatments for heavy menstrual bleeding.[31] Women who wanted medical management received their choice, as did women desiring transcervical resection of the endometrium. Those without a strong preference were randomised, and transcervical resection proved superior in both randomised and nonrandomised participants. A similar study is underway comparing short- and long-acting reversible contraception in women.[32]

COHORT MULTIPLE RANDOMISED CONTROLLED TRIAL

In 2010 Relton and colleagues introduced a variation on the partially randomised patient-preference trial.[33] The salient features include recruiting a large cohort of patients with a chronic disease (e.g., rheumatoid arthritis) and following them prospectively with regular outcome measurements. Within this cohort, random samples of eligible participants would be offered the new intervention. Their outcomes would then be compared with those in the cohort receiving usual therapy and who remain unaware of the new intervention. The consent process is intended to simulate the real-world approach to counselling and consenting patients. Of course, this design cannot be used with a placebo.

In a hypothetical cohort multiple randomised controlled trial (cmRCT), about half of the patients in an anxiety and depression service expressed willingness to join a cohort from which they could be invited into randomised trials.[34] On the other hand, clinicians were less inclined to discuss recruitment and consent. This suggests that the cmRCT approach will not skirt the problem of the reluctance of busy clinicians to recruit their patients to research.

A weakness of this approach is that consent for the trial intervention takes place after randomisation to it, as in the Zelen design.[20] This introduces the possibility of bias from participants dropping out after randomisation. Modelling suggests that an intention-to-treat analysis will have bias, and the bias will increase with refusal of the trial intervention (dilution bias).[35]

Special Populations: Reaching the Hard-to-Reach

Failure to enroll participants who are not representative of the full spectrum of persons in the target population threatens external validity. Differences in treatment response by age, gender, ethnicity, diet, and geography may be missed.[36] Exclusion from research deprives 'hard-to-reach'[37] persons of the direct personal benefits[38] of clinical trials. As a result, initiatives of the National Institutes of Health in 1993 and 1994 mandated greater participation of minorities and women in research.[39] Although progress has been made in the interim, reaching and recruiting special populations remain difficult.

Barriers to recruiting minority and poor participants are numerous. One survey catalogued 33 different hurdles to recruiting minority participants to mental health trials.[40] Reaching prospective participants can be difficult because they may be transient or living in rural areas.[41] Transportation to the study site may be impossible for those without a car or access to public transport. Language barriers and low literacy levels can make informed consent documents incomprehensible.[42] Some fear that signing an informed consent document relinquishes, rather than protects, their rights as a patient. Fear and distrust of the medical system may be abating;[39,43] awareness of the Tuskegee Syphilis Study does not appear to influence African Americans' willingness to take part in research.[44]

LANGUAGE AND CULTURAL BARRIERS

Stringent eligibility criteria impede recruitment of minorities. For example, the higher burden of comorbidities among African Americans has disqualified disproportionate numbers of potential participants.[39]

Participation by African Americans in cancer trials appears related to several factors.[44] Some have negative views of clinical research and fear of being used as a 'guinea pig'. Others are generally unfamiliar with the clinical research enterprise. Religiosity and fatalism concerning outcomes deter some from entering cancer trials. In contrast, having family members or friends who have participated in clinical research facilitates recruitment.

Recruitment at the extremes of age poses other challenges. The elderly may be deterred by limited mobility, driving restrictions, sight and hearing difficulties, or cognitive declines.[45] Moreover, the accumulating comorbidities associated with ageing can limit eligibility. The need for involvement of family or friends who serve as 'gatekeepers' who help with decisions about healthcare may add further complexity.

Minors present still other challenges and ethical considerations. For cancer trials, the likelihood of participation in National Cancer Institute-sponsored trials is inversely related to patient age: those older than 13 years are less likely to participate than are younger patients.[46] Arbitrary age limits for some trials have been questioned in this regard.[47] Social media, such as Facebook advertisements, may facilitate reaching the young.[48]

What Works?

A voluminous literature has tackled the issue of improving recruitment to trials. Regrettably, many common-sense strategies with obvious appeal have failed when formally tested.[12] This is a recurrent theme in medicine; clinical hunches without scientific validation are highly fallible.[49] Scores of recruitment tactics have been suggested, tested, and rejected.[50] Rather than reviewing this large (and largely discouraging) literature, we will focus on the few strategies that have empirical evidence of benefit.

Cochrane systematic reviews of randomised controlled trials provide the best source of evidence about interventions. Several published Cochrane reviews offer some useful tips. Treweek and his colleagues have published a full review[51] and an updated abridged version[52] of 45 trials examining strategies to improve recruitment to randomised controlled trials. Of note, these reviews also included four 'quasirandomised' trials, which we view as not random. However, more than a third of the included trials failed to describe the method of randomisation, so the actual number of randomised trials may be less than stated. Six were hypothetical trials only. Many of the trials were small, and 20 were deemed at high risk of bias.

Six main strategies were tested.[52] These included trial design, the process of informed consent, the approach to potential participants, monetary incentives, special training for the staff doing recruitment, and overall coordination of the trials. Four strategies (Panel 10.1) emerged as helpful: open-label design with participants aware of treatment, an 'opt-out' strategy of approaching all those potentially eligible, voice or text messages to nonresponders, and monetary incentives.

Concerning trial design, open-label trials in which participants knew their treatment assignment led to better recruitment than a blinded, placebo-control approach. Participants prefer to know their treatment. However, the improvement was only 20%: relative risk 1.2 (95% CI 1.1–1.4). Moreover, this open-label solution to recruitment may create more serious problems with retention (i.e., losses to follow-up) that threaten internal validity. Blinding participants to treatments aids retention. Unblinding participants, as in the open-label design, likely harms retention.

An 'opt-out' strategy to approaching patients was better than the alternative of 'opt-in'. With the 'opt-out' strategy, every potentially eligible participant was contacted unless expressly declined. Again, the benefit was limited: relative risk 1.4 (95% CI 1.1–1.8), though 'opt-out' occurs before randomisation so it should not affect internal validity.

Three trials concurred that telephone contacts improved recruitment. In two, telephone reminders to written information improved recruitment (odds ratio 2.0; 95% CI 1.0–3.7). In the third trial, investigators sent text messages with quotes from current smoking-cessation participants to prospective participants. Texting had a large effect (relative risk 35.1; 95% CI 2.1–581.5) compared with only written invitation, but the estimate was imprecise due to small numbers.

One approach with intuitive appeal was supported by level I evidence: financial incentives for participation help with recruitment. For example, in a smoking-cessation trial, adding a £5 incentive along with information and a consent form led to a 13-fold increase in recruitment. Although the confidence interval was wide (1.7–98.2).

Another Cochrane review addressed a related concern: once participants are enrolled, how can researchers promote their continuation in the trial?[53] A total of 38 trials was reviewed; most focused on questionnaire return and not participant return—an important caveat. Monetary incentives appeared to be the most useful strategy to improve return of postal or electronic questionnaires, but the benefit was weaker than that seen with recruitment to trials.[52]

Other researchers have synthesised randomised controlled trials aimed at improving recruitment. One focused on socially disadvantaged persons, the 'hard-to-reach'.[37] Nine randomised

---

PANEL 10.1 ■ Recruitment-Boosting Strategies With Empirical Support[52]

- Open-label design
- 'Opt-out' approach to potential participants
- Telephone contacts
- Financial incentives

controlled trials yielded no clear-cut recommendation. Another review focused on palliative care for those with cancer or organ failure.[54] The useful strategies included memory aids, contacting the potential participant in advance, and an opt-out approach to contacting patients about the trial.

Two reviews have examined the willingness of clinicians to recruit participants. A Cochrane review of the incentives and disincentives involved identified no randomised controlled trials of this question.[55] Eleven observational studies of various types were found. Clinicians complained that trials added to their burden of work. Some found recruiting to be embarrassing, and others feared the discussion would undermine the doctor–patient relationship. A survey of physicians involved with six pragmatic trials[56] concurred that recruitment to trials can be difficult, both emotionally and intellectually. The study reported that surgeons, in particular, had trouble expressing the clinical uncertainty that justifies performing a formal trial.

One systematic review examined the cost-effectiveness of recruitment strategies.[57] Three tactics proved to be cost-effective: financial incentives, direct contact with prospective participants, and medical referrals to trials.

The Way Ahead

Social media and hand-held devices have revolutionised contemporary communication. Nearly all adults in the United States use the Internet, and most are engaged with Facebook, Twitter, LinkedIn, Craigslist, or Instagram.[58] These media are now being harnessed to bolster recruitment to trials. For example, Facebook has been the principal recruiting tool for some trials among HIV patients. An attractive feature of this approach is the low cost.[59,60]

Researchers are developing applications that will help potential participants find relevant trials. One example is the National Library of Medicine Pharmaceutical Product Development's Clinical Trials app (http://www.clinicaltrials.com/industry/clinicaltrials_mobile.htm, accessed 16 May 2017). A search for 'clinical trials' in the Apple App Store yields numerous apps created by universities, government agencies, and pharmaceutical companies. The list is likely to expand quickly in the years ahead.

Recruitment to randomised controlled trials may be too important to be left to medicine. An alternative view is that business models should guide the process.[61] Using several clinical trials as examples, the authors explained how 'building brand value, product and market planning, making the sale, and maintaining engagement' may be germane. They noted, however, the need for empirical evidence of usefulness of this approach.

Trialists at York University have proposed a novel solution: embed studies of recruitment approaches into ongoing randomised clinical trials.[62] Rather than decrying the poor state of knowledge about what works, they suggest harnessing the large volume of ongoing trials by comparing recruitment strategies as a routine element. Although they acknowledge that the sample sizes involved may be insufficient to detect small but important improvements, bias-free assessments, even if imprecise, can help. Resistance to this approach includes reluctance of the principal investigator to agree, added complexity, and distraction from the main objective of the ongoing trial. The UK Medical Research Council is sponsoring such research,[63] and we view this as a promising direction for the future.

Conclusion

Slow recruitment to randomised trials is a widespread problem. As a result, many trials fall short of their intended sample size. To skirt this problem, alternative approaches have been developed, such as the partially randomised patient-preference trial. Empirical evidence suggests that open-label designs, 'opt-out' strategies, telephone contacts, and financial incentives improve recruitment. Use of social media and smart phones may become important recruitment tools in the future.

References

1. McDonald, A.M., Knight, R.C., Campbell, M.K., et al., 2006. What influences recruitment to randomised controlled trials? A review of trials funded by two UK funding agencies. Trials 7, 9.
2. Sully, B.G., Julious, S.A., Nicholl, J., 2013. A reinvestigation of recruitment to randomised, controlled, multicenter trials: a review of trials funded by two UK funding agencies. Trials 14, 166.
3. Toerien, M., Brookes, S.T., Metcalfe, C., et al., 2009. A review of reporting of participant recruitment and retention in RCTs in six major journals. Trials 10, 52.
4. Bernardez-Pereira, S., Lopes, R.D., Carrion, M.J., et al., 2014. Prevalence, characteristics, and predictors of early termination of cardiovascular clinical trials due to low recruitment: insights from the ClinicalTrials.gov registry. Am. Heart J. 168, 213–219. e1.
5. Kasenda, B., von Elm, E., You, J., et al., 2014. Prevalence, characteristics, and publication of discontinued randomized trials. JAMA 311, 1045–1051.
6. Chalmers, I., 1990. Underreporting research is scientific misconduct. JAMA 263, 1405–1408.
7. Halpern, S.D., Karlawish, J.H., Berlin, J.A., 2002. The continuing unethical conduct of underpowered clinical trials. JAMA 288, 358–362.
8. Chalmers, I., 2013. Acknowledging and researching treatment uncertainties in paediatric practice: an ethical imperative. Arch. Dis. Child. Educ. Pract. Ed. 98, 132–133.
9. Djulbegovic, B., Kumar, A., Glasziou, P.P., et al., 2012. New treatments compared to established treatments in randomized trials. Cochrane Database Syst. Rev. 10, MR000024.
10. Rothwell, P.M., 2006. Factors that can affect the external validity of randomised controlled trials. PLoS Clin Trials 1, e9.
11. Ulmer, M., Robinaugh, D., Friedberg, J.P., Lipsitz, S.R., Natarajan, S., 2008. Usefulness of a run-in period to reduce drop-outs in a randomized controlled trial of a behavioral intervention. Contemp. Clin. Trials 29, 705–710.
12. Fletcher, B., Gheorghe, A., Moore, D., Wilson, S., Damery, S., 2012. Improving the recruitment activity of clinicians in randomised controlled trials: a systematic review. BMJ Open 2, e000496.
13. Lasagna, L., 1979. Problems in publication of clinical trial methodology. Clin. Pharmacol. Ther. 25, 751–753.
14. Ederer, F., 1975. Practical problems in collaborative clinical trials. Am. J. Epidemiol. 102, 111–118.
15. Gross, C.P., Mallory, R., Heiat, A., Krumholz, H.M., 2002. Reporting the recruitment process in clinical trials: who are these patients and how did they get there? Ann. Intern. Med. 137, 10–16.
16. Schulz, K.F., Altman, D.G., Moher, D., CONSORT Group, 2010. CONSORT 2010 statement: updated guidelines for reporting parallel group randomised trials. BMJ 340, c332.
17. Thoma, A., Farrokhyar, F., Mc Knight, L., Bhandari, M., 2010. Practical tips for surgical research: how to optimize patient recruitment. Can. J. Surg. 53, 205–210.
18. Robinson, E.J., Kerr, C.E., Stevens, A.J., et al., 2005. Lay public's understanding of equipoise and randomisation in randomised controlled trials. Health Technol. Assess. 9, 1–192. iii-iv.
19. Montalvo, W., Larson, E., 2014. Participant comprehension of research for which they volunteer: a systematic review. J. Nurs. Scholarsh. 46, 423–431.
20. Zelen, M.A., 1979. New design for randomized clinical trials. N. Engl. J. Med. 300, 1242–1245.
21. Altman, D.G., Whitehead, J., Parmar, M.K., Stenning, S.P., Fayers, P.M., Machin, D., 1995. Randomised consent designs in cancer clinical trials. Eur. J. Cancer 31A, 1934–1944.
22. Adamson, J., Cockayne, S., Puffer, S., Torgerson, D.J., 2006. Review of randomised trials using the post-randomised consent (Zelen's) design. Contemp. Clin. Trials 27, 305–319.
23. Ellenberg, S.S., 1984. Randomization designs in comparative clinical trials. N. Engl. J. Med. 310, 1404–1408.
24. Hawkins, J.S., 2004. The ethics of Zelen consent. J. Thromb. Haemost. 2, 882–883.
25. American College of Obstetricians and Gynecologists, 2004. Ethics in Obstetrics and Gynecology, Second ed. American College of Obstetricians and Gynecologists, Washington, D.C.
26. Schellings, R., Kessels, A.G., ter Riet, G., Knottnerus, J.A., Sturmans, F., 2006. Randomized consent designs in randomized controlled trials: systematic literature search. Contemp. Clin. Trials 27, 320–332.
27. Olschewski, M., Scheurlen, H., 1985. Comprehensive Cohort Study: an alternative to randomized consent design in a breast preservation trial. Methods Inf. Med. 24, 131–134.
28. Schmoor, C., Olschewski, M., Schumacher, M., 1996. Randomized and non-randomized patients in clinical trials: experiences with comprehensive cohort studies. Stat. Med. 15, 263–271.

29. Brocklehurst, P., 1997. Partially randomised patient preference trials. Br. J. Obstet. Gynaecol. 104, 1332–1335.

30. Henshaw, R.C., Naji, S.A., Russell, I.T., Templeton, A.A., 1993. Comparison of medical abortion with surgical vacuum aspiration: women's preferences and acceptability of treatment. BMJ 307, 714–717.

31. Cooper, K.G., Grant, A.M., Garratt, A.M., 1997. The impact of using a partially randomised patient preference design when evaluating alternative managements for heavy menstrual bleeding. Br. J. Obstet. Gynaecol. 104, 1367–1373.

32. Hubacher, D., Spector, H., Monteith, C., Chen, P.L., Hart, C., 2015. Rationale and enrollment results for a partially randomized patient preference trial to compare continuation rates of short-acting and long-acting reversible contraception. Contraception 91, 185–192.

33. Relton, C., Torgerson, D., O'Cathain, A., Nicholl, J., 2010. Rethinking pragmatic randomised controlled trials: introducing the "cohort multiple randomised controlled trial" design. BMJ 340, c1066.

34. Richards, D.A., Ross, S., Robens, S., Borglin, G., 2014. The DiReCT study — improving recruitment into clinical trials: a mixed methods study investigating the ethical acceptability, feasibility and recruitment yield of the cohort multiple randomised controlled trials design. Trials 15, 398.

35. Pate, A., Candlish, J., Sperrin, M., Van Staa, T.P., GetReal Work Package 2, 2016. Cohort Multiple Randomised Controlled Trials (cmRCT) design: efficient but biased? A simulation study to evaluate the feasibility of the Cluster cmRCT design. BMC Med. Res. Methodol. 16, 109.

36. Hughson, J.A., Woodward-Kron, R., Parker, A., et al., 2016. A review of approaches to improve participation of culturally and linguistically diverse populations in clinical trials. Trials 17, 263.

37. Bonevski, B., Randell, M., Paul, C., et al., 2014. Reaching the hard-to-reach: a systematic review of strategies for improving health and medical research with socially disadvantaged groups. BMC Med. Res. Methodol. 14, 42.

38. McCann, S.K., Campbell, M.K., Entwistle, V.A., 2010. Reasons for participating in randomised controlled trials: conditional altruism and considerations for self. Trials 11, 31.

39. Nicholson, L.M., Schwirian, P.M., Groner, J.A., 2015. Recruitment and retention strategies in clinical studies with low-income and minority populations: progress from 2004–2014. Contemp. Clin. Trials 45, 34–40.

40. Waheed, W., Hughes-Morley, A., Woodham, A., Allen, G., Bower, P., 2015. Overcoming barriers to recruiting ethnic minorities to mental health research: a typology of recruitment strategies. BMC Psychiatry 15, 101.

41. Tanner, A., Kim, S.H., Friedman, D.B., Foster, C., Bergeron, C.D., 2015. Promoting clinical research to medically underserved communities: current practices and perceptions about clinical trial recruiting strategies. Contemp. Clin. Trials 41, 39–44.

42. Paskett, E.D., Reeves, K.W., McLaughlin, J.M., et al., 2008. Recruitment of minority and underserved populations in the United States: the Centers for Population Health and Health Disparities experience. Contemp. Clin. Trials 29, 847–861.

43. Salman, A., Nguyen, C., Lee, Y.H., Cooksey-James, T., 2016. A review of barriers to minorities' participation in cancer clinical trials: implications for future cancer research. J. Immigr. Minor. Health 18, 447–453.

44. Rivers, D., August, E.M., Sehovic, I., Lee Green, B., Quinn, G.P., 2013. A systematic review of the factors influencing African Americans' participation in cancer clinical trials. Contemp. Clin. Trials 35, 13–32.

45. Ridda, I., MacIntyre, C.R., Lindley, R.I., Tan, T.C., 2010. Difficulties in recruiting older people in clinical trials: an examination of barriers and solutions. Vaccine 28, 901–906.

46. Whelan, J.S., Fern, L.A., 2008. Poor accrual of teenagers and young adults into clinical trials in the UK. Lancet Oncol. 9, 306–307.

47. Fern, L.A., Lewandowski, J.A., Coxon, K.M., Whelan, J., National Cancer Research Institute Teenage and Young Adult Clinical Studies Group, UK, 2014. Available, accessible, aware, appropriate, and acceptable: a strategy to improve participation of teenagers and young adults in cancer trials. Lancet Oncol. 15, e341–e350.

48. Cui, Z., Seburg, E.M., Sherwood, N.E., Faith, M.S., Ward, D.S., 2015. Recruitment and retention in obesity prevention and treatment trials targeting minority or low-income children: a review of the clinical trials registration database. Trials 16, 564.

49. Egger, M., Pauw, J., Lopatatzidis, A., Medrano, D., Paccaud, F., Smith, G.D., 2000. Promotion of condom use in a high-risk setting in Nicaragua: a randomised controlled trial. Lancet 355, 2101–2105.

50. Foy, R., Parry, J., Duggan, A., et al., 2003. How evidence based are recruitment strategies to randomized controlled trials in primary care? Experience from seven studies. Fam. Pract. 20, 83–92.
51. Treweek, S., Pitkethly, M., Cook, J., et al., 2010. Strategies to improve recruitment to randomised controlled trials. Cochrane Database Syst. Rev., MR000013.
52. Treweek, S., Lockhart, P., Pitkethly, M., et al., 2013. Methods to improve recruitment to randomised controlled trials: Cochrane systematic review and meta-analysis. BMJ Open 3, e002360.
53. Brueton, V.C., Tierney, J.F., Stenning, S., et al., 2014. Strategies to improve retention in randomised trials: a Cochrane systematic review and meta-analysis. BMJ Open 4, e003821.
54. Boland, J., Currow, D.C., Wilcock, A., et al., 2015. A systematic review of strategies used to increase recruitment of people with cancer or organ failure into clinical trials: implications for palliative care research. J. Pain Symptom Manag. 49, 762–772. e5.
55. Rendell, J.M., Merritt, R.D., Geddes, J.R., 2007. Incentives and disincentives to participation by clinicians in randomised controlled trials. Cochrane Database Syst. Rev., MR000021.
56. Donovan, J.L., de Salis, I., Toerien, M., Paramasivan, S., Hamdy, F.C., Blazeby, J.M., 2014. The intellectual challenges and emotional consequences of equipoise contributed to the fragility of recruitment in six randomized controlled trials. J. Clin. Epidemiol. 67, 912–920.
57. Huynh, L., Johns, B., Liu, S.H., Vedula, S.S., Li, T., Puhan, M.A., 2014. Cost-effectiveness of health research study participant recruitment strategies: a systematic review. Clin. Trials 11, 576–583.
58. Rosa, C., Campbell, A.N., Miele, G.M., Brunner, M., Winstanley, E.L., 2015. Using e-technologies in clinical trials. Contemp. Clin. Trials 45, 41–54.
59. Valdez, R.S., Guterbock, T.M., Thompson, M.J., et al., 2014. Beyond traditional advertisements: leveraging Facebook's social structures for research recruitment. J. Med. Internet Res. 16, e243.
60. Khatri, C., Chapman, S.J., Glasbey, J., et al., 2015. Social media and internet driven study recruitment: evaluating a new model for promoting collaborator engagement and participation. PLoS One 10, e0118899.
61. McDonald AM, Treweek S, Shakur H, et al., 2011. Using a business model approach and marketing techniques for recruitment to clinical trials. Trials 12, 74.
62. Adamson, J., Hewitt, C.E., Torgerson, D.J., 2015. Producing better evidence on how to improve randomised controlled trials. BMJ 351, h4923.
63. Rick, J., Graffy, J., Knapp, P., et al., 2014. Systematic techniques for assisting recruitment to trials (START): study protocol for embedded, randomized controlled trials. Trials 15, 407.

CHAPTER 11

Sample Size Calculations in Randomised Trials: Mandatory and Mystical

Investigators should properly calculate sample sizes before the start of their randomised trials and adequately describe the details in their published report. In these *a priori* calculations, determining the effect size to detect (e.g., event rates in treatment and control groups) reflects inherently subjective clinical judgements. Furthermore, these judgements greatly affect sample size calculations. We question the branding of trials as unethical on the basis of an imprecise sample size calculation process. So-called underpowered trials might be acceptable if investigators use methodological rigour to eliminate bias, properly report to avoid misinterpretation, and always publish results to avert publication bias. Some shift of emphasis from a fixation on sample size to a focus on methodological quality would yield more trials with less bias. Unbiased trials with imprecise results trump no results at all.

Sample size calculations for randomised trials seem unassailable. Indeed, investigators should properly calculate sample sizes and adequately describe the key details in their published report. Research methodologists describe the approaches in books and articles. Protocol committees and ethics review boards require adherence. CONSORT reporting guidelines clearly specify the reporting of sample size calculations.[1,2] Everyone agrees. An important impetus to this unanimity burst on the medical world more than a quarter of a century ago. A group of researchers, led by Tom Chalmers, published a landmark article detailing the lack of statistical power in so-called negative randomised trials published in premier general medical journals.[3] In Chalmers' long illustrious career, he published hundreds of articles. This article on sample size and power received many citations. Paradoxically, that troubled him.[4] He regarded it as the most damaging paper that he had ever coauthored. Why? We will describe his concerns later, so stay tuned.

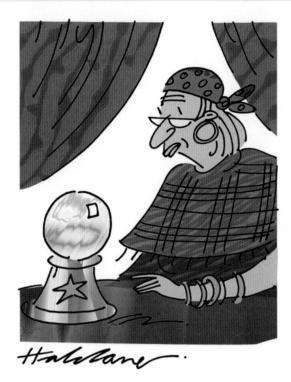

Components of Sample Size Calculations

Calculating sample sizes for trials with dichotomous outcomes (e.g., sick versus well) requires four components: type I error (α), power, event rate in the control group, and a treatment effect of interest (or analogously an event rate in the treatment group). These basic components persist through calculations with other types of outcomes, except other assumptions can be necessary. For example, with quantitative outcomes and a typical statistical test, investigators might assume a difference between means and a variance for the means. One other component of sample size calculations is the allocation ratio for the probability of assignment to the treatment groups. Throughout this chapter, we have assumed that ratio to be 1:1, which means the probability of assignment to the two groups is equal. Most medical researchers choose this 1:1 allocation ratio for their trials. Although a 1:1 allocation ratio usually maximises trial power, ratios up to 2:1 minimally reduce the power.[5-8] In Chapter 12, we discuss the implications of altering the allocation ratio on trial costs, power, and sample size.

In clinical research, hypothesis testing risks two fundamental errors (Panel 11.1). First, researchers can conclude that two treatments differ when, in fact, they do not. This type I error (α) measures the probability of making this false-positive conclusion. Conventionally, α is most frequently set at 0.05, meaning that investigators desire a less than 5% chance of making a false-positive conclusion. Second, researchers can conclude that two treatments do not differ when, in fact, they do (i.e., a false-negative conclusion). This type II error (β) measures the probability of this false-negative conclusion. Conventionally, investigators set β at 0.20, meaning that they desire less than a 20% chance of making a false-negative conclusion.

PANEL 11.1 ■ **Definition of Error Types**

Type I Error (α)
The probability of detecting a statistically significant difference when the treatments are in reality equally effective (i.e., the chance of a false-positive result).

Type II Error (β)
The probability of not detecting a statistically significant difference when a difference of a given magnitude in reality exists (i.e., the chance of a false-negative result).

Power (1 − β)
The probability of detecting a statistically significant difference when a difference of a given magnitude really exists.

Power derives from β error. Mathematically, it is the complement of β (i.e., 1 − β) and represents the probability of avoiding a false-negative conclusion. For example, for β = 0.20, the power would be 0.80, or 80%. Stated alternatively, power represents the likelihood of detecting a difference (as significant, with $p < α$), assuming a difference of a given magnitude exists. For example, a trial with a power of 80% has an 80% chance of detecting a difference between two treatments if a real difference of assumed magnitude exists in the population.

Admittedly, understanding α error, β error, and power can be a challenge. Convention, however, usually guides investigators for inputs into sample size calculations. The other inputs cause lesser conceptual difficulties but produce pragmatic problems.[9,10] Investigators estimate the true event rates in the treatment and control groups as inputs. Usually, we recommend estimating the event rate in the population and then determining a treatment effect of interest. For example, investigators estimate an event rate of 10% in the controls. They then would estimate an absolute change (e.g., an absolute reduction of 3%), a relative change (e.g., a relative reduction of 30%), or simply estimate a 7% event rate in the treatment group. Using these assumptions, investigators calculate sample sizes. Standard texts describe the procedures encompassing, for example, binary, continuous, and time-to-event measures.[6,11,12] Commonly, investigators use sample size and power software (preferably with guidance from a statistician). Most hand calculations diabolically strain human limits, even for the easiest formula, such as we offer in Panel 11.2. In this chapter, we address sample size and power for the most commonly used design, a parallel group randomised superiority trial. With this design, investigators seek to find whether one treatment is superior to another. Inability to demonstrate superiority fails to demonstrate equivalence. In contrast, investigators can undertake a noninferiority trial, which strives to establish whether a new treatment is not worse than a standard (reference) treatment by more than a tolerable amount.[13] Noninferiority of the new treatment relative to the standard treatment interests investigators because the new treatment has some other benefit, such as greater accessibility, reduced cost, less invasiveness, fewer adverse effects, or greater ease of administration. Noninferiority trials are much less commonly conducted in medicine, and we do not address calculating sample sizes for them in this chapter. However, we recommend the CONSORT extension paper on equivalence and noninferiority trials for interested readers.[13]

Effect of Selecting α Error and Power

The conventions of α = 0.05 and power = 0.80 usually suffice. However, other assumptions make sense depending on the topic studied. For example, if a standard prophylactic antibiotic for hysterectomy is effective with few side effects, in a trial of a new antibiotic we might set α error lower (e.g., 0.01) to reduce the chances of a false-positive conclusion. We might even consider lowering the power below 0.80 because of our reduced concern about missing an effective treatment because an effective safe treatment already exists. By contrast, if an investigator tests a standard prophylactic antibiotic against a cheap safe vitamin supplement, the balance changes. Little harm could come from making an α error so setting it at 0.10 might make sense.[12] However, if this cheap easy intervention produced benefit, we would not want to miss it. Thus investigators might increase power to 0.99.

Different assumptions about α error and power directly change sample sizes. Reducing α and increasing power both increase the sample: for example, reducing α from 0.05 to 0.01 generates about a 70% increase in trial size at power $= 0.50$ and a 50% increase at power $= 0.80$ (Panel 11.3). At $\alpha = 0.05$, increasing power from 0.50 to 0.80 yields a twofold increase in trial size and from 0.50 to 0.99 almost a fivefold increase (see Panel 11.3). Choices of α and power thus produce different sample sizes and trial costs.

Some investigators use one-sided tests for α error to reduce estimated sample sizes. We discourage that approach. Although we have assumed two-sided tests thus far, one-sided tests might indeed make sense in view of available biological knowledge. However, that decision should not affect sample size estimation. We suggest the same standard of evidence irrespective of whether a one-sided or two-sided test is assumed.[12] Thus, a one-sided $\alpha = 0.025$ yields the same level of evidence as a two-sided $\alpha = 0.05$. Using a one-sided test in sample size calculations to reduce required sample sizes stretches credulity.

PANEL 11.2 ■ The Simplest, Approximate Sample Size Formula for Binary Outcomes, Assuming $\alpha = 0.05$, Power $= 0.90$, and Equal Sample Sizes in the Two Groups

n The sample size of each of the groups
p_1 The event rate in the treatment group (not in formula, but implied when R and p_2 are estimated)
p_2 The event rate in the control group
R The risk ratio (p_1/p_2):

$$n = \frac{10.51\left[(R+1) - p_2\left(R^2 + 1\right)\right]}{p_2(1-R)^2}$$

For example, we estimate a 10% event rate in the control group ($p_2 = 0.10$) and determine that the clinically important difference to detect is a 40% reduction ($R = 0.60$) with the new treatment at $\alpha = 0.05$ and power $= 0.90$. (*Note:* $R = 0.60$ equates to an event rate in the treatment group of $p_1 = 0.06$, i.e. $R = 6\%/10\%$)

$$n = \frac{10.51\left[(0.60+1) - 0.10\left(0.60^2 + 1\right)\right]}{0.10(1-0.60)^2}$$

$n = 961.665 \approx 962$ in each group (PASS software version 6.0 (NCSS, Kaysville, UT)) with a more accurate formula yields 965)

This formula accommodates alternate α levels and power by replacing 10.51 with the appropriate value from the following table.

	Power (1 – β)		
α (Type I Error)	0.80	0.90	0.95
0.05	7.85	10.51	13.00
0.01	11.68	14.88	17.82

PANEL 11.3 ■ Approximate Relative Trial Sizes for Different Levels of α and Power				
	Power $(1 - \beta)$			
α (Type I Error)	**0.50**	**0.80**	**0.90**	**0.99**
0.05	100	200	270	480
0.01	170	300	390	630
0.001	280	440	540	820

Estimation of Population Parameters

For some investigators, estimation of population parameters (e.g., event rates in the treatment and control groups) has mystical overtones. Some researchers scoff at this notion, because estimating the parameters is the aim of the trial: needing to do it before the trial seems ludicrous. The key point, however, is that they are not estimating the population parameters *per se* but the treatment effect they deem worthy of detecting. That is a big difference.

Usually, investigators start by estimating the event rate in the control group. Sometimes scant data lead to unreliable estimates. For example, we needed to estimate an event rate for pelvic inflammatory disease in users of intrauterine devices in a family planning population in Nairobi, Kenya. Government officials estimated 40%; the clinicians at the medical centre thought that estimate was much too high and instead suggested 12%. We conservatively planned on 6%, but the placebo group in the actual randomised trial yielded 1.9%.[14] The first estimate was off by more than 20-fold, which enormously affects sample size calculations.

Published reports can provide an estimate of the endpoint in the control group. Usually, however, they incorporate a host of differences, such as dissimilar locations, eligibility criteria, endpoints, and treatments. Nevertheless, some information on the control group usually exists. That becomes the starting point.

In a trial on prevention of fever after hysterectomy, data assumed to be reasonably good show that 10% of women have febrile morbidity after the standard prophylactic antibiotic. That becomes the event rate for the control group. Estimation of the effect size of interest should reflect both clinical acumen and the potential public-health effect. This important aspect should not default to a statistician. The decision process proceeds by accumulating clinical background knowledge. Assume that the standard antibiotic costs US $10 for prophylaxis and incurs few side effects. The new antibiotic costs US $400 for prophylaxis and has more side effects but a broader range of coverage. These and probably many more pragmatic and clinical factors bear on the decision process. In view of the 10% event rate for fever in the control group, and knowing the clinical background, would we be interested in detecting a 10% reduction to 9%; a 20% reduction to 8%; a 30% reduction to 7%; a 40% reduction to 6%; a 50% reduction to 5%; and so forth? Determining the difference to detect reflects inherently subjective clinical judgements. No right answer exists. We could say that a 30% reduction is worthwhile to detect, but another investigator might decide on a 50% reduction.

The importance of estimating the treatment effect size of interest has been appropriately recognized. A major effort on this topic is called the DELTA (Difference ELicitation in TriAls) project. Guidance on specification of a treatment effect size (which DELTA refers to as a target difference in the primary outcome) for a two-group parallel randomised trial was created using the results of a systematic review and surveys.[15-17] Additionally, a list of reporting items for protocols and trial reports was generated.[16] With all their efforts so far, the group still realizes that better guidance is needed for researchers and funders regarding specification and reporting of this aspect of trial design.[15]

These parameter assumptions for the treatment effect size enormously influence sample size calculations.[9] Keeping the assumptions for the control group constant, halving the effect size necessitates a greater than fourfold increase in trial size. Similarly, quartering the effect size requires a greater than 16-fold increase in trial size. Stated alternatively, sample sizes rise by the inverse square of the effect size reduction (which statisticians call a quadratic relation). For example, in view of our initial parameter estimates of 10% in the control group and 6% in the intervention group, and $\alpha = 0.05$ and power $= 0.90$, about 965 participants would be necessary in each group (see Panel 11.2). Halving the effect size, thereby altering the intervention group estimate to 8%, requires a more than fourfold increase in sample size to 4301. Quartering the effect size, thereby altering the intervention group estimate to 9%, necessitates a more than 18-fold increase in trial size to 18,066 per group. Small changes in effect size generate large changes in trial size.

The need for huge trial sizes with low event rates frustrates investigators. That frustration partly stems from a lack of understanding that, with binary endpoints, numerator events drive trial power rather than denominators. For example, assume $\alpha = 0.05$ and a desired 40% reduction in the outcome event rate. A trial of 2000 participants (1000 assigned to the treatment group and 1000 to the control) with a control group event rate of 10% would provide similar power to a trial of 20,000 participants (10,000 assigned to each group) with a control group event rate of 1%. Both trials would need a similar number of numerator events (about 160) for roughly 90% power.

Low Power With Limited Available Participants

What happens when sample size software (in view of an investigator's diligent estimates) yields a trial size that exceeds the number of available participants? Frequently, investigators then calculate backwards and estimate that they have low power (e.g., 0.40) for their available participants. This practice may be more the rule than the exception.[18] Some methodologists advise clinicians to abandon such a low-power study. Many ethics review boards deem a low-power trial unethical.[19-21] Chalmers' early paper on the lack of power in published trials contributed to this response, which brings us back to our opening paragraphs. He felt his group's article fuelled these overreactions.[4] Chalmers eventually stated that so-called underpowered trials can be acceptable because they could ultimately be combined in a meta-analysis.[4,22] This view seems unsupported by many statisticians, surprisingly even those in favour of small trials.[18] Nevertheless, we agree with Chalmers' view, which undoubtedly will draw the ire of many statisticians and ethicists. Our support attaches three caveats.

First, the trial should be methodologically strong, thus eliminating bias. Unfortunately, the adequate-power mantra frequently overwhelms discussion on other methodological aspects. For example, inadequate randomisation usually yields biased results. Those biased results cannot be salvaged even if a huge sample size generates great precision.[23-26] By contrast, if investigators design and implement a trial properly, that trial essentially yields an unbiased estimate of effect, even if it has lower power (and precision). Moreover, because the results are unbiased, the trial could be combined with similar unbiased trials in a meta-analysis. Indeed, this idea, especially when incorporated into prospective meta-analyses,[27,28] is akin to multicentre trials (Chapter 21).

Second, authors must report their methods and results properly to avoid misinterpretation. If they report the trial results properly using interval estimation, the wide confidence intervals around the estimated treatment effect would accurately depict the low power. Reporting of confidence intervals represents a worthwhile contribution and avoids 'the absence of evidence is not evidence of absence' problem wrought by simplistic $p > 0.05$ conclusions.[29-31]

Third, low-powered trials must be published irrespective of their results, thereby becoming available for meta-analysis. Publication bias (which more accurately might be called 'nonpublication bias') constitutes the strongest argument against underpowered trials.[32,33] Publication bias emerges when published trials do not represent all trials undertaken, usually because reports with statistically significant results tend to be submitted and published more frequently than those with indeterminate results. Low-powered trials contribute to the problem because they more generally yield an indeterminate result. Not publishing completed trials is called both unscientific and unethical in the scientific literature.[34-36] Condemnation of all underpowered trials and prevention of their conduct, however, thwarts important research. Journal editors directly tackled the real culprit of publication bias as they now require registration before trial initiation.[37] This represents a substantial solution to publication bias, because trial registration schemes catalogue ongoing trials such that their results will not be lost.[37] Furthermore, large systematic review enterprises, most notably the Cochrane Collaboration, scour unpublished work to reduce publication bias.

Proclamations of underpowered trials being unethical strike us as a bit odd for at least two reasons. First, preoccupation with sample size overshadows the more pertinent concerns of elimination of bias. Second, how can a process rife with subjectivity fuel a black–white decision on its ethics? With that subjectivity, basing trial ethics on statistical power seems simplistic and misplaced. Indeed, because investigators estimate sample size based on rough guesses, if deeming the implementation of low-power trials as unethical is taken to a logical extreme, then the world will have no trials because sample size determination would always be open to question. 'Statements that it is unethical to embark on controlled trials unless an arbitrarily defined level of statistical power can be assured make no sense if the alternative is acquiescence in ignorance of the effects of healthcare interventions.'[35] Edicts that underpowered trials are unethical challenge reason and, furthermore, disregard that sometimes potential participants desire involvement in trials.[38]

Sample Size Samba

Investigators sometimes perform a 'sample size samba' to achieve adequate power. The dance involves retrofitting of the parameter estimates (in particular, the treatment effect worthy of detection) to the number of available participants.[39,40] This practice seems fairly common in our experience and in that of others.[39] Moreover, funding agencies, protocol committees, and even ethics review boards might encourage this backward process. It represents an operational solution to a real problem. In view of the circumstances, we do not judge harshly the samba, because it probably has facilitated the conduct of many important studies. Moreover, it truly depicts estimates of the sample sizes necessary given the provided assumptions. Nevertheless, the process emphasises the inconsistencies in the 'underpowered trials are unethical' argument: a proposed trial is unethical before the 'samba' and becomes ethical thereafter simply by shifting the estimate of effect size. All trials have an infinite number of powers, and low power is relative.

Sample Size Modification

With additional available participants and resource flexibility, investigators could consider a sample size modification strategy, which would alleviate some of the difficulties with rough guesses used in the initial sample size calculations. Usually, modifications lead to increased sample sizes,[41] so investigators should have access to the participants and the funding to accommodate the modifications.

Approaches to modification rely on revision of the event rate, the variance of the endpoint, or the treatment effect.[42-45] Importantly, any sample size modifications at an interim stage of a trial should hinge on a prespecified plan that avoids bias. The sponsor or steering committee should describe in the protocol a comprehensive plan for the timing and method of the potential modifications.[41]

Futility of *post hoc* Power Calculations

A trial yields a treatment effect and confidence interval for the results. The power of the trial is expressed in that confidence interval. Hence the power is no longer a meaningful concern.[9,12,39,46] Nevertheless, after trial completion, some investigators do power calculations on statistically nonsignificant trials using the observed results for the parameter estimates. This exercise has specious appeal but tautologically yields an answer of low power.[12,39] In other words, this ill-advised exercise answers an already answered question.

What Should Readers Look for in Sample Size Calculations?

Readers should find the *a priori* estimates of sample size. Indeed, in trial reports, confidence intervals appropriately indicate the power. However, sample size calculations still provide important information. First, they specify the primary endpoint, which safeguards against changing outcomes and claiming a large effect on an outcome not planned as the primary outcome.[47] Second, knowing the planned size alerts readers to potential problems. Did the trial encounter recruitment difficulties? Did the trial stop early because of a statistically significant result? If so, the authors should provide a formal statistical stopping rule[48] (Chapter 20). If they did not use a formal rule, then multiple looks at the data inflated the α.[6,41] Similar problems can be manifested in larger-than-planned sample sizes. Providing planned sizes, however arbitrary, lays the groundwork for transparent reporting.

Low reported power or unreported sample size calculations usually are not a fatal flaw. Low power can reflect a lack of methodological knowledge, but it may just indicate an inadequate number of potential participants. Sample size calculations, even with low power, still provide the vital information described previously.

What if authors neglect mentioning *a priori* sample size calculations or provide calculations but neglect to provide all the necessary assumptions? Unfortunately, such inadequate reporting on sample size happens frequently in the literature. For example, inadequate reporting happened in about half of the published reports in the high-impact-factor general medical journals,[49] and in over 62% of analgesic trials.[50] Readers should cautiously interpret the results because of missing information. Moreover, neglecting to report, or incompletely reporting, sample size calculations suggests a methodological naiveté that might portend other problems. Nevertheless, readers should be most concerned with systematic errors (bias) hidden by investigators. Authors failing to report poor randomisation, inadequate allocation concealment, deficient blinding, or defective participant retention hide inadequacies that could cause major bias.[51-55] (see Chapters 12–17). Thus readers should ascribe less concern to perceived inadequate sample size for two substantial reasons: first, it does not cause bias and, second, any random error produced transparently surfaces in the confidence intervals and *p* values. The severest problems for readers are the systematic errors that are not revealed. In other words, readers should not totally discount a trial simply because of low power, but they should carefully weigh its value accordingly. The value resides in the context of other research, either past or future.[56]

Readers should find all assumptions underlying any sample size calculation: type I error (α), power (or β), event rate in the control group, and a treatment effect of interest (or analogously, an event rate in the treatment group). A statement that 'we calculated necessary sample sizes of 120 in each group at α = 0.05 and power = 0.90' is almost meaningless, because it neglects the estimates for the effect size and control group event rate. Even small trials have high power to detect huge treatment effects.

Readers should also examine the assumptions for the sample size calculation. For example, they might believe that a smaller effect size is more worthy than the planned effect size. Therefore, they would recognize the lower power of the trial relative to their preferred effect size.

Conclusion

Statistical power is an important notion, but it should be stripped of its ethical bellwether status. We question the branding of trials as unethical based solely on an inherently subjective, imprecise sample size calculation process. We endorse planning for adequate power, and we salute the huge trials of the ISIS-4 ilk that randomised over 58,000 participants;[57] indeed, more large trials should be undertaken. However, if the scientific world insisted solely on large trials, many important questions in medicine would languish unanswered. Some shift of emphasis from a fixation on sample size to a focus on methodological quality would yield more trials with less bias. Unbiased trials with imprecise results trump no results at all.

References

1. Schulz, K.F., Altman, D.G., Moher, D., 2010. CONSORT 2010 statement: updated guidelines for reporting parallel group randomised trials. BMJ 340, c332.
2. Moher, D., Hopewell, S., Schulz, K.F., et al., 2010. CONSORT 2010 explanation and elaboration: updated guidelines for reporting parallel group randomised trials. J. Clin. Epidemiol. 63, e1–37.
3. Freiman, J.A., Chalmers, T.C., Smith, H.J., Kuebler, R.R., 1978. The importance of beta, the type II error and sample size in the design and interpretation of the randomized control trial. Survey of 71 "negative" trials. N. Engl. J. Med. 299, 690–694.
4. Sackett, D.L., Cook, D.J., 1993. Can we learn anything from small trials? Ann. N. Y. Acad. Sci. 703, 25–31. discussion 31–32.
5. Dumville, J.C., Hahn, S., Miles, J.N., Torgerson, D.J., 2006. The use of unequal randomisation ratios in clinical trials: a review. Contemp. Clin. Trials 27, 1–12.
6. Pocock, S., 1983. Clinical Trials: A Practical Approach. Wiley, Chichester, UK.
7. Torgerson, D.J., Campbell, M.K., 2000. Use of unequal randomisation to aid the economic efficiency of clinical trials. BMJ 321, 759.
8. Peckham, E., Brabyn, S., Cook, L., Devlin, T., Dumville, J., Torgerson, D.J., 2015. The use of unequal randomisation in clinical trials—an update. Contemp. Clin. Trials 45, 113–122.
9. Noordzij, M., Tripepi, G., Dekker, F.W., Zoccali, C., Tanck, M.W., Jager, K.J., 2010. Sample size calculations: basic principles and common pitfalls. Nephrol. Dial. Transplant. 25, 1388–1393.
10. Kelly, P.J., Webster, A.C., Craig, J.C., 2010. How many patients do we need for a clinical trial? Demystifying sample size calculations. Nephrology (Carlton) 15, 725–731.
11. Meinert, C., 1986. Clinical Trials: Design, Conduct, and Analysis. Oxford University Press, New York.
12. Piantadosi, S., 1997. Clinical Trials: A Methodologic Perspective. John Wiley & Sons, New York, NY.
13. Piaggio, G., Elbourne, D.R., Pocock, S.J., Evans, S.J., Altman, D.G., 2012. Reporting of noninferiority and equivalence randomized trials: extension of the CONSORT 2010 statement. JAMA 308, 2594–2604.
14. Sinei, S.K., Schulz, K.F., Lamptey, P.R., et al., 1990. Preventing IUCD-related pelvic infection: the efficacy of prophylactic doxycycline at insertion. Br. J. Obstet. Gynaecol. 97, 412–419.
15. Cook, J.A., Julious, S.A., Sones, W., et al., 2017. Choosing the target difference ('effect size') for a randomised controlled trial—DELTA2 guidance protocol. Trials 18, 271.
16. Cook, J.A., Hislop, J., Altman, D.G., et al., 2015. Specifying the target difference in the primary outcome for a randomised controlled trial: guidance for researchers. Trials 16, 12.
17. Cook, J.A., Hislop, J.M., Altman, D.G., et al., 2014. Use of methods for specifying the target difference in randomised controlled trial sample size calculations: Two surveys of trialists' practice. Clin. Trials 11, 300–308.
18. Matthews, J.N., 1995. Small clinical trials: are they all bad? Stat. Med. 14, 115–126.
19. Edwards, S.J., Lilford, R.J., Braunholtz, D., Jackson, J., 1997. Why "underpowered" trials are not necessarily unethical. Lancet 350, 804–807.
20. Halpern, S.D., Karlawish, J.H., Berlin, J.A., 2002. The continuing unethical conduct of underpowered clinical trials. JAMA 288, 358–362.
21. Lilford, R.J., 2002. The ethics of underpowered clinical trials. JAMA 288, 2118–2119.
22. Chalmers, T.C., Levin, H., Sacks, H.S., Reitman, D., Berrier, J., Nagalingam, R., 1987. Meta-analysis of clinical trials as a scientific discipline. I: Control of bias and comparison with large co-operative trials. Stat. Med. 6, 315–328.
23. Peto, R., 1999. Failure of randomisation by "sealed" envelope. Lancet 354, 73.
24. Schulz, K.F., Chalmers, I., Hayes, R.J., Altman, D.G., 1995. Empirical evidence of bias. Dimensions of methodological quality associated with estimates of treatment effects in controlled trials. JAMA 273, 408–412.
25. Schulz, K.F., 1995. Subverting randomization in controlled trials. JAMA 274, 1456–1458.
26. Savovic, J., Jones, H.E., Altman, D.G., et al., 2012. Influence of reported study design characteristics on intervention effect estimates from randomized, controlled trials. Ann. Intern. Med. 157, 429–438.
27. Walker, M.D., 1989. Atrial fibrillation and antithrombotic prophylaxis: a prospective meta-analysis. Lancet 1, 325–326.
28. Turok, D.K., Espey, E., Edelman, A.B., et al., 2011. The methodology for developing a prospective meta-analysis in the family planning community. Trials 12, 104.
29. Altman, D.G., Bland, J.M., 1995. Absence of evidence is not evidence of absence. BMJ 311, 485.

30. Detsky, A.S., Sackett, D.L., 1985. When was a "negative" clinical trial big enough? How many patients you needed depends on what you found. Arch. Intern. Med. 145, 709–712.

31. Lilford, R.J., Thornton, J.G., Braunholtz, D., 1995. Clinical trials and rare diseases: a way out of a conundrum. BMJ 311, 1621–1625.

32. Dickersin, K., 1997. How important is publication bias? A synthesis of available data. AIDS Educ. Prev. 9, 15–21.

33. Dickersin, K., Chan, S., Chalmers, T.C., Sacks, H.S., Smith, H.J., 1987. Publication bias and clinical trials. Control. Clin. Trials 8, 343–353.

34. Chalmers, I., 1990. Underreporting research is scientific misconduct. JAMA 263, 1405–1408.

35. Chalmers, I., 2002. Cardiotocography v Doppler auscultation. All unbiased comparative studies should be published. BMJ 324, 483–485.

36. Antes, G., Chalmers, I., 2003. Under-reporting of clinical trials is unethical. Lancet 361, 978–979.

37. De Angelis, C., Drazen, J.M., Frizelle, F.A., et al., 2004. Clinical trial registration: a statement from the International Committee of Medical Journal Editors. Lancet 364, 911–912.

38. Chalmers, I., 1995. What do I want from health research and researchers when I am a patient? BMJ 310, 1315–1318.

39. Goodman, S.N., Berlin, J.A., 1994. The use of predicted confidence intervals when planning experiments and the misuse of power when interpreting results. Ann. Intern. Med. 121, 200–206.

40. Peipert, J.F., Metheny, W.P., Schulz, K., 1995. Sample size and statistical power in reproductive research. Obstet. Gynecol. 86, 302–305.

41. DeMets, D.L., Ellenberg, S.S., Fleming, T.R., 2002. Data Monitoring Committees in Clinical Trials. John Wiley & Sons Ltd., Chichester.

42. Wang, S.J., Hung, H.M., Tsong, Y., Cui, L., 2001. Group sequential test strategies for superiority and non-inferiority hypotheses in active controlled clinical trials. Stat. Med. 20, 1903–1912.

43. Cui, L., Hung, H.M., Wang, S.J., 1999. Modification of sample size in group sequential clinical trials. Biometrics 55, 853–857.

44. Lehmacher, W., Wassmer, G., 1999. Adaptive sample size calculations in group sequential trials. Biometrics 55, 1286–1290.

45. Wittes, J., Brittain, E., 1990. The role of internal pilot studies in increasing the efficiency of clinical trials. Stat. Med. 9, 65–71. discussion 71–72.

46. Fayers, P.M., Machin, D., 1995. Sample size: how many patients are necessary? Br. J. Cancer 72, 1–9.

47. Chan, A.W., Hrobjartsson, A., Haahr, M.T., Gøtzsche, P.C., Altman, D.G., 2004. Empirical evidence for selective reporting of outcomes in randomized trials: comparison of protocols to published articles. JAMA 291, 2457–2465.

48. Schulz, K.F., Grimes, D.A., 2005. Multiplicity in randomised trials II: subgroup and interim analyses. Lancet 365, 1657–1661.

49. Charles, P., Giraudeau, B., Dechartres, A., Baron, G., Ravaud, P., 2009. Reporting of sample size calculation in randomised controlled trials: review. BMJ 338, b1732.

50. McKeown, A., Gewandter, J.S., McDermott, M.P., et al., 2015. Reporting of sample size calculations in analgesic clinical trials: ACTTION systematic review. J. Pain 16, 199–206.e1-7.

51. Schulz, K.F., Grimes, D.A., 2002. Unequal group sizes in randomised trials: guarding against guessing. Lancet 359, 966–970.

52. Schulz, K.F., Grimes, D.A., 2002. Sample size slippages in randomised trials: exclusions and the lost and wayward. Lancet 359, 781–785.

53. Schulz, K.F., Grimes, D.A., 2002. Blinding in randomised trials: hiding who got what. Lancet 359, 696–700.

54. Schulz, K.F., Grimes, D.A., 2002. Allocation concealment in randomised trials: defending against deciphering. Lancet 359, 614–618.

55. Schulz, K.F., Grimes, D.A., 2002. Generation of allocation sequences in randomised trials: chance, not choice. Lancet 359, 515–519.

56. Clarke, M., Alderson, P., Chalmers, I., 2002. Discussion sections in reports of controlled trials published in general medical journals. JAMA 287, 2799–2801.

57. ISIS-4 (Fourth International Study of Infarct Survival) Collaborative Group, 1995. ISIS-4: a randomised factorial trial assessing early oral captopril, oral mononitrate, and intravenous magnesium sulphate in 58,050 patients with suspected acute myocardial infarction. Lancet 345, 669–685.

CHAPTER 12

Generation of Allocation Sequences in Randomised Trials: Chance, Not Choice

The randomised controlled trial sets the gold standard of clinical research. However, randomisation persists as perhaps the least understood aspect of a trial. Moreover, anything short of proper randomisation courts selection and confounding biases. Researchers should spurn all systematic, nonrandom methods of allocation. Trial participants should be assigned to comparison groups based on a random process. Simple (unrestricted) randomisation, analogous to repeated fair coin-tossing, is the most basic of sequence generation approaches. Furthermore, no other approach, irrespective of its complexity and sophistication, surpasses simple randomisation for prevention of bias. Investigators should, therefore, use this method more often than they do, and readers should expect and accept disparities in group sizes. Several other complicated restricted randomisation procedures limit the likelihood of undesirable sample size imbalances in the intervention groups. The most frequently used restricted sequence generation procedure is blocked randomisation. If this method is used, investigators should randomly vary the block sizes and use large block sizes, particularly in an unblinded trial. Other restricted procedures, such as urn randomisation, combine beneficial attributes of simple and restricted randomisation by preserving most of the unpredictability while achieving some balance. The effectiveness of stratified randomisation depends on use of a restricted randomisation approach to balance the allocation sequences for each stratum. Generation of a proper randomisation sequence takes little time and effort but affords big rewards in scientific accuracy and credibility. Investigators should devote appropriate resources to sequence generation in properly randomised trials and to reporting their methods clearly.

... having used a random allocation, the sternest critic is unable to say when we eventually dash into print that quite probably the groups were differentially biased through our predilections or through our stupidity.[1]

PANEL 12.1 ■ History of Randomised Controlled Trials

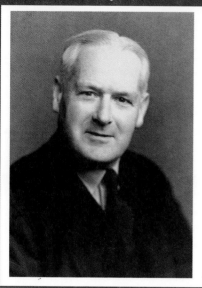

The controlled trial gained increasing recognition during the 20th century as the best approach for assessment of healthcare and prevention alternatives. R.A. Fisher[2] developed randomisation as a basic principle of experimental design in the 1920s and used the technique predominantly in agricultural research. The successful adaptation of randomised controlled trials to healthcare took place in the late 1940s, largely because of the advocacy and developmental work of Sir Austin Bradford Hill while at the London School of Hygiene and Tropical Medicine.[3] His efforts culminated in the first experimental[4] and published[5] use of random numbers to allocate trial participants. Soon after, randomisation emerged as crucial in securing unbiased comparison groups.

Austin Bradford Hill (1954)

Until recently, investigators shunned formally controlled experimentation when designing trials (Panel 12.1).[2-5] Now, however, the randomised controlled trial sets the methodological standard of excellence in medical research (Panel 12.2).[3,6] The unique capability of randomised controlled trials to reduce bias depends on investigators being able to implement their principal bias-reducing

---

PANEL 12.2 ■ Benefits of Randomisation

Proper implementation of a randomisation mechanism affords at least three major advantages.

1. **It eliminates bias in treatment assignment.**

   Comparisons of different forms of health interventions can be misleading unless investigators take precautions to ensure that their trial comprises unbiased comparison groups relative to prognosis. In controlled trials of prevention or treatment, randomisation produces unbiased comparison groups by avoiding selection and confounding biases. Consequently, comparison groups are not prejudiced by selection of particular patients, whether consciously or not, to receive a specific intervention. The notion of avoiding bias includes eliminating it from decisions on entry of participants to the trial, as well as eliminating bias from the assignment of participants to treatment, once entered. Investigators need to properly register each participant immediately on identification of eligibility for the trial, but without knowledge of the assignment. The reduction of selection and confounding biases underpins the most important strength of randomisation. Randomisation prevails as the best study design for investigating small or moderate effects.[6]

2. **It facilitates blinding (masking) of the identity of treatments from investigators, participants, and assessors, including the possible use of a placebo.[3]**

   Such manoeuvres reduce bias after random assignment and would be difficult, perhaps even impossible, to implement if investigators assigned treatments by a nonrandom scheme.

3. **It permits the use of probability theory to express the likelihood that any difference in outcome between treatment groups merely indicates chance.**

technique—randomisation. Although random allocation of trial participants is the most fundamental aspect of a controlled trial,[7] it unfortunately remains perhaps the least understood.[8,9]

In this chapter we describe the rationale behind random allocation and its related implementation procedures. Randomisation depends primarily on two interrelated but separate processes (i.e., generation of an unpredictable randomised allocation sequence and concealment of that sequence until assignment occurs [allocation concealment]). Here, we focus on how such a sequence can be generated. In Chapter 14 we address allocation concealment.

What to Look for With Sequence Generation
NONRANDOM METHODS MASQUERADING AS RANDOM

Ironically, many researchers have decidedly nonrandom impressions of randomisation.[8-11] They often mistake haphazard approaches and alternate assignment approaches as random.[11,12] Some medical researchers even view approaches antithetical to randomisation, such as assignment to intervention groups based on preintervention tests, as quasirandom.[13] Quasirandom, however, resembles quasipregnant, in that they both elude definition. Indeed, anything short of proper randomisation opens limitless contamination possibilities. Without properly done randomisation, selection and confounding biases seep into trials.[7,14]

Researchers sometimes cloak, perhaps unintentionally, nonrandom methods in randomised clothing. They think that they have randomised by a method that, when described, is obviously not random. Methods such as assignment based on date of birth, case record number, date of presentation, or alternate assignment are not random, but rather systematic occurrences. Yet in a study that we did,[10] in 5% (11 of 206) of reports, investigators claimed that they had randomly assigned participants by such nonrandom methods. Furthermore, nonrandom methods are probably used much more frequently than suggested by our findings, because 63% (129 of 206) of the reports did not specify the method used to generate a random sequence.[15]

Systematic methods do not qualify as randomisation methods for theoretical and practical reasons. For example, in some populations, the day of the week on which a child is born is not entirely a matter of chance.[16] Furthermore, systematic methods do not result in allocation concealment. By definition, systematic allocation usually precludes adequate concealment, because it results in foreknowledge of treatment assignment among those who recruit participants to the trial. If researchers report the use of systematic allocation, especially if masqueraded as randomised, readers should be wary of the results, because such a mistake implies ignorance of the randomisation process. We place more credence in the findings of such a study if the authors accurately report it as nonrandomised and explain how they controlled for confounding factors. In such instances, researchers should also discuss the degree of potential selection and information biases, allowing readers to properly judge the results in view of the nonrandom nature of the study and its biases.

METHOD OF GENERATION OF AN ALLOCATION SEQUENCE

To minimise bias, participants in a trial should be assigned to comparison groups based on some chance (random) process. Investigators use many different methods of randomisation,[17-21] the most predominant of which we describe in the sections below.

With all these methods, different allocation ratios are possible. However, the allocation ratio of 1:1 (i.e., an equal probability of assignment to each group) is usually employed leading to approximately equal group sizes.[22,23] Although a 1:1 allocation ratio usually maximises trial power, ratios up to 2:1 minimally reduce the power.[17,22]

Good reasons argue for more common usage of unequal allocation. The most obvious reasons relate to costs, because within a trial the cost of each treatment often differs. If the available trial funding is fixed, using an unequal allocation ratio to randomise more participants to the cheaper treatment group facilitates a larger sample size thus increasing the power of the trial.[23-25] With a fixed total sample size available, an unequal allocation ratio can create large cost savings in a trial with minimal effect on statistical power.[22,23,25] For example, with a fixed total sample size, using a 2:1 allocation ratio instead of a 1:1 ratio in the Scandinavian simvastatin study for preventing coronary heart disease would have led to a 34% cost savings with only a modest 3% loss in power.[25]

Furthermore, unequal randomisation could help recruitment. Suppose one treatment arm is favoured by potential participants. If the trial is designed with unequal randomisation such that potential participants would have a higher likelihood of being allocated to their favoured treatment, then better recruitment likely results.

Simple (Unrestricted) Randomisation

'Elementary yet elegant' describes simple randomisation (Panel 12.3).[26] Although the most basic of allocation approaches, analogous to repeated fair coin-tossing, this method preserves complete unpredictability of each intervention assignment. No other allocation generation approach, irrespective of its complexity and sophistication, surpasses the unpredictability and bias prevention of simple randomisation.[27,28] The unpredictability of simple randomisation, however, can also be a disadvantage.[29] With small sample sizes, simple randomisation (1:1 allocation ratio) can yield highly disparate sample sizes in the groups by chance alone. For example, with a total sample size of 20, about 10% of the sequences generated with simple randomisation would yield a ratio imbalance of 3:7 or worse.[28] This difficulty is diminished as the total sample size grows. Probability theory ensures that, in the long term, the sizes of the treatment groups will not be greatly imbalanced. For a two-arm trial, the chance of pronounced imbalance becomes negligible with trial sizes greater than 200.[28] However, interim analyses with sample sizes of less than 200 might result in disparate group sizes.

Coin-tossing, dice-throwing, and dealing previously shuffled cards represent reasonable approaches for generation of simple complete randomisation sequences. All these manual methods of drawing lots theoretically lead to random allocation schemes, but frequently become nonrandom in practice. Distorted notions of randomisation sabotage the best of intentions. Fair coin-tossing, for example, allocates randomly with equal probability to two intervention groups, but can tempt investigators to alter the results of a toss or series of tosses (e.g., when a series of heads and no tails are thrown). Many investigators do not really understand probability theory, and they perceive randomness as nonrandom. For example, the late Chicago baseball announcer Jack Brickhouse used to

---

PANEL 12.3 ■ Simple Randomisation

An almost infinite number of methods can be used to generate a simple randomisation sequence based on a random-number table.[26] For example, for equal allocation to two groups, predetermine the direction to read the table: up, down, left, right, or diagonal. Then select an arbitrary starting point (i.e., first line, 7th number):

  56 99 20 20 52 49 **05 78 58 50 62 86 52 11 88**
  31 60 26 13 69 74 80 71 48 73 72 18 60 58 20
  55 59 06 67 02 ...

For equal allocation, an investigator could equate odd and even numbers to interventions A and B, respectively. Therefore, a series of random numbers 05, 78, 58, 50, 62, 86, 52, 11, 88, 31, and so forth represents allocation to intervention A, B, B, B, B, B, B, A, B, A, and so forth. Alternatively, 00–49 could equate to A and 50–99 to B, or numbers 00–09 to A and 10–19 to B, ignoring all numbers greater than 19. Any of a myriad of options suffice, provided the assignment probabilities and the investigator adhere to the predetermined scheme.

claim that when a 0.250 hitter (someone who would have a successful hit a quarter of the time) strolled to the plate for the fourth time, having failed the previous three times, that the batsman was 'due' (i.e., that the hitter would surely get a hit). However, Jack's proclamation 'he is due' portrayed a nonrandom interpretation of randomness. Similarly, a couple who have three boys and want a girl often think that their fourth child will certainly be a girl, yet the probability of them actually having a girl is still about 50%.

A colleague regularly demonstrated distorted views of randomisation with his graduate school class. He would have half his class develop allocation schemes with a proper randomisation method, and get the other half to develop randomisation schemes based on their personal views of randomisation. The students who used a truly random method would frequently have long consecutive runs of one treatment or the other. Conversely, students who used their own judgement would not. Class after class revealed their distorted impressions of randomisation.

Moreover, manual methods of drawing lots are more difficult to implement and cannot be checked. Because of threats to randomness, difficulties in implementation, and lack of an audit trail, we recommend that investigators avoid use of coin-tossing, dice-throwing, or card-shuffling, despite these being acceptable methods. Whatever method is used, however, should be clearly indicated in a researcher's report. If no such description is made, readers should treat the study results with caution. Readers should have the most confidence in a sequence generation approach if the authors mention referral to either a table of random numbers or a computer random number generator, because these options represent unpredictable, reliable, easy, reproducible approaches that provide an audit trail. Many statistical software packages include random number generators and the Internet provides access as well.

Restricted Randomisation

Restricted randomisation procedures control the probability of obtaining an allocation sequence with an undesirable sample size imbalance in the intervention groups.[21] In other words, if researchers want treatment groups of equal sizes, they should use restricted randomisation.

BLOCKING

Balanced (restricted) randomisation strives for unbiased comparison groups, but also strives for comparison groups of about the same size throughout the trial.[29,30] That attribute becomes helpful when investigators plan interim analyses. The use of simple randomisation might, upon occasion, produce quite disparate sample sizes at early interim analyses. Blocking obviates that problem.

The most frequently used method of achieving balanced randomisation is by random permuted blocks (blocking).[31] For example, with a block size of six, of every six consecutively enrolled participants, three will normally be allocated to one treatment group and three to the other. However, the allocation ratio can be uneven. For example, a block size of six with a 2:1 ratio assigns four to one treatment group and two to the other in each block. This method can easily be extended to more than two treatments.

With blocking, the block size can remain fixed throughout the trial or be randomly varied. Indeed, if blocked randomisation is used in a trial that is not double blinded, the block size should be randomly varied to reduce the chances of the assignment schedule being seen by those responsible for recruitment of participants.[18,31-33] If the block size is fixed, especially if small (six participants or fewer), the block size could be deciphered in a trial that is not double blinded. With treatment allocations becoming known after assignment, a sequence can be discerned from the pattern of past assignments. Some future assignments could then be accurately anticipated, and selection bias introduced, irrespective of the effectiveness of allocation concealment. Larger block sizes (e.g., 10 or 20) rather than smaller block sizes (e.g., four or six) and random variation of block sizes help preserve unpredictability.[18,33] Investigators who do randomised controlled trials frequently use blocking. Those who report simply that they blocked, however, should make readers sceptical. Researchers should explicitly report having used blocking, the allocation ratio (usually 1:1), the random method of selection (e.g. random number table or computer random number generator), and the block size (or sizes if randomly varied).

RANDOM ALLOCATION RULE

The random allocation rule is the simplest form of restriction. For a particular total sample size, it ensures equal sizes only at the end of the trial. Usually, investigators identify a total sample size and then randomly choose a subset of that sample to assign to group A; the remainder are assigned to group B. For example, for a total study size of 200, placing 100 group A balls and 100 group B balls in a hat and drawing them randomly without replacement symbolises the random allocation rule. The sequence generation would randomly order 100 group A and 100 group B assignments. This method represents one large permuted block for the entire study, which means that balance would usually only arise at the end of the trial and not throughout.

The random allocation rule maintains many of the positive attributes of simple complete randomisation, especially for statistical analysis, but is more likely to yield a chance covariate imbalance (chance confounding). It is noteworthy that this difference becomes trivial with larger sample sizes.[28] Moreover, unpredictability suffers compared with simple complete randomisation. Particularly in a non–double-blinded trial, selection bias can be introduced through guessing of assignments (especially towards the end of the trial), but obviously not at the level of permuted-block randomisation with small block sizes.[28,34]

Investigators sometimes apply the random allocation rule by the restricted shuffled approach, which involves identifying the sample size, apportioning a number of specially prepared cards for each treatment according to the allocation ratio, inserting the cards into envelopes, and shuffling them to produce a form of random assignment without replacement.[29] Many investigators probably use this approach, but rarely call it restricted shuffled or the random allocation rule. Instead, they report use of envelopes or shuffling. Indeed, the restricted shuffled approach integrates and conflates allocation generation and concealment. Shuffling determines the allocation sequence, which is not optimum. Most importantly, the adequacy of the restricted shuffled approach pivots on proper allocation concealment with envelopes.[7,8]

BIASED COIN AND URN RANDOMISATION

Biased-coin designs achieve much the same objective as blocking but without forcing strict equality.[17,35] They therefore preserve most of the unpredictability associated with simple randomisation. Biased-coin designs alter the allocation probability during the course of the trial to rectify imbalances that might be happening (Panel 12.4). Adaptive biased-coin designs, with the urn design being the most widely studied, alter the probability of assignment based on the magnitude of the imbalance.

Biased-coin designs, including the urn design, appear infrequently in reports. They probably should, however, be used more often. Use of a computer is easier and more reliable than actually drawing balls from an urn, just as a computer is easier and more reliable than flipping a coin for simple randomisation. In unblinded trials, in which unpredictability becomes most important and the need for balance precludes simple randomisation, an urn design is especially useful. The unpredictability of urn designs surpasses permuted-block designs, irrespective of fixed or randomly varied block size approaches.[35] If readers encounter a biased-coin or urn design, they should consider it a proper sequence generation approach.

PANEL 12.4 ■ **Biased-Coin and Urn Randomisation**

Biased-coin approaches alter the allocation probability during the course of the trial to rectify imbalances in group numbers that might be happening. For example, investigators might use simple randomisation with equal probability of assignment (0.50/0.50 in a two-arm trial) as long as the disparity between the numbers assigned to the treatment groups remains below a prespecified limit. If the disparity reaches the limit, then investigators increase the probability of assignment to the group with the least participants (e.g., 0.60/0.40). Implemented properly, a biased-coin approach can achieve balance while preserving most of the unpredictability associated with simple randomisation.[17,35]

Adaptive biased-coin designs, with the urn design being the most widely studied, alter the probability of assignment based on the magnitude of the imbalance.[35] The urn design is designated as UD (α, β), with α being the number of blue and green balls initially and β representing the number of balls added to the urn of the opposite colour to the ball chosen (α and β being any reasonable nonnegative numbers, and, note, have no relationship to type I and type II errors). For example, in UD (2, 1), an urn contains two blue balls and two green balls—0.50/0.50 probabilities to begin ($\alpha = 2$). Balls are drawn at random and replaced for treatment assignments: blue for treatment A and green for treatment B. One additional ball ($\beta = 1$) of the opposite colour to the ball chosen is added to the urn. If a blue ball was chosen first, then two blue balls and three green balls would be in the urn after the first assignment—0.40/0.60 for the next assignment. If another blue was chosen second, then two blue balls and four green balls would be in the urn after the second assignment—0.33/0.67 for the next assignment. That drawing procedure repeats with each assignment. The allocation probabilities fluctuate with the previous assignments.

REPLACEMENT RANDOMISATION

Replacement randomisation repeats a simple randomisation allocation scheme until a desired balance is achieved. Trial investigators should establish objective criteria for replacement. For example, for a trial with 300 participants, investigators could specify that they would replace a simple randomisation scheme if the disparity between group sizes exceeds 20. If the first generated scheme's disparity exceeds 20, then they would generate an entirely new simple randomisation scheme to replace the first attempt and check it against their objective criteria for disparity. They would iterate until they have a simple randomisation scheme that meets their criteria. Although replacement randomisation seems somewhat arbitrary, it is adequate as long as it is implemented before the trial begins.[17] Moreover, it is easy to implement, ensures reasonable balance, and yields unpredictability. The main limitation of replacement randomisation is that it cannot ensure balance throughout the trial for interim analyses. Though rarely used, this approach emerged as the earliest form of restricted randomisation.[21,36]

Stratified Randomisation

Randomisation can create chance imbalances on baseline characteristics of treatment groups.[37] Investigators sometimes avert imbalances by use of prerandomisation stratification on important prognostic factors, such as age or disease severity. In such instances, researchers should specify the method of restriction (usually blocking). To reap the benefits of stratification, investigators must use a form of restricted randomisation to generate separate randomisation schedules for stratified subsets of participants defined by the potentially important prognostic factors. Stratification without restriction accomplishes nothing (i.e., placebo stratification).

Stratification in trials is methodologically valid and useful, but theoretical and pragmatic issues limit its use for those planning new trials. The added complexity of stratification yields little additional gain in large trials, because randomisation creates balanced groups anyway. Moreover, if imbalance arises, then investigators can statistically adjust on those prognostic variables (preferably preplanned).[38-40] Of greatest concern is that the added complexity of stratifying might discourage collaborators from participating in the trial or from entering participants during busy clinics, either of which affects enrolment. Thus stratification in large trials offers negligible advantages coupled with important, pragmatic disadvantages. Note one important exception, however: stratification by centre in multicentre trials promises some benefit with no added complexity to the trial implementers within each centre. Also, another potential exception arises in large multicentre trials in which investigators use central randomisation for implementation of the sequence. Central randomisation limits the practical disadvantages of stratification and some gains might be realised in centres with smaller sample sizes.

Stratification might be useful in small trials in which it can avert severe imbalances on prognostic factors. It will confer adequate balance (on the stratified factors) and probably slightly more statistical power and precision.[18] The gain from stratification becomes minimal, however, once the number of participants per group is more than 50.[18] Moreover, stratification can indirectly cause negative effects if investigators seek exact balance within small strata. To achieve that exact balance, investigators often use small, fixed block sizes, which, in turn, hurts unpredictability. Another consideration is that overall trial imbalance suffers with a large number of strata or with block sizes that are too large for the number of participants,[41] but we view that as a minor concern. Indeed, imbalance is helpful for unpredictability.

Minimisation incorporates the general notions of stratification and restricted randomisation.[17] It can be used to make small groups closely similar with respect to several characteristics. Minimisation in its strictest sense can be viewed as nonrandom,[26] but, if used, we prefer a random component. Minimisation has supporters[42-44] and detractors,[27,45,46] while others are studying it and providing suggestions for implementation.[47] In any case, investigators who use minimisation should shield trial implementers from knowledge of upcoming assignments and other information that might facilitate guessing of upcoming assignments.[17] However, this might not be possible. Moreover, minimisation balances on a limited set of known factors. Randomisation balances on all known and unknown factors. We are cautious about the use of minimisation, as are others.[27,45,46]

Separation of Generation and Implementation

Investigators often neglect, usually unintentionally, one other important element of randomised controlled trial design and reporting. With all approaches, the people who generated the allocation scheme should not be involved in ascertaining eligibility, administering treatment, or assessing outcome. Such an individual would usually have access to the allocation schedule and thus the opportunity to introduce bias.[8] Faults in this trial component might represent a crevice through which bias seeps into trials. Item 10 (Implementation) in the CONSORT statement addresses this topic.[37,48-50] Researchers should, therefore, state in reports who generated the allocation sequence, who enrolled participants, and who assigned participants. The person generating the allocation mechanism should be different from the person(s) enrolling and assigning. Nevertheless, under some circumstances, an investigator might have to generate the scheme and also enrol or assign. In such instances, the investigator should ensure the unpredictability of the assignment schedule and lock it away from everyone, particularly himself or herself.

Conclusion

Randomised controlled trials set the methodological standard of excellence in medical research. The key word is randomised, which must be done properly. Generation of a randomisation sequence takes little time and effort but affords big rewards in scientific accuracy and credibility. Investigators should devote appropriate resources to doing the generation properly and reporting their methods clearly.

References

1. Hill, A.B., 1952. The clinical trial. N. Engl. J. Med. 247, 113–119.
2. Fisher, R., 1966. The Design of Experiments. Oliver & Boyd Ltd, Edinburgh, Scotland.
3. Armitage, P., 1982. The role of randomization in clinical trials. Stat. Med. 1, 345–352.
4. Doll, R., 1998. Controlled trials: the 1948 watershed. BMJ 317, 1217–1220.
5. Medical Research Council, 1948. Streptomycin treatment of pulmonary tuberculosis. BMJ 2, 769–782.
6. Peto, R., 1987. Why do we need systematic overviews of randomized trials? Stat. Med. 6, 233–244.
7. Schulz, K.F., Chalmers, I., Hayes, R.J., Altman, D.G., 1995. Empirical evidence of bias. Dimensions of methodological quality associated with estimates of treatment effects in controlled trials. JAMA 273, 408–412.
8. Schulz, K.F., 1995. Subverting randomization in controlled trials. JAMA 274, 1456–1458.
9. Schulz, K.F., 1995. Unbiased research and the human spirit: the challenges of randomized controlled trials. CMAJ 153, 783–786.
10. Schulz, K.F., Chalmers, I., Grimes, D.A., Altman, D.G., 1994. Assessing the quality of randomization from reports of controlled trials published in obstetrics and gynecology journals. JAMA 272, 125–128.
11. Egbewale, B.E., 2014. Random allocation in controlled clinical trials: a review. J. Pharm. Pharm. Sci. 17, 248–253.
12. Grimes, D.A., 1991. Randomized controlled trials: "it ain't necessarily so". Obstet. Gynecol. 78, 703–704.
13. Grimes, D., Fraser, E., Schulz, K., 1994. Immunization as therapy for recurrent spontaneous abortion: a review and meta-analysis (letter). Obstet. Gynecol. 83, 637–638.
14. Altman, D.G., 1991. Randomisation. BMJ 302, 1481–1482.
15. Schulz, K.F., Chalmers, I., Altman, D.G., Grimes, D.A., Dore, C.J., 1995. The methodologic quality of randomization as assessed from reports of trials in specialist and general medical journals. Online J. Curr. Clin. Trials. Doc No 197:[81 paragraphs].
16. MacFarlane, A., 1978. Variations in number of births and perinatal mortality by day of week in England and Wales. Br. Med. J. 2, 1670–1673.
17. Pocock, S., 1983. Clinical Trials: A Practical Approach. Wiley, Chichester, England.
18. Meinert, C., 1986. Clinical Trials: Design, Conduct, and Analysis. Oxford University Press, New York.
19. Friedman, L., Furberg, C., DeMets, D., 1996. Fundamentals of Clinical Trials. Mosby, St. Louis.
20. Piantadosi, S., 1997. Clinical Trials: A Methodologic Perspective. John Wiley & Sons, New York, NY.
21. Lachin, J.M., 1988. Statistical properties of randomization in clinical trials. Control. Clin. Trials 9, 289–311.
22. Dumville, J.C., Hahn, S., Miles, J.N., Torgerson, D.J., 2006. The use of unequal randomisation ratios in clinical trials: a review. Contemp. Clin. Trials 27, 1–12.
23. Peckham, E., Brabyn, S., Cook, L., Devlin, T., Dumville, J., Torgerson, D.J., 2015. The use of unequal randomisation in clinical trials—an update. Contemp. Clin. Trials 45, 113–122.
24. Torgerson, D., Campbell, M., 1997. Unequal randomisation can improve the economic efficiency of clinical trials. J. Health Serv. Res. Policy 2, 81–85.
25. Torgerson, D.J., Campbell, M.K., 2000. Use of unequal randomisation to aid the economic efficiency of clinical trials. BMJ 321, 759.
26. Altman, D., 1991. Practical Statistics for Medical Research. Chapman and Hall, London.
27. Lachin, J.M., Matts, J.P., Wei, L.J., 1988. Randomization in clinical trials: conclusions and recommendations. Control. Clin. Trials 9, 365–374.
28. Lachin, J.M., 1988. Properties of simple randomization in clinical trials. Control. Clin. Trials 9, 312–326.
29. Schulz, K.F., 1998. Randomized controlled trials. Clin. Obstet. Gynecol. 41, 245–256.
30. Schulz, K.F., Grimes, D.A., 2002. Generation of allocation sequences in randomised trials: chance, not choice. Lancet 359, 515–519.
31. Higham, R., Tharmanathan, P., Birks, Y., 2015. Use and reporting of restricted randomization: a review. J. Eval. Clin. Pract. 21, 1205–1211.
32. Efird, J., 2011. Blocked randomization with randomly selected block sizes. Int. J. Environ. Res. Public Health 8, 15–20.
33. Kahan, B.C., Rehal, S., Cro, S., 2015. Risk of selection bias in randomised trials. Trials 16, 405.
34. Matts, J.P., Lachin, J.M., 1988. Properties of permuted-block randomization in clinical trials. Control. Clin. Trials 9, 327–344.

35. Wei, L.J., Lachin, J.M., 1988. Properties of the urn randomization in clinical trials. Control. Clin. Trials 9, 345–364.

36. Cox, D.R., 1958. Planning of Experiments. Wiley, New York.

37. Moher, D., Hopewell, S., Schulz, K.F., et al., 2010. CONSORT 2010 explanation and elaboration: updated guidelines for reporting parallel group randomised trials. BMJ 340, c869.

38. Moher, D., Hopewell, S., Schulz, K.F., et al., 2010. CONSORT 2010 explanation and elaboration: updated guidelines for reporting parallel group randomised trials. J. Clin. Epidemiol. 63, e1–e37.

39. Peto, R., Pike, M.C., Armitage, P., et al., 1977. Design and analysis of randomized clinical trials requiring prolonged observation of each patient. II. analysis and examples. Br. J. Cancer 35, 1–39.

40. Peto, R., Pike, M.C., Armitage, P., et al., 1976. Design and analysis of randomized clinical trials requiring prolonged observation of each patient. I. Introduction and design. Br. J. Cancer 34, 585–612.

41. Kundt, G., Glass, A., 2012. Evaluation of imbalance in stratified blocked randomization: some remarks on the range of validity of the model by Hallstrom and Davis. Methods Inf. Med. 51, 55–62.

42. Treasure, T., MacRae, K.D., 1998. Minimisation: the platinum standard for trials? Randomisation doesn't guarantee similarity of groups; minimisation does. BMJ 317, 362–363.

43. Taves, D.R., 2011. Minimization does not by its nature preclude allocation concealment and invite selection bias, as Berger claims. Contemp. Clin. Trials 32, 323.

44. Taves, D.R., 2010. The use of minimization in clinical trials. Contemp. Clin. Trials 31, 180–184.

45. Berger, V.W., 2010. Minimization, by its nature, precludes allocation concealment, and invites selection bias. Contemp. Clin. Trials 31, 406.

46. Berger, V.W., 2011. Minimization: not all it's cracked up to be. Clin. Trials 8, 443.

47. McPherson, G.C., Campbell, M.K., Elbourne, D.R., 2013. Investigating the relationship between predictability and imbalance in minimisation: a simulation study. Trials 14, 86.

48. Schulz, K.F., Altman, D.G., Moher, D., 2010. CONSORT 2010 statement: updated guidelines for reporting parallel group randomised trials. PLoS Med 7, e1000251.

49. Schulz, K.F., Altman, D.G., Moher, D., 2010. CONSORT 2010 statement: updated guidelines for reporting parallel group randomised trials. J. Clin. Epidemiol. 63, 834–840.

50. Schulz, K.F., Altman, D.G., Moher, D., 2010. CONSORT 2010 statement: updated guidelines for reporting parallel group randomised trials. BMJ 340, c332.

CHAPTER 13

Generation of Allocation Sequences in Non–Double-Blinded Randomised Trials: Guarding Against Guessing

We cringe at the pervasive notion that a randomised trial needs to yield equal sample sizes in the comparison groups. Unfortunately, that conceptual misunderstanding can lead to bias by investigators who force equality, especially if by nonscientific means. In simple, unrestricted, randomised trials (analogous to repeated coin-tossing), the sizes of groups should indicate random variation. In other words, some discrepancy between the numbers in the comparison groups would be expected. The appeal of equal group sizes in a simple randomised controlled trial is cosmetic, not scientific. Moreover, other randomisation schemes, termed restricted randomisation, force equality by departing from simple randomisation. Forcing equal group sizes, however, potentially harms the unpredictability of treatment assignments, especially when using permuted-block randomisation in non–double-blinded trials. Diminished unpredictability can allow bias to creep into a trial. Overall, investigators underuse simple randomisation and overuse fixed-block randomisation. For non–double-blinded trials larger than 200 participants, investigators should use simple randomisation more often and accept moderate disparities in group sizes. Such unpredictability reflects the essence of randomness. We endorse the generation of mildly unequal group sizes and encourage an appreciation of such inequalities. For non–double-blinded randomised controlled trials with a sample size of less than 200 overall or within any principal stratum or subgroup, urn randomisation enhances unpredictability compared with blocking. A simpler alternative, our mixed randomisation approach, attains unpredictability within the context of the currently understood simple randomisation and permuted-block methods. Simple randomisation contributes the unpredictability whereas permuted-block randomisation contributes the balance, but avoids the perfect balance that can result in selection bias.

A tantalising phone call begins, 'I have just read a report of a randomised trial, and I found problems!' All too often, however, the discussion proceeds with 'Look at that difference in sample sizes in the groups; they are not equal. I am suspicious of this trial.' Or in planning a trial, 'What can we do to end up with equal sample sizes?' Indeed, large disparities in sample sizes not explained by chance should cause concern,[1,2] but many researchers look askance at a trial with any disparity.

We cringe at this seemingly ubiquitous notion that a randomised trial needs to yield equal sample sizes. Somehow such a notion seems embedded in many a medical researcher's psyche.

Such conceptual misunderstanding deters prevention of bias in trials. Exactly equal sample sizes in a randomised controlled trial contribute little to statistical power and potentially harm unpredictability, especially in non–double-blinded trials that use permuted-block randomisation. Unpredictability reflects the essence of randomisation because those involved cannot predict the next treatment assignment. With predictability comes bias.

Greater predictability emanates from randomisation schemes that depart from simple, unrestricted randomisation.[3,4] Such departures are termed restricted randomisation schemes.[5-7] They constrain treatment assignment schedules to yield similar or, most frequently, equal group sizes throughout the trial, assuming the most common desired allocation ratio of 1:1. The restricted randomisation schemes all sacrifice unpredictability, but that increased predictability primarily surfaces in non–double-blinded trials that use permuted blocks (Panel 13.1).[3,4,8-10]

Trialists rely on the security of unpredictability. In the past, we suggested cultivation of a tolerance for groups of unequal sample sizes in simple randomised trials.[11,12] We now suggest cultivation of a tolerance for groups of unequal sizes in restricted randomisation trials as well.

Forcing Cosmetic Credibility

Studies reported as randomised yield equal sample sizes in the comparison groups more frequently than expected.[11-13] In simple, unrestricted randomised controlled trials (analogous to repeated

---

PANEL 13.1 ■ Unpredictability in Allocation Sequences

Predictability in clinical trials breeds bias. If trial investigators identify or predict upcoming allocation assignments, they can instil selection bias. In assessment of eligibility, they could exclude a participant destined for, in their opinion, the wrong group. Moreover, various manoeuvres allow them to channel participants with a better prognosis to the experimental group and those with a poorer prognosis to the control group, or vice versa.[5,10] Irrespective of the reasons for doing so, experimenters bias the comparison. Clinicians might revere predictability in caring for patients, but they must understand that predictability spawns bias in clinical trials.

Trial investigators can guess the next assignments by subverting the allocation concealment mechanism (e.g., by holding translucent envelopes to a light bulb).[9,10] However, proper allocation concealment usually prevents this subversion. Alternatively, with permuted-block randomisation, trial investigators can sometimes predict the next assignments by noting a pattern of past assignments.[3,4,7,8,10] For example, in a non–double-blinded trial with a block size of four, if a trial investigator notes that the sample size in the two groups equilibrates after every four participants, then many future assignments can be predicted.[3,4,8] For example, if the sequence ABA materialises in a block of four, B would necessarily be the next assignment, or if the sequence BB materialises, AA would be the next two assignments.

In non–double-blinded trials, all intervention allocations become known after assignment, even with proper allocation concealment. Thus if a pattern to the allocation sequence exists, the trial investigator can discern it and predict some future assignments. However, if no pattern exists, or if the pattern is indiscernible, the allocation sequence is unpredictable. Therefore knowledge of past assignments would not help in prediction of future assignments. Unpredictability is essential in non–double-blinded randomised trials.[3]

Proper allocation concealment before assignment and proper blinding of all involved in the trial after assignment shields knowledge of past assignments and thereby prevents prediction of future assignments. Proper blinding diminishes the need for unpredictability. Even in supposedly blinded trials, however, blinding after assignment is not always successful. If trial investigators perceive quickly developing, clinically obvious side effects that reveal the intervention assigned, for instance, blinding might not prevent predictions.

coin-tossing), the relative sizes of comparison groups should indicate random variation. In other words, some discrepancy between the numbers in the comparison groups would be expected. However, analyses of reports of trials in general and specialist medical journals showed that researchers too frequently reported equal sample sizes of the comparison groups (defined as exactly equal or as equal as possible in view of an odd number total sample size).[11,12] In the specialist journals, the disparity of sample sizes in the comparison groups deviated from expected $(p < 0.001)$ and produced equal group sizes in 54% of the simple randomised (unrestricted) trials.[11] This result was higher than that in blocked trials (36%), and blocked trials aspire for equality. Moreover, results of a similar analysis of the dermatology literature showed that an even higher 71% of simple randomised trials reported essentially equal group sizes.[13]

Why would investigators seek equal or similar sample sizes in comparison groups? We feel many investigators strive for equal sample sizes as an end in itself. The lure of the so-called cosmetic credibility of equal sizes seems apparent. Sadly, that cosmetic credibility also appeals to readers. Striving for equal sample sizes with simple randomisation, however, reflects a methodological *non sequitur.*

The high proportion of equal group sizes noted previously represents pronounced aberrations from chance occurrences and suggests nonrandom manipulations of assignments to force equality. Other logical explanations seem plausible, but probably do not account for the degree of aberration witnessed.[11,13] Such tinkering with assignments creates difficulties by directly instilling selection bias into trials. We hope to remove some of those difficulties by dispelling the misunderstanding behind the drive for exactly equal sizes.

Beyond the issue of nonrandom manipulations of assignments, however, we will concentrate on the potential bias introduced by balancing group sizes with valid restricted randomisation methods, primarily permuted-block randomisation, that produce equal group sizes throughout the trial. Unfortunately, methods used to ensure equal sample sizes can facilitate correct future predictions of treatment assignments, allowing bias to infiltrate.

Unequal Group Sizes in Restricted Trials

The method of restricted randomisation is used to balance sample sizes. That balance usually enhances statistical power and addresses any time trends that might exist in treatment efficacy and outcome measurement during the course of a trial.[14,15] Moreover, restricted randomisation within strata becomes essential for investigators to attain the benefits of stratification.[7,16] Thus reasonable scientific justification lends support to restriction.

For restriction to be effective, however, it need not yield exactly equal sample sizes. The power of a trial is not sensitive to slight deviations from equality of the sample sizes.[6] Thus restricted approaches that produce similar sizes would yield power, time trend, and stratification benefits much the same as those restricted randomisation approaches that produce equal sizes.

Equal sample sizes, however, can have negative consequences. The predominant restricted randomisation method is random permuted blocks (blocking). Such an approach effectively attains the goals of equal sample sizes in the comparison groups overall (and, if stratified, within strata). Moreover, the method generates equal sample sizes after every block. With that attribute, however, comes the disadvantage of predictability.[10,14]

Predictability, particularly, becomes a major weakness in a non–double-blinded trial. We define a double-blinded trial as one in which the treatment is hidden from participants, investigators, and outcome assessors. In virtually all non–double-blinded trials, some investigators become aware of the treatment. Thus even with adequate allocation concealment, treatment assignments become known after assignment. With that information, trial investigators can unravel the fixed block size (presumably the organisers initially shielded all block size information from them) and then anticipate when equality of the sample sizes will arise (see Panel 13.1) A sequence can be discerned from the pattern of past assignments and then some future assignments could be accurately anticipated.[3,4]

Hence selection bias could seep in, irrespective of the effectiveness of allocation concealment.[3,4,7,10] The same difficulty to a lesser degree might be true in a double-blinded trial in which obvious, perceptible side effects materialise quickly.

Although empirical evidence indicates that selection bias exists in randomised trials,[5] do those who implement trials actually try to anticipate future assignments? We have many anecdotal reports of such anticipation, and some researchers actually conducted a study. In questioning clinicians and research nurses, 16% admitted to trying to predict treatment allocations.[17] As expected, they did it by keeping a log of all the previous assignments in the trial.[17] Furthermore, we suspect that the 16% who admit this process represent a minimal estimate. The actual percentage that do it is probably higher.

Randomised controlled trials become prone to unravelling of block sizes when the block size remains fixed throughout the trial, especially if the block size is small (e.g., six or fewer participants). Hence if investigators use blocked randomisation, they should randomly vary the block size to lower the chances of an assignment schedule being inferred by those responsible for recruitment and assignment.[7,10,18]

Random block sizes, however, are no panacea. Even with random variation of block sizes, blocking still generates equal sample sizes many times throughout a trial. Indeed, based on a modification of a model that measures inherent predictability of intervention assignments with certainty, random block sizes, at best, decrease but do not eliminate the potential for selection bias.[14,19] In other words, random block sizes help to reduce, but in some instances might not eliminate, selection bias. Permuted-block randomisation, even with random block sizes, presents trial recruiters with opportunities to anticipate some assignments.

Alternatives in Non–Double-Blinded Trials

For non–double-blinded randomised controlled trials with an overall sample size of more than 200 (an average sample size of 100 in two groups) and within each planned subgroup or stratum, we recommend simple randomisation.[20] It provides perfect unpredictability, thereby eliminating that aspect of selection bias due to the generation of the allocation sequence. Moreover, simple randomisation also provides the least probability for chance bias of all the generation procedures,[6] and it enables valid use of virtually all standard statistical software. With sample sizes greater than 200, simple randomisation normally yields only mild disparities in sample sizes between groups. The cut-off of 200, however, is merely an overall guideline. Individual investigators might want to judge their particular acceptable levels of disparity.[21] Another caveat centres on potential interim analyses done on sample sizes of less than 200 (i.e., before investigators reach total sample size). Greater relative disparities in treatment group sizes could materialise in those instances, although we feel those costs are more than offset by the gains in unpredictability from simple randomisation.

For non–double-blinded randomised controlled trials with a sample size of less than 200 overall or within any principal stratum or subgroup of a stratified trial, we recommend a restricted randomisation procedure. The urn design[7] functions especially well to promote balance without forcing it.[22] It tends to balance more in the important early stages of a trial and then approach simple randomisation as the trial size increases. This attribute becomes useful with uncertain overall trial sizes, or more likely, uncertain stratum sizes in a stratified trial. It also proves useful in trials that might be ended due to sequential monitoring of treatment effects. Urn designs usually have adequate balancing properties while still being less susceptible to selection bias than permuted-block designs[7,20] (see Chapter 12).

With these desirable properties come caveats. Some statisticians recommend use of permutation tests with urn randomisation designs. Permutation tests are assumption-free statistical tests of the equality of treatments.[6,22] Unfortunately, they usually are not available for urn designs in standard statistical software.[22] That adds analytical complexity for researchers and statisticians. However, if no major time trends on the outcome variables exist, use of standard statistical analyses from widely available software on trials that use urn randomisation would normally yield similar results to permutation tests.[22] Moreover, with standard statistical analyses, investigators can easily obtain confidence intervals for common measures of effect.

Of interest, a number of more complex designs have performed well. The Big Stick Design, the biased-coin design with imbalance tolerance, and the Ehrenfest urn design all perform better than blocking at achieving balance between groups with less predictability.[23] The maximal procedure is also less predictable than blocking while preserving balance.[24,25] Yet, these well-performing designs, along with the aforementioned urn randomisation design, appear infrequently, if at all, in reports. For example, in a review of randomisation methods used in trials published in four high-impact-factor general medical journals, almost 90% used a restricted method, and 90% of those used blocking with all the remainder using minimisation.[4] No authors reported using any of these well-performing, complex designs.[4]

Perhaps an impediment to widespread usage pertains to the conceptual complexities of urn randomisation and these other designs; they are more difficult to understand than simple or permuted-block randomisation. 'It is not clear why trialists still predominantly favour permuted blocks over other designs, although simplicity may be a significant factor'.[4] Whatever the reasons, these well-performing but more complicated designs languish in obscurity.

Mixed Randomisation

Researchers should have an unpredictable randomisation approach to use in non–double-blinded trials until they feel comfortable with urn randomisation or other approaches that enhance unpredictability.[26] We suggest an approach that builds on the existing knowledge that trialists have on simple randomisation and blocking. We propose a restricted randomisation method that should approach the unpredictability of urn randomisation overall while exceeding its unpredictability for small sample sizes, but without its real and perceived complexities. Our proposed approach promotes balance but not the perfect balance we feel can lead to predictability and selection bias.

Our solution mixes simple randomisation with permuted-block randomisation. Simple randomisation contributes the unpredictability to the approach whereas permuted-block randomisation contributes the balance. Our mixed approach begins with an uneven block generated by a replacement randomisation procedure (Panels 13.2 and 13.3).[27-30] Then, in its simplest form, standard permuted blocks of varying size follow. The replacement randomisation sequence would establish inequality initially and make any anticipation of assignments improbable throughout the remainder of the trial.

Replacement randomisation is basically simple randomisation, with a slight twist (see Chapter 12). Because investigators should aim for an uneven block, they would select a prespecified inequality in the sample sizes of the allocated groups. Then they would prepare an allocation sequence by simple randomisation and check the disparity in sample sizes against their prespecified inequality. If the disparity in sample sizes meets or exceeds their prespecified disparity, then that simple randomisation allocation sequence suffices for the first uneven block. If not, then a whole new simple randomisation list is generated to replace the previous one. They would iterate until a simple randomisation sequence meets or exceeds their prespecified disparity (see Panel 13.2). The block size of the first uneven block could be odd or even overall and could be of most any total size, although we conceive of it usually falling in the range of 5 to 16.

Our basic approach creates an initial imbalance in a trial. Replacement randomisation represents just one approach to creating it. Another choice might be to select from random imbalanced permuted blocks or several variations on that theme (Douglas G. Altman, personal communication, 2001). Another excellent easy approach, if investigators can accept variation in the disparity, would

---

PANEL 13.2 ■ Mixed Randomisation Steps

Step 1: Generate one uneven block by replacement randomisation for the first participants.

    A. Identify block size for the first uneven block. The block size can be odd or even and of any reasonable size, but usually in the range of 5 to 16.

    B. Select a prespecified inequality in the sample sizes of the allocated groups for the first uneven block.

    C. Generate a simple randomisation sequence (e.g., with a table of random numbers or a computer random number generator).

    D. Inspect resultant sequence of assignments for matching or exceeding the desired prespecified inequality from Step 1B earlier.

    E. If sufficiently unequal distribution of As and Bs, proceed to Step 2; if not, go back to Step 1C earlier (iterate).

Step 2: Generate random permuted blocks for subsequent participants.

    A. Select block sizes for the permuted blocks. Longer block sizes, such as 10 to 20, are more unpredictable than shorter block sizes, such as 2 to 4. Longer block sizes should be preferred, unless an investigator needs approximate balance in a small trial or a small stratum of a trial. For example, an investigator might select block sizes of 8, 10, 12, and 14 as options.

    B. Generate random permuted blocks, randomly varying the block size as described in many texts.[27–30]

    C. Decide if an additional uneven block or simple randomisation block is to be interspersed in the trial. If not, complete the required sample size with random permuted blocks. Otherwise, identify a point at which to interject an uneven block or a simple randomised sequence.

    D. If interjecting another uneven block by replacement randomisation, proceed back to Step 1. If interjecting a simple random sequence, proceed to Step 3.

Step 3: Generate a simple random sequence for interjection after a set of permuted blocks

    A. Identify the size of this simple random sequence. The size can be odd or even and of any reasonable size, but usually in the range of 5 to 16. We suggest an odd number to ensure some imbalance.

    B. Generate a simple random sequence of the chosen size as suggested earlier.[7,30]

    C. Proceed to Step 2B.

---

involve setting the overall first block size at an odd number, which ensures at least some disparity, and just using simple randomisation (without replacement randomisation).

Identification of an acceptable prespecified inequality for the first block is quite insensitive. Power remains robust up to about a 2:1 ratio for the total sample sizes in the treatment groups.[6,20] Investigators need only create much smaller inequalities than that, particularly in small strata in a stratified trial. Ensuring unpredictability will probably happen as much from small inequalities as large inequalities. Moreover, inequalities can actually slightly increase power in addition to offering enhanced unpredictability. For example, in tests for proportions or life tables, the maximum power is attained with unequal treatment group sizes.[6]

After the first uneven block, investigators should proceed as in normal permuted-block randomisation (see Panels 13.2 and 13.3). We suggest that they randomly vary the block size and use as long a block size as practicable for greater unpredictability.[7] For added unpredictability, investigators could also intersperse additional uneven blocks generated with replacement randomisation throughout the trial. For example, another uneven block could be interjected after a permuted block surpasses the next 50 participants (using the whole block, which means that the next uneven block would likely begin beyond 50). Alternatively, for these interspersed blocks, investigators could just use simple randomisation. That would be slightly easier, likely provide additional unpredictability, and also provide a richer set of potential allocation sequences. Other potential options for these interspersed uneven blocks exist (e.g., imbalanced permuted blocks), but they extend beyond the range of this chapter.

PANEL 13.3 ■ Example of Mixed Randomisation

The randomisation scheme (see the table on page 148) required an overall sample size of 100, based on power calculations. The investigator decided on a first uneven block size of 10 and prespecified an inequality of at least four participants between treatment A and treatment B in that first uneven block. The investigator then proceeded to use replacement randomisation by successively selecting a simple random sequence[7] of 10 until that process yielded a sequence of 10 assignments with either treatment A or treatment B having at least four extra participants. That sequence was B, A, B, B, B, A, B, B, A, B (actually, three treatment As and seven treatment Bs). Then the investigator decided to randomly vary the permuted-block sizes between 6, 8, 10, and 12, as described in many sources.[27–30] That could simply be continued over the remainder of the study, but this investigator decided to interject a simple randomised sequence of five assignments after a whole permuted block passed the 40th participant. The block sizes randomly selected were, in order, 12, 8, and 10. The simple randomised sequence beginning with the 41st participant was B, A, B, A, A. After that simple randomised sequence, the investigator again proceeded with random permuted blocks of 6, 8, 10, or 12, with the first randomly selected block size of 8. We depicted the allocation sequence and the total cumulative assignments by treatment for the first 53 assignments.

For analysis, we suggest use of standard statistical analyses with readily available statistical software (i.e., the simpler approach). Slightly greater credibility for hypothesis testing might be gained with design-based permutation tests,[14] but we favour the estimates with confidence intervals that standard statistical analyses produce.[20] We also agree with the acceptability of ignoring blocking in the analysis. This straightforward approach usually produces slightly conservative results in trials that use blocking if a time trend on the outcome exists but otherwise produces similar results to an analysis that incorporates blocking.[14]

Those issues, however, pale in comparison to the potential effects of selection bias that could arise in the absence of unpredictability. Once selection bias infiltrates a trial, it becomes embedded and usually prevails undetected, except in limited situations where investigators might use an innovative detection approach.[31] Moreover, empirical evidence points towards substantial selection biases.[5,10,32,33] However, the discussions of standard statistical analyses versus permutation tests or unblocked analyses versus blocked analyses from trials with permuted-block randomisation focus on seemingly smaller increments of p values or power. Irrespective of the analysis method chosen, the interpretation from a trial in many instances would be the same. More importantly, unlike selection bias, investigators have a straightforward remedy. If a journal editor or statistical reviewer insists on a different approach, investigators can usually retreat to a blocked analysis or a permutation test. In sum, investigators should use their energy to focus on prevention of biases in the design and implementation of their trial, with an unpredictable allocation sequence being an integral part of that effort.

Although mixed randomisation is much simpler and more understandable than urn randomisation and the other more complex designs, some investigators have endorsed mixed randomisation but opined that even it is too complex.[34] They applied the Blackwell-Hodges model for evaluation of the unpredictability of treatment assignments and found that the performance of permuted-block randomisation with a block size of 36 was similar to that of our mixed randomisation approach.[34] We applaud their work and, as clearly stated in Chapter 12, certainly endorse large block sizes to increase unpredictability. We also endorse simplicity and agree that block sizes of 36 are appropriate for larger trials. However, block sizes of 36 are inappropriate for smaller trials or large trials with stratified randomisation that require balance in smaller strata. Those are the situations for which we developed mixed randomisation.

Thus investigators conducting non–double-blinded trials should consider using our mixed randomisation approach. It is conceptually easier to understand and pragmatically simpler to implement than the urn design and other more complex designs developed to prevent selection bias with restricted randomisation. Moreover, investigators have had success in using mixed randomisation.[35–38] In any case, in non–double-blinded randomised trials, some approach should be used to

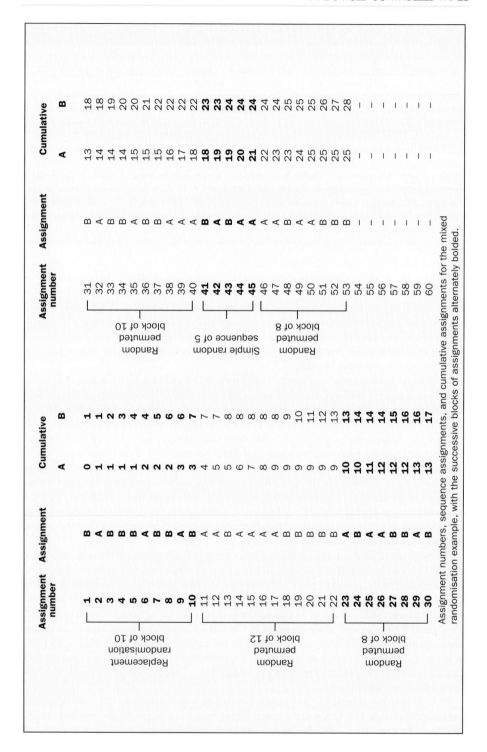

Assignment numbers, sequence assignments, and cumulative assignments for the mixed randomisation example, with the successive blocks of assignments alternately bolded.

prevent selection bias. Unfortunately, a recent review of nonblinded trials in four high-impact-factor general medical journals found few trials using techniques that would reduce the risk of selection bias.[3] The authors concluded, 'Many trials which did provide details on the randomisation procedure were at risk of selection bias due to a [sic] poorly chosen randomisation methods. Techniques to reduce the risk of selection bias should be more widely implemented'.[3]

Full Disclosure in the Protocol?

Provision of explicit details of the randomisation scheme in the protocol might facilitate deciphering of the allocation sequence, thus undermining the process. We recommend that researchers do not fully describe their generation scheme in their research protocol and investigators manual.[39-41] They would have to describe any stratification plans, but those implementing the trial should be kept ignorant of the full details of the method to generate the allocation sequence.

Some funding authorities require more documentation to ensure that researchers know proper randomisation methods. Appropriate rationale and references might suffice. If the funding agency requires more specifics, a researcher should provide a separate generation of the allocation sequence plan to the funders that will not be shared with those enrolling participants. However, in the final trial report, researchers should fully document the randomisation approach.[16,42-44]

Conclusion

Investigators underuse simple randomisation and overuse fixed-block randomisation. They do so because they inadequately appreciate the importance of unpredictability and overvalue equal treatment group sizes. Simple randomisation is totally unpredictable, implements easily, and enables use of standard statistical analysis software. For non–double-blinded trials larger than 200 participants, investigators should use it more and tolerate, if not celebrate, the disparity in group sizes. Such unpredictability reflects the essence of randomness.

For non–double-blinded randomised controlled trials smaller than about 200 participants overall or within any principal stratum or subgroup, the urn design enhances unpredictability compared with blocking. Our mixed randomisation method, however, attains unpredictability within the context of the currently understood simple and permuted-block randomisation methods. We urge researchers to use our method, at least in non–double-blinded trials.

Why add complexity to implementation of trials? The answer resides in the overriding importance of protecting the integrity of randomisation. Proper randomisation minimises bias more than any other methodological aspect of a trial: 'When the randomisation leaks, the trial's guarantee of lack of bias runs down the drain.'[45] Those involved in trials go to great pains to decipher randomisation schemes. Accordingly, researchers who design trials must take equally great pains to thwart those efforts.

References

1. Keirse, M.J.N.C., 1994. Electronic monitoring: who needs a trojan horse? Birth 21, 111–113.
2. Cates, W.J., Grimes, D.A., Schulz, K.F., Ory, H.W., Tyler Jr., C.W., 1978. World Health Organization studies of prostaglandins versus saline as abortifacients. A reappraisal. Obstet. Gynecol. 52, 493–498.
3. Kahan, B.C., Rehal, S., Cro, S., 2015. Risk of selection bias in randomised trials. Trials 16, 405.
4. Higham, R., Tharmanathan, P., Birks, Y., 2015. Use and reporting of restricted randomization: a review. J. Eval. Clin. Pract. 21, 1205–1211.

5. Schulz, K.F., Chalmers, I., Hayes, R.J., Altman, D.G., 1995. Empirical evidence of bias. Dimensions of methodological quality associated with estimates of treatment effects in controlled trials. JAMA 273, 408–412.

6. Lachin, J.M., 1988. Statistical properties of randomization in clinical trials. Control Clin. Trials 9, 289–311.

7. Schulz, K.F., Grimes, D.A., 2002. Generation of allocation sequences in randomised trials: chance, not choice. Lancet 359, 515–519.

8. Egbewale, B.E., 2014. Random allocation in controlled clinical trials: a review. J. Pharm. Pharm. Sci. 17, 248–253.

9. Schulz, K.F., Grimes, D.A., 2002. Allocation concealment in randomised trials: defending against deciphering. Lancet 359, 614–618.

10. Schulz, K.F., 1995. Subverting randomization in controlled trials. JAMA 274, 1456–1458.

11. Schulz, K.F., Chalmers, I., Grimes, D.A., Altman, D.G., 1994. Assessing the quality of randomization from reports of controlled trials published in obstetrics and gynecology journals. JAMA 272, 125–128.

12. Altman, D.G., Doré, C.J., 1990. Randomisation and baseline comparisons in clinical trials. Lancet 335, 149–153.

13. Adetugbo, K., Williams, H., 2000. How well are randomized controlled trials reported in the dermatology literature? Arch. Dermatol. 136, 381–385.

14. Matts, J.P., Lachin, J.M., 1988. Properties of permuted-block randomization in clinical trials. Control Clin. Trials 9, 327–344.

15. Peto, R., Pike, M.C., Armitage, P., et al., 1976. Design and analysis of randomized clinical trials requiring prolonged observation of each patient. I. Introduction and design. Br. J. Cancer 34, 585–612.

16. Moher, D., Hopewell, S., Schulz, K.F., et al., 2010. CONSORT 2010 explanation and elaboration: updated guidelines for reporting parallel group randomised trials. BMJ 340, c869.

17. Brown, S., Thorpe, H., Hawkins, K., Brown, J., 2005. Minimization—reducing predictability for multicentre trials whilst retaining balance within centre. Stat. Med. 24, 3715–3727.

18. Efird, J., 2011. Blocked randomization with randomly selected block sizes. Int. J. Environ. Res. Public Health 8, 15–20.

19. Tamm, M., Cramer, E., Kennes, L.N., Heussen, N., 2012. Influence of selection bias on the test decision. A simulation study. Methods Inf. Med. 51, 138–143.

20. Lachin, J.M., Matts, J.P., Wei, L.J., 1988. Randomization in clinical trials: conclusions and recommendations. Control Clin. Trials 9, 365–374.

21. Lachin, J.M., 1988. Properties of simple randomization in clinical trials. Control Clin. Trials 9, 312–326.

22. Wei, L.J., Lachin, J.M., 1988. Properties of the urn randomization in clinical trials. Control Clin. Trials 9, 345–364.

23. Zhao, W., Weng, Y., Wu, Q., Palesch, Y., 2012. Quantitative comparison of randomization designs in sequential clinical trials based on treatment balance and allocation randomness. Pharm. Stat. 11, 39–48.

24. Berger, V.W., Ivanova, A., Knoll, M.D., 2003. Minimizing predictability while retaining balance through the use of less restrictive randomization procedures. Stat. Med. 22, 3017–3028.

25. Zhao, W., Berger, V.W., Yu, Z., 2018. The asymptotic maximal procedure for subject randomization in clinical trials. Stat. Methods Med. Res. 27 (7), 2142–2153

26. Berger, V.W., Ivanova, A., Wei, E.Y., Knoll, M.A.D., 2001. An alternative to the complete randomized block procedure. Control Clin. Trials 22, 43S.

27. Friedman, L., Furberg, C., DeMets, D., 1996. Fundamentals of Clinical Trials. Mosby, St. Louis.

28. Pocock, S., 1983. Clinical Trials: A Practical Approach. Wiley, Chichester, UK.

29. Meinert, C., 1986. Clinical Trials: Design, Conduct, and Analysis. Oxford University Press, New York.

30. Altman, D., 1991. Practical Statistics for Medical Research. Chapman and Hall, London.

31. Berger, V.W., Exner, D.V., 1999. Detecting selection bias in randomized clinical trials. Control Clin. Trials 20, 319–327.

32. Moher, D., Pham, B., Jones, A., et al., 1998. Does quality of reports of randomised trials affect estimates of intervention efficacy reported in meta-analyses? Lancet 352, 609–613.

33. Savovic, J., Jones, H.E., Altman, D.G., et al., 2012. Influence of reported study design characteristics on intervention effect estimates from randomized, controlled trials. Ann. Intern. Med. 157, 429–438.

34. Kundt, G., 2005. An alternative proposal for "Mixed randomization" by Schulz and Grimes. Methods Inf. Med. 44, 572–576.

35. Lee, C.E., Kilgour, A., Lau, Y.K., 2012. Efficacy of walking exercise in promoting cognitive-psychosocial functions in men with prostate cancer receiving androgen deprivation therapy. BMC Cancer 12, 324.

36. Simcock, R., Fallowfield, L., Monson, K., et al., 2013. ARIX: a randomised trial of acupuncture v oral care sessions in patients with chronic xerostomia following treatment of head and neck cancer. Ann. Oncol. 24, 776–783.

37. McCaskey, M.A., Schuster-Amft, C., Wirth, B., de Bruin, E.D., 2015. Effects of postural specific sensorimotor training in patients with chronic low back pain: study protocol for randomised controlled trial. Trials 16, 571.

38. Hafner, P., Bonati, U., Rubino, D., et al., 2016. Treatment with L-citrulline and metformin in Duchenne muscular dystrophy: study protocol for a single-centre, randomised, placebo-controlled trial. Trials 17, 389.

39. Chan, A.W., Tetzlaff, J.M., Altman, D.G., Dickersin, K., Moher, D., 2013. SPIRIT 2013: new guidance for content of clinical trial protocols. Lancet 381, 91–92.

40. Chan, A.W., Tetzlaff, J.M., Altman, D.G., et al., 2013. SPIRIT 2013 statement: defining standard protocol items for clinical trials. Ann. Intern. Med. 158, 200–207.

41. Chan, A.W., Tetzlaff, J.M., Gøtzsche, P.C., et al., 2013. SPIRIT 2013 explanation and elaboration: guidance for protocols of clinical trials. BMJ 346, e7586.

42. Schulz, K.F., Altman, D.G., Moher, D., 2010. CONSORT 2010 statement: updated guidelines for reporting parallel group randomized trials. Ann. Intern. Med. 152, 726–732.

43. Schulz, K.F., Altman, D.G., Moher, D., 2010. CONSORT 2010 statement: updated guidelines for reporting parallel group randomised trials. BMJ 340, c332.

44. Moher, D., Hopewell, S., Schulz, K.F., et al., 2010. CONSORT 2010 Explanation and Elaboration: updated guidelines for reporting parallel group randomised trials. J. Clin. Epidemiol. 63, e1–37.

45. Mosteller, F., Gilbert, J.P., McPeek, B., 1980. Reporting standards and research strategies for controlled trials: agenda for the editor. Controlled Clin. Trials 1, 37–58.

CHAPTER 14

Allocation Concealment in Randomised Trials: Defending Against Deciphering

Proper randomisation rests on adequate allocation concealment. An allocation concealment process keeps clinicians and participants unaware of upcoming assignments. Without it, even properly developed random allocation sequences can be subverted. Within this concealment process, the crucial unbiased nature of randomised controlled trials collides with their most vexing implementation problems. Proper allocation concealment frequently frustrates clinical inclinations, which annoys those who do the trials. Randomised controlled trials are anathema to clinicians. Many involved with trials will be tempted to decipher assignments, which subverts randomisation. For some implementing a trial, deciphering the allocation scheme might frequently become too great an intellectual challenge to resist. Whether their motives indicate innocent or pernicious intents, such tampering undermines the validity of a trial. Indeed, inadequate allocation concealment leads to exaggerated estimates of treatment effect, on average, but with scope for bias in either direction. Trial investigators will be crafty in any potential efforts to decipher the allocation sequence, so trial designers must be just as clever in their design efforts to prevent deciphering. Investigators must effectively immunise trials against selection and confounding biases with proper allocation concealment. Furthermore, investigators should report baseline comparisons on important prognostic variables. Hypothesis tests of baseline characteristics, however, are superfluous and could be harmful if they lead investigators to suppress reporting any baseline imbalances.

The reason that the Medical Research Council's controlled trial of streptomycin for pulmonary tuberculosis should be regarded as a landmark is thus not, as is often suggested, because random number tables were used to generate the allocation schedule… Rather it is because of the clearly described precautions that were taken to conceal the allocation schedule from those involved in entering patients.[1]

Generation of an unpredictable randomised allocation sequence represents the first crucial element of randomisation in a randomised controlled trial.[2-5] Implementation of the sequence, while concealing it at least until patients have been assigned to their groups (allocation concealment), is the important second element,[2-4,6,7] without which randomisation collapses in a trial.

As a direct consequence of randomisation, the first table in most reports of randomised controlled trials describes the baseline characteristics of the comparison groups.[8-11] Researchers should describe their trial population and provide baseline comparisons of their groups so that readers can assess their comparability.[8-11] In this chapter we focus on proper approaches to allocation concealment and to reporting of baseline characteristics.

Allocation Concealment

Researchers have many misconceptions with respect to allocation concealment. Proper allocation concealment secures strict implementation of a random allocation sequence without foreknowledge of treatment assignments. Allocation concealment refers to the technique used to implement the sequence,[2,3] not to generate it. Nevertheless, some people discuss allocation concealment with digressions into flipping coins or use of random number tables. Those digressions amount to methodological *non sequiturs*; allocation concealment is distinct from sequence generation. Furthermore, some investigators confuse allocation concealment with blinding of treatments.[2,3,6,7,12]

Without adequate allocation concealment, even random, unpredictable assignment sequences can be undermined.[2,3,7,13,14] Knowledge of the next assignment could lead to the exclusion of certain patients based on their prognosis because they would have been allocated to the perceived inappropriate group. Moreover, knowledge of the next assignment could lead to direction of some participants to perceived proper groups, which can easily be accomplished by delaying a participant's entry into the trial until the next appropriate allocation appears. Avoidance of such bias depends on the prevention of foreknowledge of treatment assignment. Allocation concealment shields those who admit participants to a trial from knowing the upcoming assignments. The decision to accept or reject a participant should be made, and informed consent should be obtained, in ignorance of the upcoming assignment.[2,15]

IMPORTANCE OF ALLOCATION CONCEALMENT

Results of empirical investigations[7,16-22] have shown that trials that used inadequate or unclear allocation concealment, compared with those that used adequate concealment, yielded up to 40% larger estimates of treatment effect. The badly done trials tended to exaggerate treatment effects, although the opposite can happen.[7,21,22] Moreover, the worst concealed trials yielded greater heterogeneity in results (i.e., the results fluctuated extensively above and below the estimates from better studies).[7] These findings provide empirical evidence that inadequate allocation concealment allows bias to seep into trials.

Indeed, having a randomised (unpredictable) sequence should make little difference without adequate allocation concealment. Assume that investigators generate an adequate allocation sequence with a random number table. They then, however, post that sequence on a bulletin board, so that anyone involved in the trial could see the upcoming assignments. Similarly, the allocation sequence could be implemented through placing method indicator cards in translucent envelopes. This inadequate allocation concealment process could be deciphered by simply holding the envelopes to a bright light (Fig.14.1). With both the bulletin board and the envelopes, those responsible for admitting participants could detect the upcoming treatment assignments and then channel individuals with a better prognosis to the experimental group and those with a poorer prognosis to the control group or vice versa. Bias could easily be introduced, despite an adequate randomised sequence.[2,3,13]

Researchers should, therefore, ensure both adequate sequence generation and adequate allocation concealment in randomisation schemes.[2,3,6-11] A mistake in either could compromise

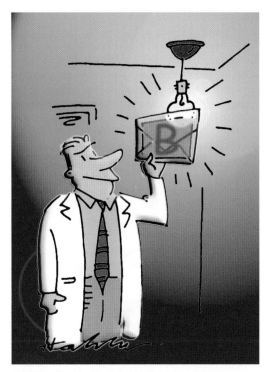

Fig. 14.1   Deciphering the allocation concealment scheme.

randomisation, resulting in incorrect results. For example, results of a trial could reveal a large treatment effect that only reflects a biased allocation procedure, or they could reveal no effect when in reality a harmful one prevails. Moreover, the results of such a trial can be more damaging than similar results from an explicitly observational research study.[23] Biases are usually assumed and acknowledged in observational studies, and the statistical analysis and eventual interpretation attempt to take those biases into account. Conversely, studies labelled as randomised are frequently assumed to be free of bias, and commonly inadequate reporting masks the deficiencies they might have.[8-11]

Consequently, the credibility of randomised controlled trials lends support to faster and greater changes in clinical or preventive management, which, if based on a compromised study, squanders scarce health resources, or even worse, harms people's health. Thus the well-deserved credibility of randomised controlled trials produces an indirect liability. Wrong judgements emanate easily from improperly randomised trials.

PERSONAL ACCOUNTS OF DECIPHERING

Findings of empirical investigations[7,16-22] suggest that investigators sometimes undermine randomisation, though they rarely document such subversions. Nevertheless, when investigators responded anonymously to queries during epidemiological workshops, many did relate instances in which allocation schemes had been sabotaged.[13]

The individual accounts of such instances describe a range of simple to intricate operations.[13] Most allocation concealment schemes were deciphered by investigators simply because the methods were inadequate. Investigators admitted, for instance, altering enrolment or allocations to particular study groups after decoding future assignments, which were either posted on a bulletin board or visible through translucent envelopes held up to bright lights. Some also related opening unsealed assignment envelopes, sensing the differential weight of envelopes, or simply opening unnumbered envelopes until they found a desired treatment.

Investigators had a harder time deciphering the better allocation concealment schemes.[13] Nevertheless, eventually someone described circumventing virtually every type of scheme. For example, some physicians took sequentially numbered, opaque, sealed envelopes to the hot light (an intense incandescent bulb) in the radiology department for deciphering of assignments. In studies using central randomisation, trial investigators related ringing the central number and asking for the next several assignments all at once; they received them in at least a couple of circumstances. In trials with sequentially numbered drug containers, someone described deciphering assignments based on the appearance of the container labels. Another had stopped trying to decipher a drug container scheme until she saw an attending physician, late at night, ransacking the office files of the principal investigator for the allocation list. Suggesting her methodological naivety and innocence, she first thought of the attending physician's cleverness and not of the probability that such action would bias the trial.

Although investigators theoretically understand the need for unbiased research, they sometimes fail to maintain impartiality once they are involved in a trial. Researchers might want certain patients to benefit from one of the treatments or the trial results to confirm their beliefs. Thus certain trial procedures in properly done randomised controlled trials frustrate clinical inclinations, which annoys those doing the trial.[13,24,25]

Some scientists aim to deliberately sabotage their results. However, many attempts at decoding the randomisation sequence simply indicate an absence of knowledge of the scientific ramifications of such actions. Furthermore, for some, the deciphering of the allocation scheme might frequently become too great an intellectual challenge to resist. As Oscar Wilde wrote, 'The only way to get rid of temptation is to yield to it.' Whether their motives are innocent or not, however, such tampering undermines the validity of a trial. Investigators must recognise the inquisitiveness of human nature and institute methodological safeguards. Proper allocation concealment will deter subversion, in effect, immunising trials against selection and confounding biases.[3,13,24,25]

To develop a proper allocation scheme takes time, effort, and thought. Investigators cannot simply delegate this task without thoroughly examining the final product. Trial investigators will be crafty in any potential efforts to decipher the allocation sequence, so trial designers must be just as clever in their design efforts to prevent deciphering.

WHAT TO LOOK FOR WITH ALLOCATION CONCEALMENT

Researchers consider certain approaches to allocation concealment as adequate: sequentially numbered, opaque, sealed envelopes (SNOSE); pharmacy controlled; numbered or coded containers; central randomisation (e.g., by telephone to a trials office); or other method whose description contained elements convincing of concealment, such as a secure computer-assisted method.[6,7,26] These criteria establish minimum methodological standards, yet they are met by only about a quarter of trials.[6,26] Consequently, in assessment of allocation concealment from published reports, readers will be fortunate to find such standards reasonably met (Panel 14.1).[27-36] Realistically, however, those minimum standards should be exceeded. If researchers provide descriptions that incorporate not only the minimum standards, but also elements of more rigorous standards, readers can have more confidence that selection and confounding biases have been averted (see Panel 14.2).

Methods that use envelopes are more susceptible to manipulation through human ingenuity than other approaches and are therefore considered a less-than-ideal method of concealment.[37] If investigators use envelopes, they should diligently develop and monitor the allocation process to preserve concealment. In addition to use of sequentially numbered, opaque, sealed envelopes,

---

PANEL 14.1 ■ Descriptions of Allocation Concealment

Identical ampullas were prepared containing either 1 ml dexamethasone (Krka, Vital Pharma Nordic, Novo Mesto, Slovenia) 4 mg/ml or 1 ml placebo (0·9 per cent saline); the solutions were transparent and identical. According to a computer-generated block randomization list, 120 identical sequentially numbered containers were prepared containing either 2 × 1 ml 4 mg/ml dexamethasone or 2 × 1 ml placebo. The randomization code was kept separately at the Hospital Pharmacy of the Capital Region of Denmark.[27]

Allocation concealment was ensured by keeping the randomization lists in the care of one of the investigators (TS) who was not involved in the clinical part of the study. Independent pharmacists dispensed the study medications into identical, sequentially numbered containers according to randomization lists.[28]

Central randomisation (by telephone) was stratified by centre.[29]

Patients were randomised centrally by the Centre for Digestive Diseases after screening in a 1:1 ratio to either faecal microbiota transplantation or placebo, using a preestablished computer-generated randomisation list...[30]

Patients were centrally allocated (1:1) to azithromycin or identical-looking placebo using concealed random allocation from a computer-generated random numbers table with permuted blocks of 4 or 6 and stratification for centre and past smoking. Stenlake Compounding Pharmacy (Bondi Junction, Sydney, NSW, Australia) formulated the study drug and matching placebo tablets. Study packs were labelled with the allocated randomisation number and bottle numbers.[31]

Immediately after randomization and for 14 days, the research pharmacists prepared reconstituted opaque bags of micafungin or placebo according to the randomization list and provided it to the site for infusion.[32]

Pharmacy-controlled randomization was used to conceal the random allocation of treatment using random number tables. This was performed by different team participants (BA, BS), who were neither directly involved in patient registration nor in assessing the outcomes. The formulation codes were broken only after complete results were obtained from all the participating patients on completion of treatment period.[33]

Allocation to treatment groups was... concealed using central randomisation generated by the clinical trials unit. The responsible senior statistician was not involved in study conduct or monitoring. Patients, investigators, and study personnel were masked to treatment assignments during the study; we used subsequently opened sealed, opaque, sequentially numbered envelopes containing the allocation information.[34]

Randomisation was done using sequentially numbered, opaque sealed envelopes, to be opened in consecutive order.[35]

The allocation sequence was concealed from the researcher (JR) enrolling and assessing participants in sequentially numbered, opaque, sealed and stapled envelopes. Aluminium foil inside the envelope was used to render the envelope impermeable to intense light. To prevent subversion of the allocation sequence, the name and date of birth of the participant was written on the envelope and a video tape made of the sealed envelope with participant details visible. Carbon paper inside the envelope transferred the information onto the allocation card inside the envelope and a second researcher (CC) later viewed video tapes to ensure envelopes were still sealed when participants' names were written on them. Corresponding envelopes were opened only after the enrolled participants completed all baseline assessments and it was time to allocate the intervention.[36]

---

they should ensure that the envelopes are numbered in advance, opened sequentially, and only after the participant's name and other details are written on the appropriate envelope.[38] We also recommend use of pressure-sensitive or carbon paper inside the envelope, which transfers such information to the assigned allocation and thus creates a valuable audit trail. Cardboard or aluminium foil placed inside the envelope further inhibits detection of assignments via hot lights.

Pharmacies can also engender both allocation concealment and sequence generation difficulties. Although reports in which the assignment was made by the pharmacy have generally been classified as having used an acceptable allocation concealment mechanism,[6,7,26] compliance of pharmacists with proper randomisation methods in these trials is unknown. The precautions they took should have been reported. We are aware of instances in which pharmacists have violated assignment schedules.[13] For instance, a pharmacy within a prominent American medical school handled randomisation assignment for a drug trial. During the course of the trial, over a weekend, the pharmacy

PANEL 14.2 ■ Minimum and Expanded Criteria for Adequate Allocation Concealment Schemes

Minimum Description of Adequate Allocation Concealment Scheme	*Additional Descriptive Elements That Provide Greater Assurance of Allocation Concealment*
Sequentially numbered, opaque, sealed envelopes (SNOSE)	Envelopes are opened sequentially only after participant details are written on the envelope
	Pressure-sensitive or carbon paper inside the envelope transfers that information to the assignment card (creates an audit trail)
	Cardboard or aluminium foil inside the envelope renders the envelope impermeable to intense light
Sequentially numbered containers	All of the containers were sealed, tamper-proof, equal in weight, and similar in appearance
Pharmacy controlled	Indications that the researchers developed, or at least validated, a proper randomisation scheme for the pharmacy
	Indications that the researchers instructed the pharmacy in proper allocation concealment
Central randomisation	The mechanism for contact (e.g., telephone, fax, or e-mail), the stringent procedures to ensure enrolment before randomisation, and the thorough training for those individuals staffing the central randomisation office
Automated assignment system	Convincing description that the system is secure, computer-assisted, and/or web-based, and must enable allocation concealment by strict preservation of the assignments until enrolment is assured and confirmed

ran out of one of the two drugs being compared and therefore allocated the other drug to all newly enrolled participants to avoid slowing recruitment. We are aware of another pharmacy that randomised patients by alternate assignment. Investigators should not assume that pharmacists and others involved in their trials know about the methods of randomised controlled trials. Investigators must ensure that their research partners adhere to proper trial procedures. Beyond the minimum criteria, readers would gain additional confidence if investigators indicate that they instructed or checked the allocation mechanism of the pharmacy.

The use of sequentially numbered containers prevents foreknowledge of treatment assignment, but only if investigators take proper precautions. Beyond the minimum criteria, authors of trial reports should specify further details of the methods. Assurances that all of the containers were tamper-proof, equal in weight, and similar in appearance, and that some audit trail had been established (such as writing the names of participants on the empty bottles or containers) would help readers to assess whether randomisation was likely to have been concealed successfully. Similarly, although central randomisation continues to be an excellent allocation concealment approach, effective trial procedures need to be established and followed. Researchers should at least specify the mechanism for contact (e.g., telephone, fax, or e-mail), the stringent procedures to ensure enrolment before randomisation, and the thorough training of individuals at the central randomisation office. All these details should be addressed when doing a trial and when writing a trial report.[8-11,13]

Other methods might suffice for adequate allocation concealment. Readers should look for descriptions that contain elements convincing of concealment. For example, a secure computer-assisted method, perhaps web-based, might enable allocation concealment by preservation of assignments until enrolment is assured and confirmed. Indeed, automated assignment systems are likely to become more common.[39,40] However, a simple computer system that merely stores assignments or naively shields assignments could turn out to be as transparent as tacking a randomisation list to a bulletin board. In describing an allocation concealment mechanism, investigators should display knowledge of the rationale behind allocation concealment and how their method met the standards.

Researchers frequently fail to report even the barest of descriptions of allocation concealment, preventing readers from assessing randomised controlled trials. Reviews published before 2000 yielded dire levels of reporting. As examples, the mechanism used to allocate interventions was omitted in reports of 93% of trials in dermatology,[41] 89% of trials in rheumatoid arthritis,[42] 48% of trials in obstetrics and gynaecology journals,[6] and 45% of trials in general medical journals.[26] Unfortunately, those examples represent the norm. In 177 reviews assessing the quality of reporting of RCTs published just between 1987 to 2007, the reporting was consistently found deficient.[43] Two studies provide the best general estimates,[44,45] because they examined a random sample of all trial reports indexed in PubMed. In those two studies, allocation concealment was not described in about three-quarters of trial reports.

Fortunately, the situation is improving as more medical journals are adopting a reporting guideline for randomised controlled trials.[8-11,46] Moreover, the guideline improves reporting. A systematic review found 50 studies that evaluated the effect of CONSORT on the quality of reporting of RCTs.[47] The results demonstrate that CONSORT leads to improved reporting, but the improvements appear moderate. Ample room for improvement remains beyond the current gains (see Chapter 22). Moreover, an important byproduct of reporting guidelines is that, with reporting guideline impetus, more investigators might design and do sound trials.

Baseline Comparisons

Although randomisation eliminates systematic bias, it does not necessarily produce perfectly balanced groups with respect to prognostic factors. Differences due to chance remain in the intervention groups (i.e., chance maldistribution). Statistical tests, however, account for these chance differences. The process of randomisation underlies significance testing and is independent of prognostic factors, known and unknown.[48]

Nevertheless, researchers should present distributions of baseline characteristics by treatment group in a table (Panel 14.3). Such information describes the hypothetical population from which their trial arose and allows readers to see the possibilities of generalisation to other populations.[49] Furthermore, it allows physicians to infer the results to particular patients.[10,11]

A table of baseline characteristics also allows readers to compare the trial groups at baseline on important demographic and clinical characteristics. The common, inappropriate use of hypothesis tests (e.g., p values in the tables) to compare characteristics concerns us, however.[6,26,50,51] Such tests assess the probability that differences observed could have happened by chance. In properly randomised trials, however, any observed differences have, by definition, occurred by chance. 'Such a procedure is clearly absurd', as Altman states.[51]

PANEL 14.3 ■ Example of a Reasonably Reported Table of Baseline Characteristics

Characteristic	Antibiotic Group (n = 116)	Placebo Group (n = 129)
Age (mean ± SD) (years)	30.2 ± 5.2	31.1 ± 5.9
Weight (median [25th, 75th percentiles]) (kg)	64 (55, 82)	65 (56, 85)
Nulliparous (number, %)	62 (53%)	63 (49%)
Previous pelvic inflammatory disease (number, %)	24 (21%)	28 (22%)

Hypothesis tests on baseline characteristics might not only be unnecessary but also harmful. Researchers who use hypothesis tests to compare baseline characteristics report fewer significant results than expected by chance.[6,26] One plausible explanation for this discrepancy is that some investigators might have decided not to report significant differences, believing that by withholding that information they would increase the credibility of their reports. Not only are hypothesis tests superfluous, but they can be harmful if they indirectly lead investigators to suppress reporting baseline imbalances.

WHAT TO LOOK FOR WITH BASELINE CHARACTERISTICS

Investigators should report baseline comparisons on important prognostic variables. Readers should look for comparisons based on consideration of the prognostic strength of the variables measured and the magnitude of any chance imbalances that have occurred, rather than statistical significance tests at baseline.[51] A table provides an efficient format of presenting baseline characteristics (see Panel 14.3).[8-11] Researchers should present continuous variables, such as age and weight, with an average and a measure of variability, usually a mean and standard deviation. If the data distribute asymmetrically, however, a median and a percentile range (i.e., interquartile range) would provide better descriptions. Variability should not be described by standard errors and confidence intervals, because they are inferential rather than descriptive statistics. Numbers and proportions should be reported for categorical variables.

In the analysis, the statistical tests on the outcomes account for any chance imbalances. Nevertheless, controlling for chance imbalances, if properly planned and done, might produce a more precise result.[52] Researchers should present any adjusted analyses and describe how and why they decided to adjust for certain covariates.

Conclusion

Proper randomisation remains the only way to avoid selection and confounding biases. The crucial unbiased nature of randomised controlled trials paradoxically coincides with their most vexing implementation problems. Randomised controlled trials antagonise human beings by frustrating their clinical inclinations. Thus many involved with trials will be tempted to undermine randomisation if afforded the opportunity to decipher assignments. To minimise the effect of this human tendency, trialists must devote meticulous attention to concealment of allocation schemes. Proper randomisation hinges on adequate allocation concealment.

References

1. Chalmers, I., 2001. Comparing like with like: some historical milestones in the evolution of methods to create unbiased comparison groups in therapeutic experiments. Int. J. Epidemiol. 30, 1156–1164.
2. Viera, A.J., Bangdiwala, S.I., 2007. Eliminating bias in randomized controlled trials: importance of allocation concealment and masking. Fam. Med. 39, 132–137.
3. Pandis, N., 2012. Randomization. Part 3: allocation concealment and randomization implementation. Am. J. Orthod. Dentofac. Orthop. 141, 126–128.
4. Pandis, N., Polychronopoulou, A., Eliades, T., 2011. Randomization in clinical trials in orthodontics: its significance in research design and methods to achieve it. Eur. J. Orthod. 33, 684–690.
5. Schulz, K.F., Grimes, D.A., 2002. Generation of allocation sequences in randomised trials: chance, not choice. Lancet 359, 515–519.
6. Schulz, K.F., Chalmers, I., Grimes, D.A., Altman, D.G., 1994. Assessing the quality of randomization from reports of controlled trials published in obstetrics and gynecology journals. JAMA 272, 125–128.
7. Schulz, K.F., Chalmers, I., Hayes, R.J., Altman, D.G., 1995. Empirical evidence of bias. Dimensions of methodological quality associated with estimates of treatment effects in controlled trials. JAMA 273, 408–412.

8. Schulz, K.F., Altman, D.G., Moher, D., 2010. CONSORT 2010 statement: updated guidelines for reporting parallel group randomised trials. BMJ 340, c332.
9. Schulz, K.F., Altman, D.G., Moher, D., 2010. CONSORT 2010 statement: updated guidelines for reporting parallel group randomized trials. Ann. Intern. Med. 152, 726–732.
10. Moher, D., Hopewell, S., Schulz, K.F., et al., 2010. CONSORT 2010 explanation and elaboration: updated guidelines for reporting parallel group randomised trials. J. Clin. Epidemiol. 63, e1–37.
11. Moher, D., Hopewell, S., Schulz, K.F., et al., 2010. CONSORT 2010 explanation and elaboration: updated guidelines for reporting parallel group randomised trials. BMJ 340, c869.
12. Schulz, K.F., Chalmers, I., Altman, D.G., 2002. The landscape and lexicon of blinding in randomized trials. Ann. Intern. Med. 136, 254–259.
13. Schulz, K.F., 1995. Subverting randomization in controlled trials. JAMA 274, 1456–1458.
14. Pocock, S., 1983. Clinical Trials: A Practical Approach. Wiley, Chichester, UK.
15. Chalmers, T.C., Levin, H., Sacks, H.S., Reitman, D., Berrier, J., Nagalingam, R., 1987. Meta-analysis of clinical trials as a scientific discipline. I: Control of bias and comparison with large co-operative trials. Stat. Med. 6, 315–328.
16. Armijo-Olivo, S., Saltaji, H., da Costa, B.R., Fuentes, J., Ha, C., Cummings, G.G., 2015. What is the influence of randomisation sequence generation and allocation concealment on treatment effects of physical therapy trials? A meta-epidemiological study. BMJ Open 5, e008562.
17. Savovic, J., Jones, H.E., Altman, D.G., et al., 2012. Influence of reported study design characteristics on intervention effect estimates from randomized, controlled trials. Ann. Intern. Med. 157, 429–438.
18. Moher, D., Pham, B., Jones, A., et al., 1998. Does quality of reports of randomised trials affect estimates of intervention efficacy reported in meta-analyses? Lancet 352, 609–613.
19. Kjaergard, L.L., Villumsen, J., Gluud, C., 2001. Reported methodologic quality and discrepancies between large and small randomized trials in meta-analyses. Ann. Intern. Med. 135, 982–989.
20. Jüni, P., Altman, D.G., Egger, M., 2001. Systematic reviews in health care: assessing the quality of controlled clinical trials. BMJ 323, 42–46.
21. Odgaard-Jensen, J., Vist, G.E., Timmer, A., et al., 2011. Randomisation to protect against selection bias in healthcare trials. Cochrane Database Syst. Rev. MR000012.
22. Kunz, R., Vist, G., Oxman, A.D., 2007. Randomisation to protect against selection bias in healthcare trials. Cochrane Database Syst. Rev. MR000012.
23. Torgerson, D.J., Roberts, C., 1999. Understanding controlled trials. Randomisation methods: concealment. BMJ 319, 375–376.
24. Schulz, K.F., 1995. Unbiased research and the human spirit: the challenges of randomized controlled trials. CMAJ 153, 783–786.
25. Schulz, K.F., 1996. Randomised trials, human nature, and reporting guidelines. Lancet 348, 596–598.
26. Altman, D.G., Doré, C.J., 1990. Randomisation and baseline comparisons in clinical trials. Lancet 335, 149–153.
27. Kleif, J., Kirkegaard, A., Vilandt, J., Gogenur, I., 2017. Randomized clinical trial of preoperative dexamethasone on postoperative nausea and vomiting after laparoscopy for suspected appendicitis. Br. J. Surg. 104, 384–392.
28. Siponen, M., Huuskonen, L., Kallio-Pulkkinen, S., Nieminen, P., Salo, T., 2017. Topical tacrolimus, triamcinolone acetonide, and placebo in oral lichen planus: a pilot randomized controlled trial. Oral Dis. 23, 660–668.
29. Sabate, M., Brugaletta, S., Cequier, A., et al., 2016. Clinical outcomes in patients with ST-segment elevation myocardial infarction treated with everolimus-eluting stents versus bare-metal stents (EXAMINATION): 5-year results of a randomised trial. Lancet 387, 357–366.
30. Paramsothy, S., Kamm, M.A., Kaakoush, N.O., et al., 2017. Multidonor intensive faecal microbiota transplantation for active ulcerative colitis: a randomised placebo-controlled trial. Lancet 389, 1218–1228.
31. Gibson, P.G., Yang, I.A., Upham, J.W., et al., 2017. Effect of azithromycin on asthma exacerbations and quality of life in adults with persistent uncontrolled asthma (AMAZES): a randomised, double-blind, placebo-controlled trial. Lancet 390, 659–668.
32. Timsit, J.F., Azoulay, E., Schwebel, C., et al., 2016. Empirical micafungin treatment and survival without invasive fungal infection in adults with ICU-acquired sepsis, Candida colonization, and multiple organ failure: the EMPIRICUS randomized clinical trial. JAMA 316, 1555–1564.
33. Kumar, R., Dogra, S., Amarji, B., et al., 2016. Efficacy of novel topical liposomal formulation of cyclosporine in mild to moderate stable plaque psoriasis: a randomized clinical trial. JAMA Dermatol. 152, 807–815.

34. Villiger, P.M., Adler, S., Kuchen, S., et al., 2016. Tocilizumab for induction and maintenance of remission in giant cell arteritis: a phase 2, randomised, double-blind, placebo-controlled trial. Lancet 387, 1921–1927.

35. Wachter, R., Groschel, K., Gelbrich, G., et al., 2017. Holter-electrocardiogram-monitoring in patients with acute ischaemic stroke (Find-AFRANDOMISED): an open-label randomised controlled trial. Lancet Neurol. 16, 282–290.

36. Radford, J.A., Landorf, K.B., Buchbinder, R., Cook, C., 2006. Effectiveness of low-Dye taping for the short-term treatment of plantar heel pain: a randomised trial. BMC Musculoskelet. Disord. 7, 64.

37. Meinert, C., 1986. Clinical Trials: Design, Conduct, and Analysis. Oxford University Press, New York.

38. Bulpitt, C., 1983. Randomised Controlled Clinical Trials. Martinus Nijhoff, The Hague, The Netherlands.

39. Dorman, K., Saade, G.R., Smith, H., Moise, K.J., Jr., 2000. Use of the World Wide Web in research: randomization in a multicenter clinical trial of treatment for twin-twin transfusion syndrome. Obstet. Gynecol. 96, 636–639.

40. Haag, U., 1998. Technologies for automating randomized treatment assignment in clinical trials. Drug Inf. J. 118, 7–11.

41. Adetugbo, K., Williams, H., 2000. How well are randomized controlled trials reported in the dermatology literature? Arch. Dermatol. 136, 381–385.

42. Gøtzsche, P.C., 1989. Methodology and overt and hidden bias in reports of 196 double-blind trials of nonsteroidal antiinflammatory drugs in rheumatoid arthritis. Control. Clin. Trials 10, 31–56.

43. Dechartres, A., Charles, P., Hopewell, S., Ravaud, P., Altman, D.G., 2011. Reviews assessing the quality or the reporting of randomized controlled trials are increasing over time but raised questions about how quality is assessed. J. Clin. Epidemiol. 64, 136–144.

44. Chan, A.W., Altman, D.G., 2005. Epidemiology and reporting of randomised trials published in PubMed journals. Lancet 365, 1159–1162.

45. Hopewell, S., Dutton, S., Yu, L.M., Chan, A.W., Altman, D.G., 2010. The quality of reports of randomised trials in 2000 and 2006: comparative study of articles indexed in PubMed. BMJ 340, c723.

46. Moher, D., Jones, A., Lepage, L., 2001. Use of the CONSORT statement and quality of reports of randomized trials: a comparative before-and-after evaluation. JAMA 285, 1992–1995.

47. Turner, L., Shamseer, L., Altman, D.G., et al., 2012. Consolidated standards of reporting trials (CONSORT) and the completeness of reporting of randomised controlled trials (RCTs) published in medical journals. Cochrane Database Syst. Rev. 11. MR000030.

48. Fisher, R., 1966. The Design of Experiments. Oliver & Boyd Ltd, Edinburgh, Scotland.

49. Lachin, J.M., 1988. Statistical properties of randomization in clinical trials. Control. Clin. Trials 9, 289–311.

50. Senn, S., 1997. Statistical Issues in Drug Development. John Wiley & Sons Ltd, Chichester.

51. Altman, D., 1985. Comparability of randomised groups. Statistician 34, 125–136.

52. Lavori, P.W., Louis, T.A., Bailar, J.C. 3rd, Polansky, M., 1983. Designs for experiments—parallel comparisons of treatment. N. Engl. J. Med. 309, 1291–1299.

CHAPTER 15

Exclusions and Losses in Randomised Trials: Retention of Trial Participants

Proper randomisation means little if investigators cannot include all randomised participants in the primary analysis. Participants might ignore follow-up, leave town, or take acetaminophen when instructed to take aspirin. Exclusions before randomisation do not bias the treatment comparison, but they can hurt generalisability. Eligibility criteria for a trial should be clear, specific, and applied before randomisation. Readers should assess whether any of the criteria make the trial sample atypical or unrepresentative of the people in which they are interested. In principle, assessment of exclusions after randomisation is simple: none are allowed. For the primary analysis, all participants enrolled should be included and analysed as part of the original group assigned (an intent-to-treat analysis). In reality, however, losses frequently occur. Investigators should, therefore, commit adequate resources to develop and implement procedures to maximise retention of participants. Moreover, researchers should provide clear, explicit information on the progress of all randomised participants through the trial by use of, for instance, a trial profile. Investigators can also do secondary analyses on, for instance, per-protocol or as-treated participants. Such analyses should be described as secondary and nonrandomised comparisons. Mishandling of exclusions causes serious methodological difficulties. Unfortunately, some explanations for mishandling exclusions intuitively appeal to readers, disguising the seriousness of the issues. Creative mismanagement of exclusions can undermine trial validity.

Proper randomisation[1,2] means little if investigators cannot include all randomly assigned participants in their primary analysis. Hence a crucial aspect of assessing a randomised controlled trial pertains to exclusions, withdrawals, losses, and protocol deviations. How should investigators handle participants who refuse entry, ignore follow-up, leave town, or take acetaminophen when they were instructed to take aspirin? Unfortunately, many inappropriate approaches to dealing with these types of problem actually seem logical and falsely appealing. Therein lies their insidious nature, because such inappropriate approaches can result in serious biases. Here we address the effect of exclusions made before and after randomisation.

Exclusions Before Randomisation

Investigators can exclude participants before randomisation. The eventual randomised treatment comparison will remain unbiased (good internal validity), irrespective of whether researchers have well-founded or whimsical reasons for exclusion of particular individuals. However, exclusions at this stage can hurt extrapolation, the generalisability of the results (external validity). For most investigations, we therefore recommend that eligibility criteria be kept to a minimum, in the spirit of the large and simple trial.[3,4] However, some valid reasons exist for exclusion of certain participants. Individuals could, for example, have a condition for which an intervention is contraindicated, or they could be judged likely to be lost to follow-up. The trial question should guide the approach.[5] Sometimes, however, investigators impose so many eligibility criteria that their trial infers to a population of little apparent interest to anyone, and, in addition, recruitment becomes difficult. If investigators exclude too many participants, or the wrong participants, their results might not represent the people of interest, even though the randomised controlled trial might have been meticulously done (i.e., the results could be true but potentially irrelevant).

WHAT TO LOOK FOR IN EXCLUSIONS BEFORE RANDOMISATION

The eligibility criteria should indicate the population to which the investigators wish to infer. When judging the results of a trial, readers should make sure that the eligibility criteria are clear and specific. Most importantly the criteria should have been applied before randomisation. Readers should also assess whether any of the criteria make the study sample atypical, unrepresentative, or irrelevant to the people of interest. In practice, however, results from a trial will infrequently be totally irrelevant: 'most differences between our patients and those in trials tend to be quantitative (they have different ages or social classes or different degrees of risk of the outcome event or of responsiveness to therapy) rather than qualitative (total absence of responsiveness or no risk of the event)'.[6] Such qualitative differences in response are rare; thus, trials tend to have rather robust external validity.[6]

Exclusions After Randomisation

Exclusions made after randomisation threaten to bias treatment comparisons. Randomisation itself configures unbiased comparison groups at baseline. Any erosion, however, over the course of the trial from those initially unbiased groups produces bias, unless, of course, that erosion is random, which is unlikely. Consequently, for the primary analysis, methodologists suggest that results for all patients who are randomly assigned should be analysed and, furthermore, should be analysed as part of the group to which they were initially assigned.[3,4,7,8] Trialists refer to such an approach as an intent-to-treat (ITT) analysis. Simply put: once randomised, always analysed as assigned.

ITT principles underlie the primary analysis in a randomised controlled trial to avoid biases associated with nonrandom loss of participants.[7,9-13] Investigators can also do secondary analyses, preferably preplanned, based on only those participants, for example, who comply with the trial treatment protocol or who receive the treatment irrespective of randomised assignment (generally referred to as per protocol [PP], on-treatment, or as-treated analysis). Secondary analyses are acceptable as long as researchers label them as secondary and nonrandomised comparisons. Trouble brews, however, when investigators exclude participants and, in effect, present a secondary, nonrandomised comparison as the primary randomised comparison from a trial. In reality, this analysis represents a cohort study masquerading as a randomised controlled trial. Exclusion of participants from an analysis can lead to misleading conclusions (Panel 15.1).[14-17]

Researchers often do not provide adequate information on excluded participants.[7,8,18,19] Furthermore, in an older review of 249 randomised controlled trials published in major general medical journals in 1997, only 2% (5 of 249) of the reports explicitly stated that all randomly

---

PANEL 15.1 ■ A Randomised Controlled Trial of Sulfinpyrazone Versus Placebo for Prevention of Repeat Myocardial Infarction

For this trial, the researchers reported a primary analysis that compared rates of death from cardiac causes rather than from all cardiac deaths.[14,15] In their analysis, inappropriate exclusions due to eventual discovery of patient ineligibility caused a problem[16]: the investigators withdrew as ineligible seven patients who had received treatment (six in the treatment group and one in the placebo group) resulting in more patients who died being withdrawn from the treatment group than from the placebo group.

Moreover, results of a detailed audit of this trial by the US Food and Drug Administration (FDA) indicate that additional patients from the placebo group could have been declared ineligible on the basis of similar criteria, but were not.[16] Furthermore, the trial protocol did not mention exclusion of ineligible patients after entry, particularly patients who had died. The researchers also excluded two deaths in the sulfinpyrazone group and one death in the placebo group as nonanalysable because of poor compliance. However, the trial protocol did not include plans to exclude patients because of poor compliance.

Additionally, the investigators used a 7-day rule. They declared as nonanalysable any death of a patient who had not received treatment for at least 7 days or who died more than 7 days after termination of treatment. The FDA review committee did not criticise this practice strongly, principally because the protocol described the 7-day rule, and also because the rule had little overall effect on the results.

Overall, these inappropriate exclusions did, however, affect the results of the study.[16] Although the researchers initially reported a 32% reduction ($p = 0.058$) in rates of death from cardiac causes for participants who took the drug, a reanalysis showed a weaker result. When individuals judged ineligible or nonanalysable were included in the originally assigned groups, the reduction was only 21% ($p = 0.16$). It is noteworthy that only p values were provided.

We urge the use of confidence intervals in reporting results.[17] Moreover, the fallout from inappropriate exclusions, as ascertained by the FDA, cast doubt over the trial. The FDA advisory committee announced that sulfinpyrazone could not be labelled and advertised as a drug to prevent death in the critical months after a heart attack because, on close examination, the data were not as convincing as they seemed at first glance.

---

assigned participants were analysed according to the randomised group assignment.[20] About half of the reports (119 of 249) noted an ITT analysis, but many provided no details to support this claim.

More recent data on ITT analyses are not encouraging. In the 50 trials of experimental pain models, none (0%) reported using an ITT analysis.[13] Of the 123 trials of clinical pain, 47% reported using an ITT analysis and 5% reported using a modified ITT (mITT).[13] In another review of 2349 trials, 25% were classified as an ITT analysis, 14% as an mITT analysis, and 61% as not reporting an ITT analysis.[7] Moreover, the mITT classification is a misnomer in that it is decidedly not even close to an ITT analysis. 'Whatever the definition used in the ITT approach, it is clear that the analysis performed in the mITT trials is a "PP [per-protocol] analysis". It is important to underline that the authors of mITT studies inappropriately used the term "ITT" because in reality, the analyses they performed were substantially "PP analyses", which can confuse the reader'.[7] PP analyses, sometimes called 'as-treated' or 'on-treatment' analyses, represent distinctly non-ITT analyses in that they are nonrandomised comparisons. Indeed, the mITT trials displayed larger treatment effects than ITT trials, which supports the view that mITT trials represent nonrandomised, biased comparisons.[9]

Additionally, researchers frequently do not report anything with respect to exclusions.[8] Left in this information void, many readers deduce that certain trials used ITT principles and had no exclusions. We call this scenario 'no apparent exclusions'. Readers commonly view trials with no apparent exclusions as less biased, when in fact unreported exclusions probably occurred in many of them. Indeed, trials with no apparent exclusions were methodologically weaker than those reporting at least some exclusions.[8,21] In other words, some of the more biased trials might be mistakenly interpreted as unbiased, and many of the less biased trials as biased; we call this inconsistency 'the exclusion paradox'. Until researchers comprehensively report exclusions after randomisation, readers should be aware of this unsettling irony.

WHAT TO LOOK FOR IN EXCLUSIONS AFTER RANDOMISATION

Before we launch into attributes of proper handling of exclusions after randomisation, we should acknowledge the tenuous ground on which any such discussion rests. Reporting on exclusions is poor, with the exclusion paradox misleading readers. Investigators should provide clear, explicit information on the progress through the trial of all randomised participants, and when such information is absent, readers should be sceptical. The flow diagrams specified in the CONSORT statement provide appropriate guidelines.[22-25]

Optimally, of course, investigators would have no exclusions after randomisation and use an ITT analysis. Assessment of exclusions after randomisation is simple: none are allowed. All participants enrolled should be analysed as part of the original group assigned. Clinical research is not normally that simple, but the principle holds. One pragmatic hint for minimising exclusions after randomisation involves randomly assigning individuals at the last possible moment. If randomisation takes place when the participant is first identified, but before treatment is initiated, then any exclusions arising before treatment still become exclusions after randomisation. Investigators can address this potential difficulty by delaying randomisation until immediately before treatment begins.[26]

If investigators report exclusions after randomisation, those exclusions should be carefully scrutinised because they could bias comparisons. Exclusions arise after randomisation for several reasons, including discovery of patient ineligibility; post-randomisation, pretreatment outcome; deviation from protocol; and losses to follow-up.

Discovery of Participant Ineligibility

In some trials, participants are enrolled and later discovered not to have met the eligibility criteria. Exclusions at this point could seriously bias the results, because discovery is probably not random. For example, participants least responsive to treatment or who have side effects might draw more attention and, therefore, might be more likely to be judged ineligible than other study participants. Alternatively, a physician who had treatment preferences for certain participants might withdraw individuals from the trial if they were randomly assigned to what he or she believes to be the wrong group.

Participants discovered to be ineligible should remain in the trial. An exception could be made if establishment of eligibility criteria is difficult. In such instances, investigators could obtain the same information from each patient at time of randomisation and have it centrally reviewed by an outside source, blinded to the assigned treatment. That source, whether a person or group, could then withdraw patients who did not satisfy the eligibility criteria, presumably in an unbiased way.

Post-Randomisation, Pretreatment Outcome

Researchers sometimes report exclusion of participants on the basis of outcomes that happen before treatment has begun or before the treatment could have had an effect. For example, in a clinical trial of a specific drug's effect on death rates, investigators withdrew as nonanalysable data on all patients who died after randomisation but before treatment began or before they had received at least 7 days of treatment. This winnowing seems intuitively attractive, because none of the deaths can then be attributable to treatment. But the same argument could be made for excluding data on all patients in a placebo group who died during the entire study interval, because, theoretically, none of these deaths could have been related to treatment. This example illustrates the potential for capriciousness in addressing post-randomisation, pretreatment outcomes.

Randomisation tends to balance the nonattributable deaths in the long run. Any tinkering after randomisation, even if done in the most scientific and impartial manner, cannot improve upon that attribute but can hurt it. More importantly, this meddling sometimes serves as a *post hoc* rationale for inappropriate exclusions.

Post hoc rationalisation arises when investigators observe the results and then frame rules that favour their hypotheses. Assume that an investigator postulates that a drug used for treatment reduced the death rate associated with a particular condition. After analysis of data, however, the investigator notes that 14 deaths in the treatment group and two deaths in the placebo group arose before treatment had begun or before the drug had been taken for at least 7 days. She then rationalises the deaths as unrelated to treatment and withdraws them from analysis. Such a response would seriously bias her results, even though her reasoning in the report would likely seem logical.

Imposed *a priori*, such rules only complicate trial implementation; imposed *a posteriori*, they lead to biased and invalid results. In assessment of randomised controlled trials, identification of when researchers stipulated rules usually proves impossible. We prefer to find, in reports of randomised controlled trials, that investigators did not allow any withdrawal of participants after randomisation. The data of all randomised patients should be analysed. Planned or unplanned, the exclusion of nonanalysable outcomes on grounds of efficiency is not a generally accepted practice in the analysis of a randomised clinical trial.[27]

Protocol Deviations

Deviations from assigned treatment happen in many trials. Some investigators suggest that participants who deviate substantially from the allotted treatment should be excluded in the final analysis or should be included only up to the point of deviation. Although this approach seems attractive, it has a serious flaw: 'the group which deviates from one protocol and the group which deviates from the other protocol may be so different … that the treatment comparison in the remaining patients will be severely biased'.[4]

For example, suppose investigators want to know if prophylactic amoxicillin, given by mouth, reduces complications from dental operations. They randomly allocate participants to receive antibiotics or placebo (Fig. 15.1). Unfortunately, 25% of the patients in the antibiotic group deviate from the protocol and do not take their antibiotics. In effect, these deviates receive the same treatment (i.e., nothing) as the placebo group. Should the investigators exclude them from analysis? Alternatively, should investigators merge them with the placebo group and compare them with the compliant patients in the antibiotic group who adhered to the protocol? Some investigators opt for one of these speciously attractive options.

For the primary analysis, however, neither option proves acceptable. The two treatment groups would no longer be comparable. The participants who did not take antibiotics might have been in better health or less concerned about possible complications. In either instance, they were probably less susceptible to morbidity. If investigators exclude the deviates, the antibiotic group will contain only the more susceptible; thus the treatment comparison would be biased. If investigators include the deviates in the placebo group, then not only will those left in the antibiotic group be more susceptible to febrile morbidity, but the placebo group will have been infiltrated with less susceptible patients; thus the treatment comparison would be even more biased. Those who deviated could be sicker rather than healthier; it does not matter. The point remains that the treatment comparison would be systematically biased.

All protocol deviations should be followed up, and their data should be analysed with the group to which they were originally assigned. In our example, the deviates from the antibiotic group should remain with the antibiotic group. Similarly, any deviates in the placebo group should remain

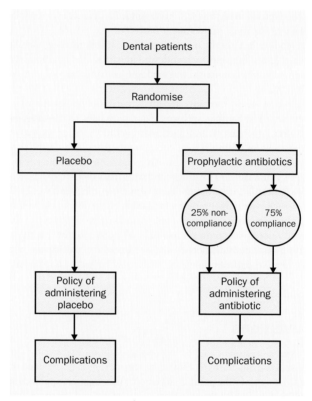

Fig. 15.1 Schematic of randomised dental patients, accounting for their compliance with treatment during the trial.

in that group. Despite what happened during the course of the trial, investigators should compare the group randomly allocated to antibiotics with the group allocated to placebo. This approach, in addition to being unbiased, will provide a pragmatic answer to the question of primary clinical interest (i.e., does the policy of giving prophylactic antibiotics for dental operations prevent complications?). Thus if researchers report excluding protocol deviates, or if they report moving protocol deviates from one group to another group, the resultant treatment comparison should be considered biased, analogous to an observational study.

Loss to Follow-Up and Retention

Losses to follow-up are perhaps the most vexing of the proffered reasons for exclusions after randomisation. Participants might move or might refuse to continue participating in the trial. Participants lost to follow-up could still be included in the analysis if outcome information could be obtained from another source, such as gathering data from a national death registry. Such opportunities, however, rarely arise. Without outcomes from those lost to follow-up, investigators have little choice but to exclude them from the analysis. Any losses damage internal validity, but differential rates of loss among comparison groups cause major damage. Hence investigators must minimise their losses to follow-up. We consider follow-up rates and retention rates as synonymous.

Minimisation of loss in some trials exudes difficulties. Investigators should commit adequate attention and resources to develop and implement procedures to minimise losses.[12] Although many procedures tend to be unique and site-specific, others pertain to many circumstances.[28-32] For example, investigators might exclude patients before randomisation if deemed likely to be lost to follow-up. Alternatively, they could obtain contact information to locate lost participants and hire special follow-up personnel who visit unresponsive participants. Providing monetary incentives might not only be ethically necessary for compensation, but also might increase retention.[33] Clearly, ample evidence indicates that clinical researchers should use many retention strategies involving several topical areas to boost the retention of participants.[32,34,35] Indeed, studies yielding high retention rates '... included specialized and persistent teams and utilized tailored strategies specific to their cohort and individual participants. Studies' written protocols and published manuscripts often did not reflect the varied strategies employed and adapted through the duration of study. Appropriate retention strategy use requires cultural sensitivity'.[36] A good roadmap developed for surgery applies to many other specialties.[30] Sometimes simple, singular approaches have little effect.[37]

Some investigators add innovative twists that cultivate high follow-up rates. One approach uses a large number of conveniently placed follow-up clinics.[30,38] Too often, investigators expect participants to visit a single, inconvenient location. Shortening the data-collection instrument to a manageable size caters to the participants' wishes and needs. Investigators foster follow-up by not overburdening participants. Such instruments might not only promote higher follow-up rates, but might also engender higher quality data on the main items of interest. In situations where participants lack mobile phones, provision of mobile phones and texting might be important.[39-41] Social media may also play an important role.[42] Community involvement and innovative tracking of participants adapted for the setting has been found to be important.[43] Complete elimination of loss could be impossible, but investigators too frequently profess insurmountable difficulties. Many investigators could work much harder and smarter to obtain higher follow-up rates (Panel 15.2).

What is an acceptable rate of loss to follow-up? Only one answer, 0%, ensures the benefits of randomisation. Obviously, this is unrealistic at times. Some researchers suggest a simple 5-and-20 rule of thumb, with fewer than 5% loss probably leading to little bias, greater than 20% loss

---

PANEL 15.2 ■ Some Approaches to Enhance Participant Follow-Up

- Hire a person to manage and encourage follow-up.
- Hire personnel to call participants or to visit participants at their homes or places of work, if participants are not returning for follow-up.
- Exclude before randomisation those likely to be unwilling to return.
- Exclude before randomisation those likely to move away.
- Obtain contact information to prompt participants to return for follow-up and to facilitate location of participants if they do not return (e.g., mail, telephone, and e-mail for enrolled participants, for close friends or relatives who do not live with the participant, and for the participant's family doctor).
- Obtain an identification number, such as a national healthcare number.
- Establish follow-up venues suited to participants rather than to investigators and trial implementers (e.g., more locations than just the central clinic or hospital, close to where participants live, convenient to access, and sensitive to waiting time).
- Streamline trial procedures to move participants quickly through a follow-up visit.
- Keep data collection instrument short so as to not overburden the participant.
- Provide excellent and free medical care.
- Provide monetary subsidies, primarily for time and travel costs incurred by participants.
- Provide mobile phones if participants lack access.
- Consider texting messages to participants.
- Consider using social media approaches.

potentially posing serious threats to validity, and in-between levels leading to intermediate levels of problems.[44] With sensitivity analyses and use of the worst-case scenario, a trial would be unlikely to successfully withstand challenges to its validity with losses of more than 20%.[6] Indeed, some journals refuse to publish trials with losses greater than 20%.[6]

Although the 5-and-20 rule is useful, it can oversimplify the problem in situations with infrequent outcomes. Expectations for loss to follow-up depend on various factors, such as the topic examined, the outcome event rate, and the length of follow-up. For example, if researchers examined outcomes during the first day after birth to women delivering in hospitals, we would expect no losses. If the researchers examined use of microbicides by women in Africa (who usually have no phones and sometimes lack street addresses) to prevent HIV-1 transmission over a 1-year follow-up period, however, we would expect perhaps 5% to 15% loss to follow-up, although hoping for lower. Actually, many investigators have done much worse under such circumstances with losses to follow-up over 50%. However, recent exhaustive efforts that have included establishing many follow-up facilities have yielded loss to follow-up rates of about 1.5%.[38] Another useful general rule of thumb suggests not allowing the loss to follow-up rate to exceed the outcome event rate. For example, if the outcome event rate is 3%, the loss to follow-up should not exceed 3%.

Perhaps more important than the absolute overall loss to follow-up rate is the comparative loss rates in the groups. Researchers should analyse the data for differential rates of loss in the groups. Bias could arise when losses are related to differences in unpleasantness, toxicity, or efficacy of the treatments. In any case, investigators should have recorded and analysed the outcomes from those participants lost, at least up to the point of loss.

Conclusion

Trialists should endeavour to minimise exclusions after randomisation and to conduct ITT analyses. They should also follow the CONSORT statement for reporting.[22-25] The flow diagram (trial profile) tracks the progress of participants through a trial.

For readers, nonreporting of exclusions results in interpretation difficulties, such as the exclusion paradox, which misleads readers about trial quality. Moreover, mishandling of exclusions causes serious methodological difficulties. Unfortunately, some explanations provided in reports for such difficulties intuitively appeal to readers, which disguises the seriousness of the issues. Readers must battle both inadequate reporting and their intuition to discover potential threats to validity.

References

1. Schulz, K.F., Grimes, D.A., 2002. Generation of allocation sequences in randomised trials: chance, not choice. Lancet 359, 515–519.
2. Schulz, K.F., Grimes, D.A., 2002. Allocation concealment in randomised trials: defending against deciphering. Lancet 359, 614–618.
3. Peto, R., Pike, M.C., Armitage, P., et al., 1977. Design and analysis of randomized clinical trials requiring prolonged observation of each patient. II. Analysis and examples. Br. J. Cancer 35, 1–39.
4. Peto, R., Pike, M.C., Armitage, P., et al., 1976. Design and analysis of randomized clinical trials requiring prolonged observation of each patient. I. Introduction and design. Br. J. Cancer 34, 585–612.
5. Sackett, D.L., 1983. On some prerequisites for a successful clinical trial. In: Shapiro, S.H., Louis, T.A. (Eds.), Clinical Trials: Issues and Approaches. Marcel Dekker, Inc., New York, pp. 65–79
6. Sackett, D.L., Straus, S.E., Richardson, W.S., Rosenberg, W., Haynes, R.B., 2000. Evidence-Based Medicine: How to Practice and Teach EBM. Churchill Livingstone, Edinburgh.
7. Abraha, I., Cozzolino, F., Orso, M., et al., 2017. A systematic review found that deviations from intention-to-treat are common in randomized trials and systematic reviews. J. Clin. Epidemiol. 84, 37–46.
8. Schulz, K.F., Grimes, D.A., Altman, D.G., Hayes, R.J., 1996. Blinding and exclusions after allocation in randomised controlled trials: survey of published parallel group trials in obstetrics and gynaecology. BMJ 312, 742–744.

9. Abraha, I., Cherubini, A., Cozzolino, F., et al., 2015. Deviation from intention to treat analysis in randomised trials and treatment effect estimates: meta-epidemiological study. BMJ 350, h2445.
10. Lee, Y.J., Ellenberg, J.H., Hirtz, D.G., Nelson, K.B., 1991. Analysis of clinical trials by treatment actually received: is it really an option? Stat. Med. 10, 1595–1605.
11. Lewis, J.A., Machin, D., 1993. Intention to treat—who should use ITT? Br. J. Cancer 68, 647–650.
12. Lachin, J.M., 2000. Statistical considerations in the intent-to-treat principle. Control. Clin. Trials 21, 167–189.
13. Gewandter, J.S., McDermott, M.P., McKeown, A., et al., 2014. Reporting of intention-to-treat analyses in recent analgesic clinical trials: ACTTION systematic review and recommendations. Pain 155, 2714–2719.
14. The Anturane Reinfarction Trial Research Group, 1978. Sulfinpyrazone in the prevention of cardiac death after myocardial infarction. The anturane reinfarction trial. N. Engl. J. Med. 298, 289–295.
15. The Anturane Reinfarction Trial Research Group, 1980. Sulfinpyrazone in the prevention of sudden death after myocardial infarction. The anturane reinfarction trial research group. N. Engl. J. Med. 302, 250–256.
16. Temple, R., Pledger, G.W., 1980. The FDA's critique of the anturane reinfarction trial. N. Engl. J. Med. 303, 1488–1492.
17. Grimes, D.A., Schulz, K.F., 2002. An overview of clinical research: the lay of the land. Lancet 359, 57–61.
18. DerSimonian, R., Charette, L.J., McPeek, B., Mosteller, F., 1982. Reporting on methods in clinical trials. N. Engl. J. Med. 306, 1332–1337.
19. Meinert, C.L., Tonascia, S., Higgins, K., 1984. Content of reports on clinical trials: a critical review. Control. Clin. Trials 5, 328–347.
20. Hollis, S., Campbell, F., 1999. What is meant by intention to treat analysis? Survey of published randomised controlled trials. BMJ 319, 670–674.
21. Schulz, K.F., Chalmers, I., Hayes, R.J., Altman, D.G., 1995. Empirical evidence of bias. Dimensions of methodological quality associated with estimates of treatment effects in controlled trials. JAMA 273, 408–412.
22. Schulz, K.F., Altman, D.G., Moher, D., 2010. CONSORT 2010 statement: updated guidelines for reporting parallel group randomised trials. BMJ 340, c332.
23. Schulz, K.F., Altman, D.G., Moher, D., 2010. CONSORT 2010 statement: updated guidelines for reporting parallel group randomized trials. Ann. Intern. Med. 152, 726–732.
24. Moher, D., Hopewell, S., Schulz, K.F., et al., 2010. CONSORT 2010 explanation and elaboration: updated guidelines for reporting parallel group randomised trials. J. Clin. Epidemiol. 63, e1–37.
25. Moher, D., Hopewell, S., Schulz, K.F., et al., 2010. CONSORT 2010 explanation and elaboration: updated guidelines for reporting parallel group randomised trials. BMJ 340, c869.
26. Friedman, L., Furberg, C., DeMets, D., 1996. Fundamentals of Clinical Trials. Mosby, St. Louis.
27. Meier, P., 1981. Anturane reinfarction trial. N. Engl. J. Med. 304, 730.
28. Kuang, H., Jin, S., Thomas, T., et al., 2015. Predictors of participant retention in infertility treatment trials. Fertil. Steril. 104, 1236–1243.e1-2.
29. Jiang, L., Manson, S.M., Dill, E.J., et al., 2015. Participant and site characteristics related to participant retention in a diabetes prevention translational project. Prev. Sci. 16, 41–52.
30. Kaur, M., Sprague, S., Ignacy, T., Thoma, A., Bhandari, M., Farrokhyar, F., 2014. How to optimize participant retention and complete follow-up in surgical research. Can. J. Surg. 57, 420–427.
31. Koog, Y.H., Gil, M., We, S.R., Wi, H., Min, B.I., 2013. Barriers to participant retention in knee osteoarthritis clinical trials: a systematic review. Semin. Arthritis Rheum. 42, 346–354.
32. Robinson, K.A., Dennison, C.R., Wayman, D.M., Pronovost, P.J., Needham, D.M., 2007. Systematic review identifies number of strategies important for retaining study participants. J. Clin. Epidemiol. 60, 757–765.
33. Boucher, S., Grey, A., Leong, S.L., Sharples, H., Horwath, C., 2015. Token monetary incentives improve mail survey response rates and participant retention: results from a large randomised prospective study of mid-age New Zealand women. N. Z. Med. J. 128, 20–30.
34. Gappoo, S., Montgomery, E.T., Gerdts, C., et al., 2009. Novel strategies implemented to ensure high participant retention rates in a community based HIV prevention effectiveness trial in South Africa and Zimbabwe. Contemp. Clin. Trials 30, 411–418.
35. Olds, D.L., Baca, P., McClatchey, M., et al., 2015. Cluster randomized controlled trial of intervention to increase participant retention and completed home visits in the nurse-family partnership. Prev. Sci. 16, 778–788.

36. Abshire, M., Dinglas, V.D., Cajita, M.I., Eakin, M.N., Needham, D.M., Himmelfarb, C.D., 2017. Participant retention practices in longitudinal clinical research studies with high retention rates. BMC Med. Res. Methodol. 17, 30.

37. Severi, E., Free, C., Knight, R., Robertson, S., Edwards, P., Hoile, E., 2011. Two controlled trials to increase participant retention in a randomized controlled trial of mobile phone-based smoking cessation support in the United Kingdom. Clin. Trials 8, 654–660.

38. Roddy, R.E., Zekeng, L., Ryan, K.A., Tamoufe, U., Tweedy, K.G., 2002. Effect of nonoxynol-9 gel on urogenital gonorrhea and chlamydial infection: a randomized controlled trial. JAMA 287, 1117–1122.

39. Joseph Davey, D., Nhavoto, J.A., Augusto, O., et al., 2016. SMSaude: evaluating mobile phone text reminders to improve retention in HIV care for patients on antiretroviral therapy in Mozambique. J. Acquir. Immune Defic. Syndr. 73, e23–30.

40. McCallum, G.B., Versteegh, L.A., Morris, P.S., et al., 2014. Mobile phones support adherence and retention of indigenous participants in a randomised controlled trial: strategies and lessons learnt. BMC Public Health 14, 622.

41. Finocchario-Kessler, S., Gautney, B.J., Khamadi, S., et al., 2014. If you text them, they will come: using the HIV infant tracking system to improve early infant diagnosis quality and retention in Kenya. AIDS 28 (Suppl 3), S313–S321.

42. Mychasiuk, R., Benzies, K., 2012. Facebook: an effective tool for participant retention in longitudinal research. Child Care Health Dev. 38, 753–756.

43. Idoko, O.T., Owolabi, O.A., Odutola, A.A., et al., 2014. Lessons in participant retention in the course of a randomized controlled clinical trial. BMC Res. Notes 7, 706.

44. Sackett, D.L., Richardson, W.S., Rosenberg, W., Haynes, R.B., 1997. Evidence-Based Medicine: How to Practice and Teach EBM. Churchill Livingstone, New York.

CHAPTER 16

Blinding in Randomised Trials: Hiding Who Got What

Blinding embodies a rich history spanning over two centuries. Most researchers worldwide understand blinding terminology, but confusion lurks beyond a general comprehension. Terms such as 'single blind', 'double blind', and 'triple blind' mean different things to different people. Moreover, many medical researchers confuse blinding with allocation concealment. Such confusion indicates misunderstandings of both. The term 'blinding' refers to keeping trial participants, investigators (usually healthcare providers), or assessors (those collecting outcome data) unaware of the assigned intervention, so they will not be influenced by that knowledge. Blinding usually reduces differential assessment of outcomes (information bias) but can also improve compliance and retention of trial participants while reducing biased supplemental care or treatment (sometimes called 'co-intervention'). Many investigators and readers naively consider a randomised trial as high quality simply because it is double blind, as if double blinding is the *sine qua non* of a randomised controlled trial. Although double blinding (blinding investigators, participants, and outcome assessors) indicates a strong design, trials that are not double blinded should not automatically be deemed inferior. Rather than solely relying on terminology such as 'double blinding', researchers should explicitly state who was blinded, and how. We recommend placing greater credence in results when investigators at least blind outcome assessments, except with objective outcomes, such as death, which leave little room for bias. If investigators properly report their blinding efforts, readers can judge them. Unfortunately, many articles do not contain proper reporting. If an article claims blinding without any accompanying clarification, readers should remain sceptical about its effect on bias reduction.

The rich history of blinding in clinical trials spans a couple of centuries.[1] Most researchers worldwide appreciate its meaning. Unfortunately, beyond that general appreciation lurks confusion. Terms such as 'single blind', 'double blind', and 'triple blind' mean different things to different people.[2] Moreover, many medical researchers confuse the term 'blinding' with allocation concealment. The fact that such confusion arises suggests that both terms are misunderstood. Clear theoretical and practical differences separate the two. Blinding prevents ascertainment bias and protects the sequence after allocation.[3,4] By contrast, researchers use methods of allocation concealment primarily to prevent selection bias and to protect an assignment sequence before and until allocation. Furthermore, in some trials, blinding cannot be successfully implemented, whereas allocation concealment can always be successfully implemented.[4,5]

Blinding represents an important, distinct aspect of randomised controlled trials.[3] The term 'blinding' refers to keeping trial participants, investigators (usually healthcare providers), or assessors (those collecting outcome data) unaware of an assigned intervention, so they are not influenced by that knowledge. Blinding prevents bias at several stages of a trial, although its relevance varies according to circumstance. Although initial forays into blinding might have used a blindfold,[1] the processes have now become much more elaborate. In this chapter we focus on the nomenclature, attributes, and benefits of blinding. In Chapter 17 we address implementation of blinding in randomised trials.

Potential Effects of Blinding

If participants are not blinded, knowledge of group assignment can affect responses to the intervention received.[3] Participants who know that they have been assigned to a group who will receive a new treatment might harbour favourable expectations or increased apprehension. Those assigned to standard treatment, however, might feel deprived or relieved. Despite evidence to suggest that new treatments are as likely to be worse as they are to be better than standard treatments,[6] participants probably assume that new treatments will be better than standard treatments—'new' means 'improved'. In any case, knowledge of the intervention received, and perceptions of that treatment, can affect the psychological or physical responses of the participants. Knowledge of treatment allocation can also affect compliance and retention of trial participants (Panel 16.1).

Blinding investigators—those who contribute to a broadly defined trial team including, but not limited to, trial designers, participant enrollers, randomisation implementors, healthcare providers, intervention counsellors, and routine data collectors—is also important.[3] Investigators especially pertinent to blinding include healthcare providers (such as an attending physician or nurse) and intervention counsellors (e.g., someone who delivers a behavioural prevention message) who might interact with the participants throughout the trial. If investigators are not blinded, their attitudes for or against an intervention can be directly transferred to participants.[7] Their inclinations could also be manifested in differential use of ancillary interventions of supplemental care or treatment (co-interventions), differential decisions to withdraw participants from a trial, or differential adjustments to the medication dose (see Panel 16.1). Investigators might also encourage or discourage continuation in a trial on the basis of knowledge of the intervention group assignment.

Perhaps most importantly, blinding helps to reduce differential assessment of outcomes (often called information or ascertainment bias) (see Panel 16.1). For example, if outcome assessors who

PANEL 16.1 ■ Potential Benefits Accruing Dependent on Those Individuals Successfully Blinded	
Individuals Blinded	*Potential Benefits*
Participants	Less likely to have biased psychological or physical responses to intervention
	More likely to comply with trial regimens
	Less likely to seek additional adjunct interventions
	Less likely to leave trial without providing outcome data, thus less likely lost to follow-up
Trial investigators	Less likely to transfer their inclinations or attitudes to participants
	Less likely to differentially administer co-interventions
	Less likely to differentially adjust dose
	Less likely to differentially withdraw participants
	Less likely to differentially encourage or discourage participants to continue trial
Assessors	Less likely to have biases affect their outcome assessments, especially with subjective outcomes of interest

know of the treatment allocation believe a new intervention is better than an old one, they could register more generous responses to that intervention. Indeed, in a placebo-controlled trial in patients with multiple sclerosis[8] the unblinded, but not the blinded, neurologists' assessments showed an apparent benefit of the intervention.

Subjective outcomes (e.g., pain scores) present great opportunities for bias.[3] Furthermore, some outcomes can be fraught with subjectivity (e.g., salpingitis). In general, though, blinding becomes less important to reduce observer bias as the outcomes become less subjective, because objective (hard) outcomes leave little opportunity for bias. Knowledge of the intervention would not greatly affect measurement of a hard outcome, such as death.

Lexicon of Blinding

Nonblinded (open or open label) denotes trials in which everyone involved knows who has received which interventions throughout the trial. Blinding (masking) indicates that knowledge of the intervention assignments is hidden from participants, trial investigators, or assessors.

The terminology 'single blind' usually means that one of the three categories of individuals (normally participant rather than investigator) remains unaware of intervention assignments throughout the trial.[9] A single-blind trial might also, confusingly, mean that the participant and investigator both know the intervention, but that the assessor remains unaware of it.

In a double-blind trial, participants, investigators, and assessors usually all remain unaware of the intervention assignments throughout the trial.[3] In view of the fact that three groups are kept ignorant, the terminology 'double blind' is sometimes misleading. In medical research, however, an investigator frequently also assesses, so in this instance the terminology accurately refers to two categories.

'Triple blind' usually means a double-blind trial that also maintains a blind data analysis.[10] Some investigators, however, denote trials as triple blind if investigators and assessors are distinct people and both, as well as participants, remain unaware of assignments. Investigators rarely use 'quadruple blind', but those who do use the term to denote blinding of participants, investigators, assessors, and data analysts.[11] Thus 'quintuple blind' must mean that the allocation schedule has been lost and nobody knows anything. Contrary to Mae West's claim that 'too much of a good thing can be wonderful', such is not the case with blinding.

Confused terminology of single, double, and triple blinding permeates the literature.[3] When investigators examined physician interpretations and textbook definitions of double blinding, they found 17 unique interpretations and 9 different definitions.[2] Another survey of authors who had used double blinding provided 15 different operational meanings of the term 'double blind' and 'typically felt that their preferred definition was the most widely used'.[12] Not only do investigators not define double-blind trials consistently, in particular, but they make matters worse by frequently failing to report their definitions clearly in their articles. Building on the original blindfolding efforts,[1] and the once common double-blindfold terminology,[13] we illustrate double versus single blinding (Fig. 16.1) and double versus triple blinding (Fig. 16.2). More seriously, when we use 'double blind' or its derivatives in this chapter, we mean that steps have been taken to blind participants, investigators, and assessors to group assignments. In reporting randomised controlled trials, we urge researchers to explicitly state what steps they took to keep whom blinded.

Sparse reporting on blinding, however, is common. Many authors neglect to report whether or not their trial was blinded. For example, reports of 51% of 506 trials in cystic fibrosis,[14] 33% of 196 trials in rheumatoid arthritis,[15] and 38% of 68 trials in dermatology[16] did not state whether blinding was used. If authors specifically report that their trial is blinded, many fail to report the blinding method used. In a review of blinding in reports of randomised trials of pharmacological treatments and nonpharmacological treatments, 42%[17] and 25%,[18] respectively, of trials reporting blinding did not report the method used.[17] In another review of 156 trials described as 'double blind', 26% did not provide any relevant information on who was blinded or how anyone was blinded.[12]

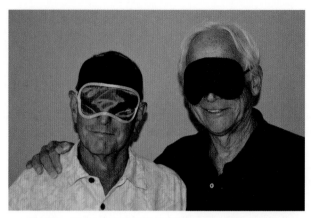

Fig. 16.1   The authors: double blinded versus single blinded.

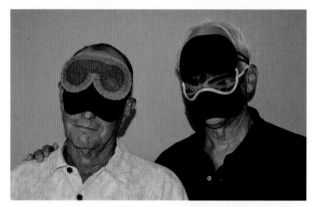

Fig. 16.2   The authors: double blinded versus triple blinded.

When researchers have reported their study as double blind, they frequently have not provided much further clarification.[15,19-21] For example, of 31 double blind trials in obstetrics and gynaecology, only 14 (45%) reports indicated the similarity of the treatment and control regimens (e.g., appearance, taste, administration) and only 5 (16%) provided statements to indicate that blinding was successful.[21] In a review of 156 articles described as 'double blind', only 2% explicitly described the blinding status of participants, healthcare providers, and outcome assessors while 56% did not describe the blinding status of any of the key categories. The remaining 42% provided only minimal information on who was blinded and how.[12] In a follow-up survey of the authors of trial articles described as 'double blind' in the literature, 19% indicated that they had not blinded either participants, investigators (healthcare providers), or outcome assessors (data collectors)[12] (i.e., they were not double blind by our definition).

Masking or Blinding?

Some people prefer the term 'masking' to 'blinding' to describe the same procedure. Masking might be more appropriate in trials that involve participants who have impaired vision, and could be less confusing in trials in which blindness is an outcome.[3] Blinding, however, conveys a strong bias-prevention message. Apparently, blinding terminology emerged when Benjamin Franklin and

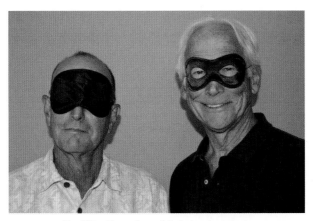

Fig. 16.3 The authors: blinded and masked.

colleagues[22] actually blindfolded participants to shield them from knowledge in their assessments of the therapeutic claims made for mesmerism. The imagery of blindfolding, a total covering of the eyes, conveys stronger bias prevention than masking, where eye holes could permit viewing (Fig. 16.3). Blinding also suggests a more secure procedure to some. The International Conference on Harmonisation (ICH) guidance,[23] for example, primarily uses blinding terminology. (The ICH is a collaboration between regulatory authorities and the pharmaceutical industry in Europe, Japan, and the United States to develop common guidelines for the design, implementation, and reporting of clinical trials.) We prefer blinding because it has a long history, maintains worldwide recognition, creates strong imagery, and permeates the ICH guidelines.[3]

Placebos and Blinding

Interventions (treatments) sometimes have no effect on the outcomes being studied.[3] When an ineffective intervention is administered to participants in the context of a well-designed randomised controlled trial, however, beneficial effects on participants' attitudes sometimes occur, which in turn affect outcomes.[10] Researchers refer to this phenomenon as the placebo effect.

A placebo refers to a pharmacologically inactive agent that investigators administer to participants in the control group of a trial.[3] The use of a placebo control group balances the placebo effect in the treatment group, allowing for independent assessment of the treatment effect. Although placebos can have a psychological effect, they are administered to participants in a trial because they are otherwise inactive. An active placebo is a placebo with properties that mimic the symptoms or side effects (e.g., dry mouth, sweating) that might otherwise reveal the identity of the pharmacologically active test treatment. Most researchers agree that placebos should be administered, whenever possible, to controls when assessing the effects of a proposed new treatment for a condition for which no effective treatment already exists.[9,10] Indeed, blinding frequently necessitates the use of placebos.

However, a proven effective standard treatment, if such exists, is usually given to the control group for comparison against a new treatment.[3] Thus investigators might compare two active treatment groups without a placebo group. Even then, however, investigators frequently attempt to achieve blinding by use of the double-dummy method, in essence two placebos.[11,24] For example, for comparison of two agents, one in a blue capsule and the other in a red capsule, the investigators would prepare blue placebo capsules and red placebo capsules. Then both treatment groups would receive a blue and a red capsule, one active and one inactive. Consult Chapter 17 for more detail on the use of placebos and the double-dummy method, which is used frequently in the medical literature.[17]

Does Blinding Prevent Bias?

Some investigators, readers, and editors overstate the importance of blinding in prevention of bias. Indeed, some consider a randomised trial as high quality if it is double blind (i.e., as if double blinding is the *sine qua non* of a randomised controlled trial).[3] Unfortunately, scientific life is not that simple. A randomised trial can be methodologically sound and not be double blind or, conversely, double blind and not methodologically sound. Lasagna[13] captured that notion long ago: 'Let us examine the placebo somewhat more critically, however, because it and 'double blind' have reached the status of fetishes in our thinking and literature. The Automatic Aura of Respectability, Infallibility, and Scientific Savoir-faire which they possess for many can be easily shown to be undeserved in certain circumstances.'[13] Although double blinding suggests a strong design, it is not the primary indicator of overall trial quality. Moreover, many trials cannot be double blinded. Such trials must, therefore, be judged on overall merit rather than an inapplicable standard based on double blinding.

We do not, however, suggest that blinding is unimportant.[3] Intuitively, blinding should reduce bias, and available evidence supports that impression. Methodological investigations tend to show that double blinding prevents bias[4,25-27] but some indicate that it is less important, on average, in prevention of bias than is adequate allocation concealment.[4,26,27]

What to Look for in Descriptions of Blinding

In general, if researchers describe a trial as double blind, readers can assume that they have avoided bias. Empirical evidence lends support to this recommendation. As suggested in the CONSORT guidelines,[28-31] however, investigators should not use only the single-blind, double-blind, or triple-blind terminology, but should also explicitly state who was blinded, and how. Moreover, if the researchers contend that the trial investigators, participants, and assessors were blinded (i.e., double blind), then they should provide information about the mechanism (e.g., capsules, tablets, film), similarity of treatment characteristics (e.g., appearance, taste, administration), and allocation schedule control (e.g., location of the schedule during the trial, when the code was broken for the analysis, and circumstances under which the code could be broken for individual instances). Such additional information can lend support to or undermine claims of double blinding (Panel 16.2).[32-42]

If researchers properly report their blinding efforts, readers can judge those efforts. Unfortunately, many articles will not contain proper reporting. If a researcher claims to have done a blinded study but does not provide accompanying clarification, readers should remain sceptical about its effect on bias reduction. For example, one trial[43] of prophylactic antibiotics claimed to be blinded, but the methods section of the report revealed that little or no blinding occurred.

Ideally, researchers should also relate whether blinding was successful. Investigators can theoretically assess the success of blinding by directly asking participants, healthcare providers, or outcome assessors which intervention they think was administered (Panel 16.3). In principle, if blinding was successful, these individuals should not be able to do better than chance when guessing the intervention, for example. In practice, however, blinding might be totally successful, but participants, healthcare providers, and outcome assessors might nevertheless guess the intervention because of ancillary information. Disproportionate levels of adverse side effects might provide strong hints as to the intervention. Irrespective of painstaking efforts to do double-blinded trials, some interventions have side effects that are so recognisable that their occurrence will unavoidably reveal the intervention received to both the participants and the healthcare providers.[11,30,31] Even more fundamental than hints from adverse effects are the hints from clinical outcomes. Researchers usually welcome large clinical effects (except perhaps in noninferiority or equivalence trials). If they arise, healthcare providers and participants would likely deduce—not always accurately, of course—that a participant with a positive outcome received the active (new) intervention

---

PANEL 16.2 ■ Descriptions of Blinding

'*All subjects and researchers remained blinded to treatment assignment until data collection and analyses were completed. …Study supplements were hard gelatin capsules that were identical in appearance and taste*'.[32]

'*The placebo tablets that will be used in the PACE Plus trial are identical in appearance and taste to their active counterparts, but do not contain the active component. All medication packaging will be identical between the 3 medication groups, except for a unique randomization number for each participant*'.[33]

'*Medications were dispensed in blister packs indicating treatment day and time. Placebo and active medications were encapsulated in gel capsules with filler to give identical weight and appearance. Blinding could only be broken if a participant experienced treatment failure or an adverse event for which an acceptable alternative treatment could not be given and knowledge of the treatment assignment was needed for clinical care*'.[34]

'*The active medication was 1 mL of triamcinolone (purchased from Bristol-Myers Squibb), 40 mg/mL, for injection. The comparator was 1 mL of 0.9% sodium chloride for injection (Hosperia Inc). Neither was mixed with local anesthetic. Both were administered every 12 weeks for 2 years. Synovial fluid ($\leq$10 mL) was aspirated prior to the injection*'.[35]

'*The treatment group (vitamin D3 + calcium group) received vitamin D3 (cholecalciferol; 2000-IU capsule, once daily) and calcium carbonate (500-mg tablet, 3 times daily) and the placebo group received identical placebos. Only the statistician and a research assistant who had no contact with participants were unblinded to group assignment. Supplements and placebos were made by Tishcon*'.[36]

'*We randomly assigned 112 of the 126 men who were screened (Figure 1) to receive alendronate, 70 mg once weekly, or matching placebo (Merck & Co. Inc., Rahway, New Jersey).… A pharmacist (who had no contact with patients) provided the assigned treatment (the study drug or placebo) to the study coordinators to give to patients*'.[37]

'*Participants, caregivers, and study staff (site investigators and trial coordinating centre staff) were masked to treatment allocation. An emergency un-blinding service was available via Sealed Envelope Ltd. The tranexamic acid (Cyklokapron injection) used in the trial was manufactured by Pfizer Ltd, Sandwich, UK. The matching placebo (sodium chloride 0·9%) was prepared by South Devon Healthcare NHS Trust, Devon, UK. Ampoules and packaging were identical in appearance. The masking was done by Brecon Pharmaceuticals Limited, Hereford, UK and involved the removal of the original manufacturer's label and replacement with the clinical trial label bearing the randomisation number, which was used as the pack identification. Apart from the randomisation number, all pack label texts were identical for tranexamic acid and placebo. Correct masking and coding of ampoules was checked by independent random testing of each batch by high-performance liquid chromatography to confirm the contents of the ampoules*'.[38]

'*No patient, research nurse, investigator, or any other medical or nursing staff in the ICU [intensive care unit] was aware of the treatment assignments for the duration of the study. All statistical analysis was also done with masking maintained. Randomisation authorities were instructed to report any suspected breach of the masking procedures. No report was filed … The drug or placebo (vehicle without active drug) was prepared for syringe pump infusion or for volumetric pump infusion in indistinguishable syringes or bags*'.[39]

'*The study was double-blinded—that is, neither the women nor the study staff, including the biostatisticians at Family Health International, knew which group was using the nonoxynol 9 film. The nonoxynol 9 film contained …The placebo film contained … The films were identical in appearance, packaging, and labeling*'.[40]

'*The doxycycline and placebo were in capsule form and identical in appearance … The randomization code was kept in the USA. [Note: The trial was conducted in Kenya.] Thus, all administration and assessments were done blinded to treatment assignment, and the investigators and patients were also blinded to the ongoing results of the study. The code was broken only after data collection had been completed*'.[41]

'*Participants and study physicians were not masked to group assignment, but both endpoint committees (one for adjudication of atrial fibrillation, and one for cerebral ischaemic events) were*'.[42] [Blinding of just the outcome assessment]

---

rather than the control (standard). If indeed the active (new) intervention materialises as helpful (highly desirable), then their deductions would be correct more often than chance guesses.[30,31,44] Irrespective of their suspicions, end-of-trial tests of blindness might actually be tests of hunches for adverse effects or efficacy.[45-47] Because of that lack of validity, the latest CONSORT reporting guidelines removed testing of blinding from its checklist.[28-31,47]

PANEL 16.3 ■ Assessment of the Success of Blinding

The success of the double-dummy blinding technique was assessed using a mixed-methods approach including the Bang Blinding Index (BBI), and semistructured qualitative interviews. By asking participants to state which treatment arm they believed themselves to have been allocated to, the BBI can be used to estimate the percentage of correct guesses (beyond the level expected by chance) in each treatment group.... The double-dummy blinding technique was implemented successfully for all patients. Data for the BBI were collected from 24 patients, and ten also did qualitative interviews. There was no difference in the rates of unblinding between the two arms. The BBI score was 0·15 in the epidural analgesia arm and 0·31 in the wound infusion catheter (WIC) arm, suggesting that 15 per cent more than expected by chance correctly guessed the treatment allocation in the epidural analgesia arm, and 31 per cent in the WIC arm (P = 0·412)'.[48]

Furthermore, individuals might be reluctant to expose any unblinding efforts by providing accurate responses to the queries; in other words, if they have deciphered group assignments, they might provide responses contrary to their deciphering findings to disguise their actions. That difficulty, along with interpretation difficulties stemming from adverse side effects and successful clinical outcomes, leads us to question the usefulness of tests of blinding in some circumstances. Investigators should carefully consider the usefulness of assessing the success of their blinding efforts, but if they proceed, should provide the results of any assessments. At the very least, they should report any failure of the blinding procedure, such as nonidentical placebo or active preparations. Published reports rarely contain assessments of blinding, but, if provided, readers should sceptically assess the information presented.

Double blinding proves difficult or impossible in many trials. For instance, surgical trials usually cannot be double blinded. Similarly, a trial that compares degrees of pain associated with sampling blood from the ear or thumb cannot be double blinded.[49] If researchers do not describe their trial as double blind or the equivalent, it could still be scientifically strong. Apart from assessment of the other methodological aspects of the trial, readers would have to assess how much bias might have ensued due to absence of blinding. Readers should identify whether anybody was blinded in the trial and what benefits might have accrued (see Panel 16.1). Indeed, blinding of outcome assessors is often possible and advisable, even in open trials.[11] For example, lesions can be photographed before and after treatment and assessed by someone not involved in the study.[11] We recommend placing greater credence in results when someone unaware of treatment assignments judges outcome measures.

Even that recommendation, however, is not absolute. As noted earlier, some hard outcomes, such as death, leave little room for ascertainment bias. In other words, blinding the assessor to hard outcomes might have little effect.

Conclusion

Blinding embodies a rich history spanning over two centuries. Most researchers worldwide understand blinding terminology, but confusion lurks beyond a general comprehension. Investigators should clearly explicate those blinded and not blinded in their trial, rather than only labelling their trial as single blind, double blind, or triple blind. Readers should expect such clarity when reading and judging a trial report.

References

1. Kaptchuk, T.J., 1998. Intentional ignorance: a history of blind assessment and placebo controls in medicine. Bull. Hist. Med. 72, 389–433.
2. Devereaux, P.J., Manns, B.J., Ghali, W.A., et al., 2001. Physician interpretations and textbook definitions of blinding terminology in randomized controlled trials. JAMA 285, 2000–2003.
3. Schulz, K.F., Chalmers, I., Altman, D.G., 2002. The landscape and lexicon of blinding in randomized trials. Ann. Intern. Med. 136, 254–259.
4. Schulz, K.F., Chalmers, I., Hayes, R.J., Altman, D.G., 1995. Empirical evidence of bias. Dimensions of methodological quality associated with estimates of treatment effects in controlled trials. JAMA 273, 408–412.
5. Schulz, K.F., Chalmers, I., Grimes, D.A., Altman, D.G., 1994. Assessing the quality of randomization from reports of controlled trials published in obstetrics and gynecology journals. JAMA 272, 125–128.
6. Chalmers, I., 1997. What is the prior probability of a proposed new treatment being superior to established treatments? BMJ 314, 74–75.
7. Wolf, S., 1950. Effects of suggestion and conditioning on action of chemical agents in human subjects — pharmacology of placebos. J. Clin. Invest. 29, 100–109.
8. Noseworthy, J.H., Ebers, G.C., Vandervoort, M.K., Farquhar, R.E., Yetisir, E., Roberts, R., 1994. The impact of blinding on the results of a randomized, placebo-controlled multiple sclerosis clinical trial. Neurology 44, 16–20.
9. Meinert, C., 1986. Clinical Trials: Design, Conduct, and Analysis. Oxford University Press, New York.
10. Pocock, S., 1983. Clinical Trials: A Practical Approach. Wiley, Chichester, England.
11. Day, S.J., Altman, D.G., 2000. Statistics notes: blinding in clinical trials and other studies. BMJ 321, 504.
12. Haahr, M.T., Hrobjartsson, A., 2006. Who is blinded in randomized clinical trials? A study of 200 trials and a survey of authors. Clin. Trials 3, 360–365.
13. Lasagna, L., 1955. The controlled trial: theory and practice. J. Chronic Dis. 1, 353–367.
14. Cheng, K., Smyth, R.L., Motley, J., O'Hea, U., Ashby, D., 2000. Randomized controlled trials in cystic fibrosis (1966-1997) categorized by time, design, and intervention. Pediatr. Pulmonol. 29, 1–7.
15. Gøtzsche, P.C., 1989. Methodology and overt and hidden bias in reports of 196 double-blind trials of non-steroidal antiinflammatory drugs in rheumatoid arthritis. Control. Clin. Trials 10, 31–56.
16. Adetugbo, K., Williams, H., 2000. How well are randomized controlled trials reported in the dermatology literature? Arch. Dermatol. 136, 381–385.
17. Boutron, I., Estellat, C., Guittet, L., et al., 2006. Methods of blinding in reports of randomized controlled trials assessing pharmacologic treatments: a systematic review. PLoS Med 3, e425.
18. Boutron, I., Guittet, L., Estellat, C., Moher, D., Hrobjartsson, A., Ravaud, P., 2007. Reporting methods of blinding in randomized trials assessing nonpharmacological treatments. PLoS Med 4, e61.
19. Mosteller, F., Gilbert, J.P., McPeek, B., 1980. Reporting standards and research strategies for controlled trials: agenda for the editor. Control Clin. Trials 1, 37–58.
20. DerSimonian, R., Charette, L.J., McPeek, B., Mosteller, F., 1982. Reporting on methods in clinical trials. N. Engl. J. Med. 306, 1332–1337.
21. Schulz, K.F., Grimes, D.A., Altman, D.G., Hayes, R.J., 1996. Blinding and exclusions after allocation in randomised controlled trials: survey of published parallel group trials in obstetrics and gynaecology. BMJ 312, 742–744.
22. Franklin, B., Bailly, J., Lavoisier, A., 1785. Rapport des commissaires chargés par le roi, de l'examen du magnetisme animal. A Nice: Chez Gabriel Floteron.
23. Department of Health and Human Services FDA, 1998. International conference on harmonisation: guidance on statistical principles for clinical trials. Fed. Regist. 63, 49583–49598.
24. Altman, D., 1991. Practical Statistics for Medical Research. Chapman and Hall, London.
25. Savovic, J., Jones, H.E., Altman, D.G., et al., 2012. Influence of reported study design characteristics on intervention effect estimates from randomized, controlled trials. Ann. Intern. Med. 157, 429–438.
26. Khan, K.S., Daya, S., Collins, J.A., Walter, S.D., 1996. Empirical evidence of bias in infertility research: overestimation of treatment effect in crossover trials using pregnancy as the outcome measure. Fertil. Steril. 65, 939–945.
27. Moher, D., Pham, B., Jones, A., et al., 1998. Does quality of reports of randomised trials affect estimates of intervention efficacy reported in meta-analyses? Lancet 352, 609–613.

28. Schulz, K.F., Altman, D.G., Moher, D., 2010. CONSORT 2010 statement: updated guidelines for report-ing parallel group randomised trials. BMJ 340, c332.

29. Schulz, K.F., Altman, D.G., Moher, D., 2010. CONSORT 2010 statement: updated guidelines for report-ing parallel group randomized trials. Ann. Intern. Med. 152, 726–732.

30. Moher, D., Hopewell, S., Schulz, K.F., et al., 2010. CONSORT 2010 explanation and elaboration: updated guidelines for reporting parallel group randomised trials. J. Clin. Epidemiol. 63, e1–37.

31. Moher, D., Hopewell, S., Schulz, K.F., et al., 2010. CONSORT 2010 explanation and elaboration: updated guidelines for reporting parallel group randomised trials. BMJ 340, c869.

32. Vaes, A.M.M., Tieland, M., de Regt, M.F., Wittwer, J., van Loon, L.J.C., de Groot, L.C.P.G.M., 2018. Dose-response effects of supplementation with calcifediol on serum 25-hydroxyvitamin D status and its metabolites: a randomized controlled trial in older adults. Clin. Nutr. 37, 808–814.

33. Schreijenberg, M., Luijsterburg, P.A., Van Trier, Y.D., et al., 2017. Efficacy of paracetamol, diclofenac and advice for acute low back pain in general practice: design of a randomized controlled trial (PACE Plus). BMC Musculoskelet. Disord. 18, 56.

34. Moran, G.J., Krishnadasan, A., Mower, W.R., et al., 2017. Effect of cephalexin plus trimethoprim-sulfamethoxazole vs cephalexin alone on clinical cure of uncomplicated cellulitis: a randomized clinical trial. JAMA 317, 2088–2096.

35. McAlindon, T.E., LaValley, M.P., Harvey, W.F., et al., 2017. Effect of intra-articular triamcinolone vs saline on knee cartilage volume and pain in patients with knee osteoarthritis: a randomized clinical trial. JAMA 317, 1967–1975.

36. Lappe, J., Watson, P., Travers-Gustafson, D., et al., 2017. Effect of vitamin D and calcium supplemen-tation on cancer incidence in older women: a randomized clinical trial. JAMA 317, 1234–1243.

37. Greenspan, S.L., Nelson, J.B., Trump, D.L., Resnick, N.M., 2007. Effect of once-weekly oral alendronate on bone loss in men receiving androgen deprivation therapy for prostate cancer: a randomized trial. Ann. Intern. Med. 146, 416–424.

38. WOMAN Trial Collaborators, 2017. Effect of early tranexamic acid administration on mortality, hyster-ectomy, and other morbidities in women with post-partum haemorrhage (WOMAN): an international, randomised, double-blind, placebo-controlled trial. Lancet 389, 2105–2116.

39. Bellomo, R., Chapman, M., Finfer, S., Hickling, K., Myburgh, J., 2000. Low-dose dopamine in patients with early renal dysfunction: a placebo-controlled randomised trial. Australian and New Zealand Intensive Care Society (ANZICS) Clinical Trials Group. Lancet 356, 2139–2143.

40. Roddy, R.E., Zekeng, L., Ryan, K.A., Tamoufe, U., Weir, S.S., Wong, E.L., 1998. A controlled trial of nonoxynol 9 film to reduce male-to-female transmission of sexually transmitted diseases. N. Engl. J. Med. 339, 504–510.

41. Sinei, S.K., Schulz, K.F., Lamptey, P.R., et al., 1990. Preventing IUCD-related pelvic infection: the effi-cacy of prophylactic doxycycline at insertion. Br. J. Obstet. Gynaecol. 97, 412–419.

42. Wachter, R., Groschel, K., Gelbrich, G., et al., 2017. Holter-electrocardiogram-monitoring in patients with acute ischaemic stroke (Find-AFRANDOMISED): an open-label randomised controlled trial. Lan-cet Neurol. 16, 282–290.

43. Baker, K.R., Drutz, H.P., Barnes, M.D., 1991. Effectiveness of antibiotic prophylaxis in preventing bac-teriuria after multichannel urodynamic investigations: a blind, randomized study in 124 female patients. Am. J. Obstet. Gynecol. 165, 679–681.

44. Quitkin, F.M., Rabkin, J.G., Gerald, J., Davis, J.M., Klein, D.F., 2000. Validity of clinical trials of anti-depressants. Am. J. Psychiatry 157, 327–337.

45. Sackett, D., Gent, M., Taylor, D., 1986. Tests for the blindness of randomized trials may not. Clin. Res. 34, 711A.

46. The Canadian Cooperative Study Group, 1978. A randomized trial of aspirin and sulfinpyrazone in threat-ened stroke. The Canadian Cooperative Study Group. N. Engl. J. Med. 299, 53–59.

47. Schulz, K.F., Altman, D.G., Moher, D., Fergusson, D., 2010. CONSORT 2010 changes and testing blindness in RCTs. Lancet 375, 1144–1146.

48. Boulind, C.E., Ewings, P., Bulley, S.H., et al., 2013. Feasibility study of analgesia via epidural versus con-tinuous wound infusion after laparoscopic colorectal resection. Br. J. Surg. 100, 395–402.

49. Carley, S.D., Libetta, C., Flavin, B., Butler, J., Tong, N., Sammy, I., 2000. An open prospective rando-mised trial to reduce the pain of blood glucose testing: ear versus thumb. BMJ 321, 20.

CHAPTER 17

Implementation of Treatment Blinding in Randomised Trials

This chapter focuses on implementation of blinding in randomised trials. Investigators use single blinding frequently with nonpharmaceutical treatments where total blinding is not possible. In those circumstances, often participants are those blinded and the treatments involve surgery or a medical device. The concept is to standardise the experiences of the participants among all the treatment groups throughout the trial. Some trials just use simple visual screening such as draping. Other trials might use complicated approaches such as sham operations in which skin incisions are made and then closed. If healthcare personnel or participants cannot be blinded, investigators should always consider blinding the outcome assessor. That form of single blinding can frequently be done.

Most double blinding involves drugs, which include vaccines and other medicinal interventions. Placebos are generally used in double-blind trials. Hospital pharmacies and pharmaceutical companies may provide valuable assistance in these blinding activities. When examining the effects of a proposed new treatment for a condition for which no effective treatment already exists, the drug and placebo must be prepared identically, such as in capsules or pills, and packaged identically, such as in bottles or blister packs. They should appear, taste, and smell the same while also being administered identically. The experiences of the control group should mimic the experiences of the treatment group.

If an accepted effective treatment exists, sometimes ethics review boards or investigators determine that it should be administered to everyone enrolled in a trial. In that circumstance, the trial compares a new treatment plus the accepted effective treatment versus the placebo plus the accepted effective treatment. Frequently, however, if an effective standard treatment exists, it is used in the control group for comparison against a new treatment. Thus trialists compare two active treatments.

Continued

In that circumstance, they usually have three options to double blind their trial. The research pharmacy could obtain the drugs in raw form and prepackage the two drugs equally, encapsulate the two standard formulation drugs in a larger capsule, or utilise a double-dummy, double-blinding approach. Frequently, investigators will encounter fewer implementation difficulties with the simpler double-dummy approach.

Introduction

Many potential benefits derive from participants, investigators, and outcome assessors not knowing the group to which the participants have been assigned. This is commonly referred to as blinding (Chapter 16). It can reduce differential assessment of outcomes (ascertainment bias) stemming from knowing the treatment group assignment of the participants being observed.[1,2] In addition, and not well appreciated, blinding may improve compliance and retention of trial participants while reducing biased supplemental care or treatment (sometimes called co-intervention).[1,2] Furthermore, empirical evidence from methodological studies indicates that indeed blinding prevents bias.[2-4]

Notably, without successful blinding, subjective outcomes pose greater opportunities for bias.[1,2] Pain-rating scales and wound-healing scores are examples. Generally, blinding becomes less important in reducing ascertainment bias as the outcomes become less subjective. Hard, objective outcomes, such as death, allow slight opportunity for ascertainment bias.

In Chapter 16 we avoided discussions of implementation. Frequently, medical researchers have a reasonable idea of how to implement blinding. At least they understand it better than how to randomise and adequately follow up participants. However, since we wrote the first edition of our book, we have noticed gaps in blinding implementation knowledge for investigators who conduct randomised trials. This chapter has been added to complement our earlier chapter by focusing on implementation of blinding in trials.

Descriptions of strategies for treatment blinding invariably refer to 'single blinding' and 'double blinding'. These terms are best avoided due to confusion over definitions, as described in the literature[5] and in Chapter 16. However, avoiding their use is nearly impossible because the terms are used ubiquitously. Moreover, they permeate the methodological literature. We believe that investigators can reasonably use those terms given that they explicitly define them in the paper in which they are used. We use the terms 'single blinding' and 'double blinding' in this chapter and clearly define them.

We seek to clarify issues around implementation of blinding. We will first address single blinding of participants, investigators, or assessors. Some approaches are described that often neglect to achieve at least some level of blinding, particularly in surgical and medical device trials. Thereafter, we will address the more complex issues surrounding double blinding. The double-dummy, double-blinded approach persists as perhaps the most confusing aspect of blinding, while actually often simplifying the process of double-blinding. The role of placebos remains misunderstood as well. Our goal is to clarify those concepts and present examples. We hope these presentations will stimulate solutions to blinding implementation issues.

Single Blinding: Participants, Investigators, or Assessors

We define single blinding as keeping trial participants, investigators (usually healthcare providers), or assessors (those determining outcome data) unaware of the assigned treatment so that they will not be influenced by that knowledge. Our definition means that one of those three categories would be blinded.

PARTICIPANTS

Typically, single blinding connotes a trial in which participants remain ignorant to the treatment received.[6] Participants usually are easier to blind than investigators. The key is to prevent the participant from knowledge of the treatment received.

As discussed in Chapter 16, several potential benefits emanate from blinding participants.[2] If blinded, participants are less likely to have biased psychological or physical responses to intervention, less likely to seek additional adjunct interventions, and less likely to leave the trial without providing outcome data, which leads to losses to follow-up. Also, they are more likely to comply with trial regimens. For example, a participant's discovery that he or she is receiving placebo and not the desired new drug can lead to disappointment and dropping out of the study.

INVESTIGATORS

Usually, single-blind trials do not refer to the investigator being blinded. Indeed, if the investigator can be blinded, then likely the participants and assessors can also be blinded. We address that situation in the later section on 'total blinding' (what others frequently call 'double blinding').

ASSESSORS

The other form of single blinding that occurs relatively frequently in the medical literature is the blinding of assessors.[7] Often, trial investigators and participants would not be blinded in this case. If the assessors are blinded, they would be less likely to have biases affect their outcome assessment, especially with subjective outcomes of interest (Chapter 16). This can be a major benefit in a trial in which participants and investigators cannot be blinded.[1,2,8,9]

IMPLEMENTATION ISSUES: PARTICIPANTS

Blinding of anyone tends to be easiest in trials of pharmaceutical agents, but these are instances where total blinding (usually referred to as double blinding) is frequently possible. We address trials involving pharmaceutical agents under the double-blinding section. In this section, we focus on nonpharmaceutical treatments (NPTs) where total blinding is generally not possible. Often, such treatments involve surgery, a medical device, or a treatment involving a collaboration among participants and investigators/caregivers such as rehabilitation, education, or psychotherapy.[7]

In many instances, investigators have difficulty blinding participants. Yet they often can achieve some level of success with thorough and often ingenious planning. The concept is to standardise the experiences of all participants among all the treatment groups in the trial. The actual treatment and its administration must be perceived as the same for those participants. Usually, investigators manipulate the experiences of the control group to mimic the experiences of the treatment group. Given the innumerable potential treatments involved, the trial blinding implementation approaches need to be customised. Although we provide some examples in this chapter, readers should consult the paper by Boutron et al. for an excellent cataloguing of methods used for blinding in NPT trials.[7]

As an example, consider a randomised trial of two different intrauterine devices (IUDs) for contraception. Blinding the clinician who inserts the IUDs would be impossible. The providers will know which IUD is inserted in each woman. However, procedures could be used that would blind the participant. A visual screening, such as a paper drape over the woman's legs, might suffice.

In another example, a randomised controlled trial examined acupressure wristbands for treating nausea and vomiting in pregnancy.[10] Those randomised to the active treatment group had the pressure beads applied to the P6 meridian point on the anterior forearms. Those assigned to the placebo group had the bead applied to the dorsal forearm, a site thought to be ineffective. Women in both groups had the same bands worn for the same duration, but with pressure applied to different spots.

In another, a trial of paracervical anaesthesia for first-trimester abortion used a sham treatment arm.[11] All participants received the same oral premedications. All then had cervical injection of buffered lidocaine 2 mL for tenaculum placement (a holding instrument on the cervix). Participants assigned to the active treatment had an additional 18 mL of buffered lidocaine injected at four sites around the cervix. Those assigned to the sham arm had a covered needle pressed against the vaginal sidewall in two sites for a similar amount of time. That sham procedure was a reasonable choice, because paracervical injection of saline as a placebo may provide anaesthesia by tissue distention.[12]

Blinding in surgical trials is difficult, and, of course, blinding the surgeon is invariably impossible. However, to blind the participant and assessor, an operation could be done on one group, and a sham operation, such as a skin incision only, could be done on the comparison group.

Indeed, in NPTs, methods for blinding of participants mainly entail 'sham procedures such as simulation of surgical procedures, attention-control interventions, or a placebo with a different mode of administration for rehabilitation or psychotherapy. Trials assessing devices reported various placebo interventions such as use of a sham prosthesis, identical apparatus (e.g., identical but inactivated machine or use of activated machine with a barrier to block the treatment), or simulation of using a device'.[7]

Although we are focusing on examples of sham surgery in the next section, much of what we discuss extends to medical device trials as well. In a survey of 123 NPT trials that reported blinding, 58% utilised a sham procedure.[7] Of note, successful blinding of participants usually enables successful blinding of assessors as well.

SHAM PROCEDURES

Sometimes investigators go to great lengths to ensure blinding of participants. For example, in a randomised trial, investigators allocated patients with osteoarthritis of the knee to arthroscopic debridement, arthroscopic lavage, or placebo surgery.[13] Those allocated to the placebo surgical group received skin incisions and underwent a simulated debridement without insertion of the arthroscope. Patients and assessors apparently were unaware of the treatment assignments. Interestingly, this trial revealed that the outcomes from arthroscopic lavage or arthroscopic debridement were not superior to the placebo procedure.[13] Sham knee incisions were invasive but were an innovative approach that probably eliminated bias.

Another randomised trial involved sham burr holes in the skull. Investigators allocated patients who had severe Parkinson disease to receive a transplant of nerve cells into the putamen bilaterally or undergo sham surgery in which burr holes were drilled in the skull with the dura not being penetrated.[14] The authors concluded that their intervention yielded some clinical benefit in younger but not older patients. In this challenging blinding design, surgeons did not know which procedure would be done until they were in the operating room. The blinded participants assessed the primary outcome.

Blinding efforts can be arduous. The two examples of sham operations presented previously were useful to reduce bias, but they were difficult to implement. Particularly in surgery trials, investigators must go to extraordinary lengths to properly blind participants.[15] Too frequently, blinding challenges investigators; they become frustrated and shun proper blinding because of difficulties. In addition, they may excuse their lack of attention to proper blinding by claiming ethical problems. However, those claims ring hollow if they never made a diligent attempt.

As with all trials, surgery trials pass through clearance with ethical review boards (ERBs), sometimes called institutional review boards (IRBs). Certainly, trials involving sham operations face higher hurdles than pharmaceutical trials. ERBs balance the need for unnecessary comparative surgeries to reduce bias against the risks to participants. Criteria for use of sham surgery controls have been proposed:[16]

- Satisfy all the general standards for ethical conduct of clinical research.
- Assure that no reasonable alternative research design exists.
- Involve a procedure for minimising the risk–benefit ratio.
- Recruit a minimum sample size to answer the trial question.
- Establish an exceptionally vigilant, independent safety monitoring board.

When an investigator or ERB decide that sham surgery is not appropriate, then a less invasive sham procedure may be warranted. For example, in a trial of laparoscopic compared with open appendectomy, an analogous approach to a sham treatment was used, although it was probably not as effective: 'At the end of each procedure, 3 wound dressings and an abdominal binder were applied to every patient to blind the patient, the nursing and the medical staff, and the independent data collector as to the nature of the procedure'.[17] The investigators used placebo wound dressings that appeared identical and were equivalently applied. In this instance, however, greater risk for bias prevails in that the incisions were not similar. Hence examining under the wound dressing could reveal the operative method. Of note the authors term this a double-blind randomised trial. However, because the operators could not be blinded, this does not fit our definition of a double-blind trial.

IMPLEMENTATION ISSUES: ASSESSORS

Consideration should be given to blinding assessors in trials. The process involves an assessor (such as a research nurse) blinded to the intervention group of the participants, who determines the outcomes of those participants. In some trials, blinding of participants makes that easier. In other trials, such as the knee-surgery trial discussed previously, the potential blinding of assessors necessitates the blinding of participants. Yet often the assessors can be blinded even if the participants are not blinded. In a study of NPT trials, the 'methods reported for blinding outcome assessors relied mainly on centralized assessment of paraclinical examinations, clinical examinations (i.e., use of video, audiotape, photography), or adjudications of clinical events'.[7] Investigators should consider blinding the outcome assessor more frequently than currently happens.[1,2,9]

As an example, consider an HIV prevention, open-label randomised trial of two highly effective, reversible methods of contraception. Injectable depot medroxyprogesterone acetate (DMPA) would be compared with a copper IUD to evaluate whether DMPA increases the risk of acquiring HIV infection. Blinding the investigators and participants would be impossible. However, with the outcome being HIV seropositivity based on a blood sample, the assessor could be blinded to the intervention group of the participants and make the outcome determination based on a blinded reading of laboratory results. Even with this hard, laboratory outcome, blinding the assessor guards against any hint of bias, which includes fraudulent assessment. 'Investigators should . . . attempt to blind the outcome assessment whenever possible'.[18]

Blinding the assessor becomes much more important with subjective outcomes. If the outcome in the previous example had been some clinical assessment of disease status, then having the outcome assessor be blinded to the treatment group of the participants would be critical to eliminating as much bias as possible. This has been done, for example, by relying on assessment of outcomes 'by a blinded adjudication committee or a blinded assessment of the extract of the case report form'.[7]

Double Blinding: Participants, Investigators, and Assessors

Total blinding means that trial participants, investigators (including healthcare providers), and assessors (those collecting outcome data) all remain oblivious to the intervention assignments throughout the trial so that they will not be influenced by that knowledge.[2] Researchers usually use the terminology 'double blind' (or less appropriately 'double masked') synonymously with 'total blinding'. However, they inconsistently define their terms. When investigators examined physician interpretations and textbook definitions of double blinding, they found 17 unique interpretations and 9 different definitions.[5] In a different survey, investigators offered 15 diverse operative meanings of the term 'double blind'.[19] Given that three groups are involved, 'double-blind' appears misleading. In medical research, however, frequently an investigator also assesses, so in that instance the terminology refers to two individuals. When we use the term 'double-blind' or its derivatives in this chapter, we mean that steps have been taken to blind all three groups: participants, investigators, and assessors. We consider 'double blinding' to be synonymous with 'total blinding'.

Of note, we would not label a trial as double blinded if any two of those three categories were blinded. For example, if participants and investigators were blinded but assessors were not, we would not label that a double-blinded trial. Similarly, if participants and assessors were blinded but investigators were not, we would not label that a double-blinded trial. In this instance the proper label would be as a blinded trial with the specification that participants and assessors were blinded. In reporting randomised trials, we urge that authors explicitly state what steps were taken to keep whom blinded, as clearly stated in the CONSORT randomised trial reporting guidelines.[20,21]

Because most double blinding involves drugs, we mainly confine our comments to such instances. Vaccines and other medicinal interventions pertain to the broad category of drugs for this discussion. Placebos are generally used in double-blind trials, and for a further discussion of placebos, please refer to Chapter 16.

Hospital pharmacies and pharmaceutical companies provide support in blinding activities. Research pharmacists, in particular, may help and should be consulted early in the trial design process.[9] In the United States, drugs used in clinical research must be stored, prepared, and dispensed by research pharmacies.[22] Although the stated aim of this Joint Commission requirement is improving patient safety, this regulation often has a net negative effect on clinical research and patient care. We were recently involved with a trial comparing an injection of lidocaine versus saline placebo in fewer than 100 patients. The requirement for the pharmacy (rather than the treating physicians) to add lidocaine or saline to syringes added several thousands of dollars to the trial's cost and delayed each participant's care by at least 20 min.

IMPLEMENTATION ISSUES: IF NO EFFECTIVE TREATMENT EXISTS

When examining the effects of a proposed new treatment for a condition for which no effective treatment already exists, double blinding necessitates a placebo control group. This situation probably occurs most frequently, as placebo alone represented over half (52%) of the control groups in a study of drug trials that reported blinding.[23] For comparison, active control alone represented 23% of the control groups and placebo plus active control represented 23%.[23]

When no effective treatment exists, use of placebo control tends to yield the least complex implementation schemes. Operationally, the drug and placebo must be prepared identically, such as in capsules or pills, and packaged identically, such as in bottles or blister packs. They should appear, taste, and smell the same while also being administered identically. They should also weigh the same and yield the same sound if shaken. Examples comparing treatments with placebo from the medical literature can be found in Chapter 16.

IMPLEMENTATION ISSUES: IF AN ACCEPTED EFFECTIVE TREATMENT EXISTS

If an accepted effective treatment exists, sometimes ERBs or investigators determine that it should be administered to everyone enrolled in the trial. In that circumstance the trial compares the new treatment plus the accepted effective treatment versus the placebo plus the accepted effective treatment. All participants receive the effective treatment, with the participants allocated to the new treatment receiving the drug and those allocated to the control group receiving the placebo. In essence the actual double blinding issues resemble the same issues described previously when no accepted effective treatment exists (i.e., a comparison of treatment versus placebo).

Treatment blinding becomes more complicated in a trial if an accepted, effective treatment exists but is not administered to all participants. That effective treatment, and not a placebo, is usually used in the control group for comparison against the new treatment. Consequently, investigators evaluate two active treatments. In that situation, they typically entertain three options to double blind their trial.

First, they could acquire the drugs in prepared and prepackaged form such that the two treatments are indistinguishable, such as in tablets, capsules, or pills. Taste and smell should also be indistinguishable, as much as possible. Participants would merely ingest one standard-sized tablet, capsule, or pill.

Often, however, this approach poses production difficulties. A logical source for indistinguishable preparation and prepackaging would be the original pharmaceutical manufacturers. However, they rarely deliver their drugs in any form other than the customary formulations.[9] Besides, even if they or another manufacturer did, producing different formulations might cause government regulatory bodies (such as the US FDA) to raise objections as to the equivalent bioavailability of the created formulations, even with drugs with approved formulations.[24] Alleviating those objections likely entails more research, more expense, and more time. This indistinguishable preparation and packaging approach frequently represents challenging production obstacles.

Second, the customary formulation drugs could be encapsulated in a larger capsule. This eases some production worries but again might prompt equivalent bioavailability concerns.[9,24] That creates additional expense and delays. Additionally, although the participants would only take one capsule, it may be so bulky that swallowing it becomes difficult.[9] Besides, some encapsulation systems permit the participant to open the capsules, thus deciphering the treatments, which defeats blinding.[24] This encapsulation method still involves production complications, poses a compliance obstacle, and presents unblinding opportunities in some cases.

Nevertheless, some investigators use encapsulation. In the following example, the investigators describe circumventing appearance and weight problems by using a filler:

Medications were dispensed in blister packs indicating treatment day and time. Placebo and active medications were encapsulated in gel capsules with filler to give identical weight and appearance. Blinding could only be broken if a participant experienced treatment failure or an adverse event for which an acceptable alternative treatment could not be given and knowledge of the treatment assignment was needed for clinical care.[25]

Third, they could utilise a double-dummy (some call 'double-placebo') design in which participants take the allocated active drug and the placebo matched to the comparison drug. The double-dummy approach first appeared in the medical literature in 1964.[26,27] It was considered 'an important methodological legacy for tackling observer bias'.[27] The trial practice entails two active drugs and two corresponding placebos. For example, in comparing two drugs, one a blue tablet and the other a red capsule, the investigators would obtain blue placebo tablets and red placebo capsules. Participants in the treatment A group would take an active blue tablet and a placebo red capsule, while the participants in the treatment B group would take a placebo blue tablet and an active red capsule. This option safeguards the double blinding at a similar level as the first option and better than the second option. Unlike the other two options, however, it does not provoke equivalent bioavailability issues. Also, it does not entail additional production problems, delays, and costs. The only disadvantage tends to be that participants take more pills, which potentially could hurt enrolment or compliance. However, when examined, investigators found minimal effect on enrolment.[24] Practically, investigators should encounter fewer difficulties with double-dummy blinding. Overall, this may be the best of the three options when an effective treatment exists, and it is used frequently.[23] In a survey of methods of blinding in reports of randomised trials assessing pharmacological treatments, 23% reported the use of the double-dummy method.[23]

Implementation Issues: Challenging Double-Dummy Situations

Thus far, we have only addressed how the double-dummy technique addresses different appearing treatments. In addition, however, it can also address different dosing schedules. The following example involves comparing two different appearing treatments, but they also have vastly different dosing schedules:

> One tablet of the herbal combination contained 80 mg horseradish root powder and 200 mg nasturtium herb powder, produced by grinding of unmodified dried plants containing isothiocyanates as the active ingredients. The comparator (co-trimoxazole) consisted of a combination of 160 mg trimethoprim and 800 mg sulfamethoxazole per tablet. Placebo tablets were identical in appearance to the respective study drug. Since both drugs have different galenic properties and treatment durations, a double-dummy technique was used to maintain blinding. The phytotherapy group received five herbal combination tablets four times per day and one placebo comparator tablet two times per day for 7 days. The antibiotic group administered five placebo herbal combination tablets four times per day for 7 days and one active comparator tablet two times per day for 3 days. For the remaining 4 days, a placebo comparator tablet was used to maintain blinding.[28]

For simplicity of presentation, our discussions thus far have focused on drugs in capsule, pill, or tablet formulations. The concepts, however, extend easily to other formulations, such as intravenous fluids and ampoules administered through injections or intravenous fluids. The following example involves comparing two infusions:

> To maintain masking, each patient received two simultaneous infusions, one active and one placebo. The placebo infusion regimen was identical to its respective active counterpart.[29]

This double-dummy approach even extends to inhalers:

> Patients received either once-daily UMEC/VI 62.5/25 µg via ELLIPTA® dry powder inhaler (DPI; delivering 55/22 µg . . .) and once-daily placebo via HandiHaler® or once-daily TIO 18 µg (delivering 10 µg . . .) via the HandiHaler® and once-daily placebo via ELLIPTA® DPI for 12 weeks. As UMEC/VI and TIO are delivered via different inhaler devices; a double-dummy design was used for dosing, where patients received two inhalers, one containing active drug and the other placebo.[30]

Moreover, the double-dummy technique applies to mixtures of these formulations. The following example represents a mixture of an intravenous treatment and a tablet treatment:

> Patients who were randomized to treatment with IV etelcalcetide and oral placebo received thrice weekly IV doses of etelcalcetide at the end of each hemodialysis session and daily oral doses of placebo tablets. Patients who were randomized to treatment with oral cinacalcet and IV placebo received daily oral doses of cinacalcet tablets, and thrice weekly IV doses of placebo at the end of each hemodialysis session. The IV study drug was administered via bolus injection into the venous line of the dialysis circuit, immediately prior to or during rinse-back after each hemodialysis session for 26 weeks.[31]

The Importance of Placebos

The use of placebos tends to be criticised. Unfortunately, some of those criticisms are unjustified. Placebos are inappropriately blamed for investigators using a placebo (inactive) treatment control group when ethically an active treatment control group should be used. Improper trial design should be blamed, not the placebo itself.[32] Indeed, we believe if an effective treatment is available, then ethically, practically, and scientifically, it should represent the control group or, alternatively, be administered to all participants. Yet scientists debate the roles of placebo-controlled trials and active-controlled trials in medicine.[33,34]

Placebos prove scientifically crucial, regardless of whether the control group is active or inactive. Placebos usually enable double blinding in randomised trials. In trials with a control group receiving no active treatment, placebos are needed for double blinding, which matches the customary pattern of placebo usage. However, as discussed previously, placebos often are obligatory if a trial compares two or more active treatments. If those treatments differ—for example, in shape, size, weight, taste, or colour—the double-dummy procedure, which uses two placebos, becomes necessary to satisfy methodological and production concerns.

Conclusion

For many NPTs, double blinding (total blinding) proves impossible. Most often, those treatments involve surgery or a medical device. Investigators should consider single blinding, which may involve sham surgery or some other sham procedure. If healthcare personnel and participants cannot be blinded, investigators should at least consider blinding the outcome assessor. That should be done more frequently than currently happens.

Most double blinding involves drugs. When an effective standard treatment exists, ERBs or investigators may determine that it should be administered to all participants. Otherwise, it is usually used in the control group for comparison against a new treatment. Thus trialists compare two active treatments. In that circumstance, they typically entertain three options to double blind their trial. They could obtain the drugs in raw form and prepackage the two drugs equally, encapsulate the two standard formulation drugs in a larger capsule, or utilise a double-dummy approach. Practically, investigators should encounter fewer difficulties with the simpler double-dummy, double-blinding approach. Often, it emerges as the best option.

References

1. Schulz, K.F., Grimes, D.A., 2002. Blinding in randomised trials: hiding who got what. Lancet 359, 696–700.
2. Schulz, K.F., Chalmers, I., Altman, D.G., 2002. The landscape and lexicon of blinding in randomized trials. Ann. Intern. Med. 136, 254–259.
3. Schulz, K.F., Chalmers, I., Hayes, R.J., Altman, D.G., 1995. Empirical evidence of bias. Dimensions of methodological quality associated with estimates of treatment effects in controlled trials. JAMA 273, 408–412.
4. Savovic, J., Jones, H.E., Altman, D.G., et al., 2012. Influence of reported study design characteristics on intervention effect estimates from randomized, controlled trials. Ann. Intern. Med. 157, 429–438.
5. Devereaux, P.J., Manns, B.J., Ghali, W.A., et al., 2001. Physician interpretations and textbook definitions of blinding terminology in randomized controlled trials. JAMA 285, 2000–2003.
6. Meinert, C., 1986. Clinical Trials: Design, Conduct, and Analysis. New York: Oxford University Press.
7. Boutron, I., Guittet, L., Estellat, C., Moher, D., Hrobjartsson, A., Ravaud, P., 2007. Reporting methods of blinding in randomized trials assessing nonpharmacological treatments. PLoS Med 4, e61.
8. Boutron, I., Altman, D.G., Moher, D., Schulz, K.F., Ravaud, P., 2017. CONSORT statement for randomized trials of nonpharmacologic treatments: a 2017 update and a CONSORT extension for nonpharmacologic trial abstracts. Ann. Intern. Med. 167, 40–47.
9. Wan, M., Orlu-Gul, M., Legay, H., Tuleu, C., 2013. Blinding in pharmacological trials: the devil is in the details. Arch. Dis. Child. 98, 656.
10. Heazell, A., Thorneycroft, J., Walton, V., Etherington, I., 2006. Acupressure for the in-patient treatment of nausea and vomiting in early pregnancy: a randomized control trial. Am. J. Obstet. Gynecol. 194, 815–820.

11. Renner, R.M., Nichols, M.D., Jensen, J.T., Li, H., Edelman, A.B., 2012. Paracervical block for pain control in first-trimester surgical abortion: a randomized controlled trial. Obstet. Gynecol. 119, 1030–1037.

12. Miller, L., Jensen, M.P., Stenchever, M.A., 1996. A double-blind randomized comparison of lidocaine and saline for cervical anesthesia. Obstet. Gynecol. 87, 600–604.

13. Moseley, J.B., O'Malley, K., Petersen, N.J., et al., 2002. A controlled trial of arthroscopic surgery for osteoarthritis of the knee. N. Engl. J. Med. 347, 81–88.

14. Freed, C.R., Greene, P.E., Breeze, R.E., et al., 2001. Transplantation of embryonic dopamine neurons for severe Parkinson's disease. N. Engl. J. Med. 344, 710–719.

15. Ergina, P.L., Cook, J.A., Blazeby, J.M., et al., 2009. Challenges in evaluating surgical innovation. Lancet 374, 1097–1104.

16. Albin, R.L., 2002. Sham surgery controls: intracerebral grafting of fetal tissue for Parkinson's disease and proposed criteria for use of sham surgery controls. J. Med. Ethics 28, 322–325.

17. Katkhouda, N., Mason, R.J., Towfigh, S., Gevorgyan, A., Essani, R., 2005. Laparoscopic versus open appendectomy: a prospective randomized double-blind study. Ann. Surg. 242, 439–448; discussion 48–50.

18. Poolman, R.W., Struijs, P.A., Krips, R., et al., 2007. Reporting of outcomes in orthopaedic randomized trials: does blinding of outcome assessors matter? J. Bone Joint Surg. Am. 89, 550–558.

19. Haahr, M.T., Hrobjartsson, A., 2006. Who is blinded in randomized clinical trials? A study of 200 trials and a survey of authors. Clin. Trials 3, 360–365.

20. Schulz, K.F., Altman, D.G., Moher, D., 2010. CONSORT 2010 statement: updated guidelines for reporting parallel group randomised trials. BMJ 340, c332.

21. Moher, D., Hopewell, S., Schulz, K.F., et al., 2010. CONSORT 2010 explanation and elaboration: updated guidelines for reporting parallel group randomised trials. J. Clin. Epidemiol. 63, e1–e37.

22. Rich, D.S., 2004. New JCAHO medication management standards for 2004. Am. J. Health Syst. Pharm. 61, 1349–1358.

23. Boutron, I., Estellat, C., Guittet, L., et al., 2006. Methods of blinding in reports of randomized controlled trials assessing pharmacologic treatments: a systematic review. PLoS Med. 3, e425.

24. Martin, B.K., Meinert, C.L., Breitner, J.C., 2002. Double placebo design in a prevention trial for Alzheimer's disease. Control. Clin. Trials 23, 93–99.

25. Moran, G.J., Krishnadasan, A., Mower, W.R., et al., 2017. Effect of cephalexin plus trimethoprim-sulfamethoxazole vs cephalexin alone on clinical cure of uncomplicated cellulitis: a randomized clinical trial. JAMA 317, 2088–2096.

26. Percy, J.S., Stephenson, P., Thompson, M., 1964. Indomethacin in the treatment of rheumatic diseases. Ann. Rheum. Dis. 23, 226–231.

27. Marusic, A., Ferencic, S.F., 2013. Adoption of the double dummy trial design to reduce observer bias in testing treatments. J. R. Soc. Med. 106, 196–198.

28. Stange, R., Schneider, B., Albrecht, U., Mueller, V., Schnitker, J., Michalsen, A., 2017. Results of a randomized, prospective, double-dummy, double-blind trial to compare efficacy and safety of a herbal combination containing Tropaeoli majoris herba and Armoraciae rusticanae radix with co-trimoxazole in patients with acute and uncomplicated cystitis. Res. Rep. Urol. 9, 43–50.

29. Follath, F., Cleland, J.G., Just, H., et al., 2002. Efficacy and safety of intravenous levosimendan compared with dobutamine in severe low-output heart failure (the LIDO study): a randomised double-blind trial. Lancet 360, 196–202.

30. Kerwin, E.M., Kalberg, C.J., Galkin, D.V., et al., 2017. Umeclidinium/vilanterol as step-up therapy from tiotropium in patients with moderate COPD: a randomized, parallel-group, 12-week study. Int. J. Chron. Obstruct. Pulmon. Dis. 12, 745–755.

31. Block, G.A., Bushinsky, D.A., Cheng, S., et al., 2017. Effect of etelcalcetide vs cinacalcet on serum parathyroid hormone in patients receiving hemodialysis with secondary hyperparathyroidism: a randomized clinical trial. JAMA 317, 156–164.

32. Senn, S., 2009. Placebo misconceptions. Am. J. Bioeth. 9, 53–54.

33. Howick, J., 2009. Questioning the methodologic superiority of 'placebo' over 'active' controlled trials. Am. J. Bioeth. 9, 34–48.

34. Miller, F.G., 2009. The rationale for placebo-controlled trials: methodology and policy considerations. Am. J. Bioeth. 9, 49–50.

CHAPTER 18

Surrogate Endpoints and Composite Outcomes: Shortcuts to Unknown Destinations

Clinical research should focus on outcomes that matter. For many reasons, that is often not the case. As the health of the population has improved, serious morbidity such as strokes has declined in frequency, and longevity has improved. Although great news for public health, this poses a growing challenge for researchers who now have fewer events to study. Prospective studies with sufficient power to find clinically important differences need to be larger, longer, or both than previously. Moreover, the pressure for regulatory bodies, such as the US Food and Drug Administration, to approve new products is relentless, given the huge economic implications for pharmaceutical companies.

In response to these problems, two workarounds have become common in clinical research: surrogate endpoints and composite endpoints. In this chapter we will review these two alternatives, discuss their advantages and disadvantages, describe some notorious examples, and generally advise against their use.

What is a Surrogate Endpoint?

As its name implies, a surrogate endpoint is a proxy or substitute for a clinical outcome of importance. Some synonyms include 'intermediate measures' and 'surrogate markers'. These endpoints are usually biological processes measured with laboratory tests of blood or body fluids or imaging studies thought to be along the causal pathway to illness.[1] Regrettably, the pathway is often a parallel track not causally involved. Examples of common surrogate endpoints include intraocular pressure as a surrogate outcome for vision loss in glaucoma[2] or blood pressure as a surrogate for myocardial infarction or stroke. In nephrology, declining glomerular filtration rate or rising creatinine or proteinuria serve as surrogates for kidney failure.[3]

Advantages of Surrogate Endpoints

Surrogate endpoints have enormous appeal to researchers conducting randomised controlled trials because of their efficiency. Rather than waiting for years to accrue sufficient numbers of clinical events (e.g., fracture, stroke, or death), the researcher can quickly and cheaply get an answer by focusing instead on a laboratory test or imaging study. Keeping trials short helps to minimise losses to follow-up and deviations from the assigned treatment. Another rationale for using surrogate endpoints is that the clinical endpoint of interest may be so expensive, invasive, or painful that a surrogate is deemed more acceptable to participants. Clinicians tend to be comfortable with surrogate endpoints, such as haemoglobin A_{1c}, which are part of routine care; short-term effects of treatment are readily observable, as opposed to late complications of diabetes. Another seductive appeal is that surrogate endpoints can give clinicians a sense of mastery over how a treatment should influence disease process.[4] As discussed later, this reassurance is often unwarranted.

Disadavantages of Surrogate Endpoints

Surrogate endpoints may not measure what is intended. Some surrogate endpoints provide ambiguous results, waste resources, and lead clinicians astray.[5] More importantly, changes in surrogate endpoints may not translate into clinical benefit.[2] Indeed, sometimes use of surrogate endpoints for clinical decisions inadvertently harms patients.

The danger of using cardiovascular drugs approved on the basis of benefit on surrogate endpoints has been well documented (Panel 18.1). In each of these examples, the drug was approved using surrogate endpoints; later studies with true clinical endpoints found that they had a paradoxical effect on survival.[4] The most notorious example was the wide use of antiarrhythmic drugs to suppress ventricular irritability after an acute myocardial infarction. This was anticipated to reduce the risk of sudden cardiac death. Indeed, drugs such an encainide and flecainide nicely suppressed premature ventricular contractions—but tripled the risk of death through unknown mechanisms.[5] More than 200,000 patients in the United States received these drugs in clinical practice, and many thousands died needlessly as a result of poor science. Poor-quality research is unethical, because it misleads clinicians and hurts patients.[6,7]

Another infamous example is the use of fluorides to treat osteoporosis. A randomised trial compared fluoride with placebo and observed the anticipated 35% increase in bone mineral density. Those given fluoride, however, had a paradoxical increase in both vertebral and nonvertebral fractures. Bones became denser but apparently more brittle.[5] Bone mineral density measures only one characteristic of bone health: bone quantity, not bone quality (the living biomatrix).

In 2004, the US Food and Drug Administration (FDA) placed a black box warning on labelling of depo-medroxyprogesterone acetate (DMPA) injections for contraception for more than 2 years of use (Fig. 18.1). A 'black box' is the most serious warning from the FDA, usually reserved for potentially life-threatening adverse effects of a drug. To our knowledge, DMPA is the only modern contraceptive never linked to a death. The warning was based on the transient effect of DMPA on bone mineral density, similar to that with breastfeeding. As in the previous fluoride example, bone mineral density was known not to be a valid predictor of fracture.[8] In response to the FDA's alarmist labelling, some gynaecologists started ordering bone mineral density tests for teenagers and began prescribing them supplemental oestrogen and bisphosphonates.[9] In contrast, the World Health Organization recommends no restrictions on DMPA for contraception (Fig. 18.2).[10] The FDA's black box warning based on an invalid surrogate endpoint has been widely criticised as not evidence-based.[11-13]

Rosiglitazone reached the market based on its lowering of haemoglobin A_{1c} in patients with type 2 diabetes; subsequent studies revealed the drug was associated with a modest increase in the risk of myocardial infarction and death from cardiovascular disease.[14] This discovery (and a subsequent

---

PANEL 18.1 ■ Examples of Drugs Approved for Use Based on Surrogate Endpoints but Later Found to Increase the Risk of Death[4]

Drug	Indication	Surrogate Endpoint
Aprotinin	High-risk cardiac surgery	Decreased need for blood transfusion
Clofibrate	Hypercholesterolaemia in healthy men	Decreased serum cholesterol
Encainide, flecainide	Ventricular irritability after myocardial infarction	Fewer premature ventricular contractions
Erythropoietin	Anaemia from chronic renal failure	Increased haemoglobin level
Flosequinan	Chronic congestive heart failure	Improved ventricular function
Ibopamine	Severe congestive heart failure	Increased exercise tolerance, decreased vascular resistance
Milrinone	Severe congestive heart failure	Increased cardiac contractility
Metoprolol	Noncardiac surgery in patients at cardiovascular risk	Decreased postoperative myocardial ischemia
Moxonidine	Congestive heart failure	Decreased plasma norepinephrine

---

Physician Information

WARNING: LOSS OF BONE MINERAL DENSITY

See full prescribing information for complete boxed warning.

Women who use Depo-Provera Contraceptive Injection (Depo-Provera CI) may lose significant bone mineral density. Bone loss is greater with increasing duration of use and may not be completely reversible.

It is unknown if use of Depo-Provera Contraceptive Injection during adolescence or early adulthood, a critical period of bone accretion, will reduce peak bone mass and increase the risk for osteoporotic fracture in later life.

Depo-Provera Contraceptive Injection should not be used as a long-term birth control method (i.e., longer than 2 years) unless other birth control methods are considered inadequate.

Fig. 18.1 USPI boxed warning for Depo-Provera CI (medroxyprogesterone acetate injection, suspension) as of December, 2017 used with the permission of Pfizer.

With regard to bone density and hormonal contraception, the World Health Organization recommends:

- Women aged 18-45 should be able to use DMPA (and other progestin-only injectables) without any limits.

Fig. 18.2 World Health Organization statement on depo-medroxyprogesterone and bone health. (Reproduced with permission of the World Health Organization.)

black box warning from the FDA) had a chilling effect on its use.[15,16] A trial of the effect of tighter control of type 2 diabetes found that reducing this surrogate endpoint led to a paradoxical increase in deaths through other mechanisms.[17]

The FDA continues to use surrogate endpoints inappropriately.[5] Multiple drug-resistant tuberculosis is a deadly infection, and the need for novel treatments is acute. In 2012 the FDA approved a new type of drug, bedaquiline, based on its effect on a surrogate endpoint of unknown validity: conversion of the patient's sputum culture from positive to negative for *Mycobacterium tuberculosis*. Instead of requiring large trials of clinical efficacy, the drug approval was based on two modest-sized trials of 47 and 161 patients, and the effect on sputum culture was not dramatic. What was dramatic was the paradoxical five fold increase in death among those who received the new drug.[15] Here the surrogate endpoint (sputum culture) trumped the true endpoint (death) for unknown reasons.[18] Nonetheless, the drug was approved despite being more lethal.

Validation of Surrogate Endpoints

As cautioned by Fleming and DeMets, 'A correlate does not a surrogate make'.[19] Decades after this warning, clinicians, researchers, and drug regulators remain largely unaware of this distinction. Two criteria must be met to validate a surrogate endpoint. First, the surrogate must correlate with the true clinical endpoint. This criterion is generally met. Second, the surrogate must fully capture the effect of the treatment on the true clinical endpoint of interest. Sadly, this criterion is almost never satisfied. To meet both criteria requires at least one prospective study using both the surrogate and true endpoints. Avoiding such a large, expensive, and time-consuming study is the rationale for using surrogates in the first place. Hence such studies are rarely done.[5]

This two-step approach to validation[20] has been challenged in recent years. As an alternative, sophisticated approaches are now being considered.[21] Meta-analysis of the literature is being considered. However, aggregation of incomplete information cannot plug the gaps.[4] Empirical evidence of validity is still needed.

A small number of surrogate endpoints have been established as valid. For patients infected with HIV, viral RNA load has been shown through several confirmatory trials with different drugs to capture the effect of treatment on disease progression and death. Other examples include haemoglobin A_{1c} as a surrogate for microvascular complications of diabetes and low-density lipoprotein cholesterol lowering as a surrogate for cardiovascular disease concerning statins.

Terminological Tangles

Terms used to describe surrogate endpoints, risk markers, and biomarkers are inconsistent and confusing. In an attempt to provide greater clarity, the National Institutes of Health promulgated suggested terminology in 2001.[22,23] Next, the Institute of Medicine (now National Academy of Medicine) weighed in with a scholarly tome of more than 300 pages.[24] More recently, the FDA and the NIH took another stab at nomenclature with a regulatory focus; it had an obligatory acronym: BEST (**B**iomarkers **E**ndpoint**S**, and other **T**ools) Resource.[25]

In the glossary of this document, surrogate endpoints are ranked by their credibility (Panel 18.2).

PANEL 18.2 ■ Suggested Definitions for Endpoints From the Food and Drug Administration and National Institutes of Health, 2016[26]

Endpoint

A precisely defined variable intended to reflect an outcome of interest that is statistically analyzed to address a particular research question. A precise definition of an endpoint typically specifies the type of assessments made, the timing of those assessments, the assessment tools used, and possibly other details, as applicable, such as how multiple assessments within an individual are to be combined.

> **PANEL 18.2 ■ Suggested Definitions for Endpoints From the Food and Drug Administration and National Institutes of Health, 2016** (Continued)
>
> ### Clinical Endpoint
>
> *A characteristic or variable that reflects how a patient [or consumer] feels, functions, or survives. Example: death.*
>
> ### Intermediate Clinical Endpoint
>
> *In a regulatory context, an endpoint measuring a clinical outcome that can be measured earlier than an effect on irreversible morbidity or mortality (IMM) and that is considered reasonably likely to predict the medical product's effect on IMM or other clinical benefit. The intermediate clinical endpoint may be a basis for full approval if the effect on the endpoint is considered clinically meaningful. It may also be a basis for accelerated approval if the IMM effect is considered critical for use of the drug or for expedited access for medical devices intended for unmet medical need for life threatening or irreversibly debilitating diseases or conditions.*
>
> *Example: Exercise tolerance has been used as an intermediate clinical endpoint in trials of device treatments for heart failure.*
>
> *Example: A treatment for preterm labor was approved based on a demonstration of delay in delivery. Under accelerated approval, the sponsor was required to conduct postmarketing studies to demonstrate improved long-term postnatal outcomes.*
>
> ### Surrogate Endpoint
>
> *An endpoint that is used in clinical trials as a substitute for a direct measure of how a patient feels, functions, or survives. A surrogate endpoint does not measure the clinical benefit of primary interest in and of itself, but rather is expected to predict that clinical benefit or harm based on epidemiologic, therapeutic, pathophysiologic, or other scientific evidence.*
>
> *From a U.S. regulatory standpoint, surrogate endpoints and potential surrogate endpoints can be characterized by the level of clinical validation:*
>
> ### Validated Surrogate Endpoint
>
> *An endpoint supported by a clear mechanistic rationale and clinical data providing strong evidence that an effect on the surrogate endpoint predicts a clinical benefit. Therefore, it can be used to support traditional approval without the need for additional efficacy information.*
>
> *Example: Hemoglobin A_{1c} (HbA_{1c}) reduction is a validated surrogate endpoint for reduction of microvascular complications associated with diabetes mellitus and has been used for the basis for approval of drugs intended to treat diabetes mellitus.*
>
> *Example: HIV-RNA reduction is a validated surrogate endpoint for human immunodeficiency virus (HIV) clinical disease control and has been used for the basis for approval of drugs intended to treat HIV.*
>
> *Example: Low-density lipoprotein (LDL) cholesterol reduction is a validated surrogate endpoint for reduction of cardiovascular events and has been used for the basis for approval of statins.*
>
> *Example: Blood pressure reduction is a validated surrogate endpoint for reduction in rates of stroke, myocardial infarction, and mortality and has been used for the basis for the approval of drugs intended to treat hypertension.*
>
> ### Reasonably Likely Surrogate Endpoint
>
> *An endpoint supported by clear mechanistic and/or epidemiologic rationale but insufficient clinical data to show that it is a validated surrogate endpoint. Such endpoints can be used for accelerated approval for drugs or expedited access for medical devices. In the case of accelerated approval for drugs, additional trial data, assessing the effect of the intervention on the clinical benefit endpoint of interest will be collected in the post-marketing setting to verify whether an effect on the reasonably likely surrogate actually predicts clinical benefit in the specific context under study.*
>
> *Example: Outcomes of 6-month follow-up treatment (i.e., sputum culture status and infection relapse rate) have been considered reasonably likely to predict the resolution of pulmonary tuberculosis and have supported accelerated approval of drugs to treat tuberculosis.*
>
> ### Candidate Surrogate Endpoint
>
> *An endpoint still under evaluation for its ability to predict clinical benefit.*

Apart from the immodest acronym, the BEST guidelines will strike some as self-serving. Under the heading 'reasonably likely' is the approval of a drug (presumably bedaquiline) based on sputum culture despite a paradoxical increased risk of death.[15,18] This approval remains puzzling.

Levels of Evidence

We have previously suggested three levels of scientific credibility for surrogate endpoints.[27] The first is science, the systematic knowledge of the world around us based on observation and experiment. The second is protoscience, which can be thought of as nascent science. Its theories and applications are based on scientific principles, including testability, but the theories have not been subjected to scrutiny. The theory of plate tectonics subsequently was confirmed by study of its mechanisms. The protoscience of alchemy led to the science of chemistry, and astrology led to astronomy.

The bottom of the hierarchy is pseudoscience. It does not adhere to scientific theories and empirical testing; instead, it relies on beliefs—often strongly held. Just as protoscience can ascend to science, it can also decline into pseudoscience. Although alchemy spawned the science of chemistry, no one today would suggest that base metals can be transformed into gold. Despite the popularity of astrology columns, no scientist would support the notion that star signs influence human events.[28]

Fleming and Powers[1] have categorised surrogate endpoints in four strata according to scientific credibility (Panel 18.3). Level 1 includes true clinical events of importance. Levels 2 to 4 are all surrogate endpoints with progressively less-established validity. Of note, only level 2 surrogates have been validated. Level 4 endpoints should be avoided in clinical trials designed to establish efficacy.

PANEL 18.3 ■ Categorisation of Outcome Measures, According to Level of Evidence Regarding Efficacy

Composite endpoints will be denoted by brackets.
Level 1 *A true clinical efficacy measure*
(*When evidence establishing risk is acceptable in the context of evidence of benefit*)
 _ Death
 _ [Death or hospitalisation], in heart failure
 _ [Death, lung transplantation, or hospitalisation for pulmonary arterial hypertension] in PAH
 _ [Cardiovascular death, stroke, or symptomatic myocardial infarction] in acute coronary syndrome
 _ [Stroke or systemic embolic event], in atrial fibrillation
 _ Progression to EDSS 7 (i.e., becoming wheelchair bound), in multiple sclerosis
 _ 15-letter loss in best corrected visual acuity, in age-related macular degeneration
 _ [Cough, dyspnoea, chest pain, or fever (if defined as symptomatic warmth and chills)],
    in community-acquired bacterial pneumonia
 _ Pain or loss of joint function, in osteoarthritis or rheumatoid arthritis
 _ Symptomatic bone fractures
 _ Pain in the area of skin lesions, in acute bacterial skin and skin structure infections
Level 2 *A validated surrogate (for a specific disease setting and class of interventions)*
(*When interventions are safe, with strong evidence that risks from off-target effects are acceptable*)
 _ HbA1c for clinical effects on long-term risk of microvascular complications, in T2DM
 _ [Death or cancer recurrence], in adjuvant colorectal cancer, with 5-fluorouracil-based regimens
 _ Systolic and diastolic blood pressure, in multiple classes of antihypertensives
 _ >40 m improvements in 6-min walk distance, in pulmonary arterial hypertension
 _ HIV infection, if the mechanisms of the HIV prevention intervention only reduce susceptibility
    rather than affecting disease progression or infectiousness should infection occur

---

PANEL 18.3 ■ Categorisation of Outcome Measures, According to Level of Evidence Regarding Efficacy (Continued)

Level 3 *A nonvalidated surrogate, yet one established to be 'reasonably likely to predict clinical benefit' (for a specific disease setting and class of interventions)*
(When interventions are safe, with evidence that risks from off-target effects are acceptable)
  _ Large and durable effects on viral load, in some treatment of HIV-infection settings
  _ Durable complete responses, in some hematologic oncology settings
  _ Large effects on progression-free survival, in some solid-tumour oncology settings
Level 4 *A correlate that is a measure of biological activity but not established to be at a higher level*
  _ CD-4, in HIV-infected patients
  _ Fever (if defined as elevated body temperature), in community-acquired bacterial pneumonia
  _ Decolonisation of VRE, in the gastrointestinal tract to prevent VRE bacteremia
  _ Decolonisation of *Staphylococcus aureus*, in preventing wound or bloodstream infections
  _ Hematocrit levels, in chemotherapy-induced anaemia or in end-stage renal disease
  _ Antibody levels and cell-mediated immune responses, in vaccines for prevention of HIV
  _ Urine GAG and urine KS, in rare-disease settings such as MPS-I, MPS-II, and MPS-IV
  _ PSA levels or prostate cancer biopsy, in prevention of prostate cancer symptoms or death
  _ Detecting asymptomatic ulcers on endoscopy, in prevention of symptomatic ulcers
  _ FEV-1 and FVC, in pulmonary diseases
  _ Silent myocardial infarction, in cardiovascular disease
  _ Asymptomatic fracture rate, in prevention of symptomatic disease
  _ Negative cultures and polymerase chain reaction tests, in treating various infectious diseases

---

EDSS, expanded disability status scale score; T2DM, type 2 diabetes mellitus; VRE, vancomycin resistant enterococci; PSA, prostate specific antigen; FEV-1, forced expiratory volume in 1 second; FVC, forced vital capacity; MPS, mucopolysaccharidosis; GAG, glycosaminoglycans; KS, keratan sulphate
Source: Fleming and Powers[1]

The Way Forward

Surrogate endpoints have a limited role in clinical research. Making clinical decisions based on unproved surrogate endpoints, whether drug regulatory approval or treatment choices, is unscientific and sometimes deadly.[5] As pointed out decades ago, clinical hunches without the check of formal scientific controls have proven to be a highly fallible compass. For diseases that slowly progress but are always lethal, such as amyotrophic lateral sclerosis, surrogate endpoints may be a reasonable option.[4] For rare diseases in which adequate sample sizes cannot be achieved, surrogate endpoints might be used, provided strong caveats are included about interpretation. In most circumstances, trials should focus on outcomes that matter.

Research using unproved surrogate endpoints is unethical for other reasons. The literature is replete with hundreds of thousands of reports on surrogate markers of unknown validity. At the time of this writing, more than 1800 reports in PubMed have studied 'oral contraception' and 'coagulation'. After this huge wasted effort, consensus exists: no coagulation test predicts which woman will suffer a rare, serious event such as venous thromboembolism.[29] This dead horse requires no further flogging, and regulatory bodies should stop requesting coagulation studies that are not predictive of anything. Because a finite amount of money and resources is available for research, every study that leads to a result incapable of interpretation has a net negative effect on health. Researchers have a fiduciary responsibility to society.

Composite Outcomes

Like surrogate endpoints, composite outcomes are usually a poor solution to the problem of inadequate statistical power. A composite outcome is a single outcome with two or more components; if a participant experiences one or more of the components, then he or she has the composite outcome.[30] By lumping individual outcomes into a composite, the number of outcome events rises—along with power. This approach is widely used in cardiovascular trials,[31] HIV trials,[32] and to a lesser extent, in other areas of research.[33] In cardiovascular research, many trials have examined the effects of drugs on several outcomes termed 'MACE' (major adverse cardiac events). These can include myocardial infarction (both lethal and not), stroke, and death.

The aggregation of outcomes into a composite is predicated on several assumptions, often not met. The components should be equal in seriousness, their frequencies should be similar, the direction of the effect for components should be consistent, and the components should have similar importance to participants.[31,34] When these criteria are not fulfilled, clinical interpretation of trial results can be difficult. A trial may have better precision stemming from larger numbers of events, but better precision offers little benefit when the target is fuzzy.

Advantages of Composite Outcomes

Composite outcomes have several appealing features. The overriding benefit is statistical efficiency; as the number of outcome events increases, the requisite sample size decreases, thus saving money and time. The relationship between sample size and power is not linear, however, as noted in Chapter 11. Assume that a trial wanted to show a 25% reduction in a serious adverse event with a frequency of 5%. With 80% power and an alpha of 0.05, more than 8000 patients would be needed (because of the infrequency of the event). To look for the same percent reduction with a frequency of 20% would require far fewer participants.[34] Efficiency results.

Use of a composite outcome obviates the need for statistical adjustment for multiple testing (Chapter 19). When many statistical tests are done, the possibility of alpha errors (false positives) increases. A composite outcome may reflect net benefit or harm to the participant. A prerequisite here is that all the components are deemed of equal importance. Finally, use of composite outcome may avoid arbitrary choices about what should be primary and secondary outcomes. If all components are deemed equally important, then all weigh equally in the composite outcome.[35]

Another potential advantage is avoiding misinterpretation of results stemming from competing risks. For example, reduction in the frequency of component A may stem from an increase in frequency of component B, which renders A impossible.[36] Competing risks are a common concern in cardiovascular trials. Assume that nonfatal myocardial infarction is the focus of a new drug trial. If the mortality rate associated with the new drug is higher than with the standard drug, fewer participants receiving the new drug will remain alive and at risk of nonfatal infarction. Thus one might incorrectly conclude that the new drug reduces the risk of nonfatal infarction because of the competing risk of death.[37]

A famous obstetrical trial examined the neuroprotective effect of intravenous magnesium sulphate given when preterm birth was anticipated.[38] One of the primary outcomes was a composite: death or cerebral palsy at age two years. The researchers were criticised for having combined components with such disparate 'economic, social, or clinical values'. The authors tactfully pointed out that a child cannot have motor dysfunction at age two if he or she is already dead.[33] Because magnesium was associated with a reduction in cerebral palsy, the researchers needed to exclude the possibility that the reduction in cerebral palsy was due to more deaths among those having received magnesium.

Disadvantages of Composite Outcomes

Composite outcomes have important limitations. The interpretation of results can be difficult if the components have differing importance to participants (qualitative heterogeneity).[37] What would a participant conclude if a drug lowered the risk of myocardial infarction while raising the risk of stroke? In another example, assume that a cardiovascular trial composite outcome included 'death or cerebral haemorrhage, or presence of new pathology Q waves in the electrocardiogram'. How would the trial be interpreted if treatment dramatically lowered the number of participants with electrocardiogram abnormalities, modestly increased strokes, and had negligible effect on death?[39] Is this drug an improvement over traditional therapy? Confusion can result when components include true clinical endpoints and surrogate endpoints lacking validation.

Some trials mislead readers when heterogeneity exists between components of different seriousness. In the DREAM trial,[40] more than 5000 participants with glucose intolerance but without cardiovascular disease were randomised to receive either rosiglitazone or placebo (Panel 18.4).

The first paragraph of the report's discussion section began this way:

This large, prospective, blinded international clinical trial shows that 8 mg of rosiglitazone daily, together with lifestyle recommendations, substantially reduces the risk of diabetes or death by 60% in individuals at high risk for diabetes.[40]

Casual readers could easily infer a 60% reduction in the risk of death, a remarkable benefit. As Panel 18.4 reveals, however, this composite outcome was driven almost entirely be the reduction in new diabetes; the effect on death was negligible. Interpretation can be challenging if the frequencies of events or relative risks for components differ (quantitative heterogeneity). Treatment effects in opposite directions render a composite outcome uninformative about the various components.

Composite outcomes must be prespecified in the study protocol.[37] Sometimes composite outcomes are cobbled together during the analysis in pursuit of statistical significance.[41] If none of the planned primary outcome measures reaches statistical significance, lumping together several outcomes can nudge a trial into the zone of statistical significance.[36] Readers should ignore reports with *post hoc* composite outcome generation. These researchers may be 'torturing the data until they speak'. This sort of cherry-picking is both inappropriate and misleading.[30]

Determining sample sizes still can be challenging. What is a clinically important difference in a composite outcome when the components vary in effect or in the direction of treatment effect? A related problem is that common, minor components, such as hospitalisation, contribute more to the composite than do the less common, more serious components such as death. The serious and highly rated outcomes contribute the least numerically toward the composite outcome because of their rarity.[36] The treatment effect on the minor event can overwhelm the effect on the more serious (Panel 18.4).

PANEL 18.4 ■ Composite and Component Outcomes in Trial of Rosiglitazone for Participants With Glucose Intolerance[40]

	Percent With Outcome		
Outcome	Rosiglitazone	Placebo	Hazard Ratio (95% CI)
Composite (incident diabetes or death)	11.6	26	0.4 (0.35–0.46)
Incident diabetes	10.6	25	0.38 (0.33–0.44)
Death	1.1	1.3	0.9 (0.55–1.5)

Composite outcomes can mislead. A new drug that led to fewer hospitalisations but more deaths might be viewed as superior to traditional therapy, thanks to the reduced composite outcome frequency compared with traditional treatment. Given the choice, most of us would prefer to be in a hospital bed than in a coffin. Stated alternatively, the relative risk for the composite outcome is more representative of the effect on the minor, more common outcomes.[34] To avoid this problem, any report with composite outcomes needs to provide outcome frequencies for each component as well.[35]

Composite Outcomes in Contemporary Research

Surveys have assessed the contemporary use of composite outcomes in clinical research; the results were not encouraging. Lim and associates surveyed all two-group randomised controlled trials that used a composite outcome in a sample of journals from 2000 to 2007.[42] In these 304 reports, the median number of components was three. The smaller the trial, the larger was the number of components in the composite outcome to boost the number of events (suspicions confirmed). Linear regression indicated that for each component added to the composite, the trial had 721 fewer participants. The distribution of composite outcome p values was asymmetrical; more than expected fell below the threshold of 0.05. This suggests either publication bias or *post hoc* construction of the composite (*p*-hacking). Death had little effect on the composite outcome in these trials; more common events, such as revascularisation, dominated the composite outcome frequency.

Another survey reviewed 40 trials with a binary composite outcome published in 2008; most were cardiovascular trials.[30] Most trials (70%) did not explain the rationale for the composite components selected. The clinical importance of components differed in most trials. Many combined hospitalisation and death as equal components. Changing definitions of the composite in various sections of the published report was common. Only 60% of reports provided results for both the composite and component outcome events. Most worrisome, most reports that found a significant effect in composite outcome falsely implied that the overall effect applied to the most important component.

Conclusion

In general, surrogate endpoints and composite outcomes should be avoided in clinical research. Surrogate endpoints need to be validated before use. Changes in clinical practice based on invalid surrogate endpoints have led to needless death and suffering. This is patently unethical.[27,29] For composite outcomes, guidelines[37,42-44] should be followed. However, in current practice, composite outcomes are often clinically irrational and insufficiently justified. Because of incomplete reporting, readers may incorrectly infer that the results apply equally to all components of the composite; this is not always the case.[40]

A medical aphorism notes that 'a difference to be a difference must make a difference'. We agree. Clinical research should focus on outcomes that matter. Worry about statistical significance is misplaced. Validity is more important than precision. Trials that are well done and free of bias that use clinically important outcomes can contribute importantly to medicine. In contrast, trials that are statistically significant but focus on an invalid surrogate endpoint or a confusing composite outcome are not only unhelpful but potentially deadly.[5] Patients deserve better from us.

References

1. Fleming, T.R., Powers, J.H., 2012. Biomarkers and surrogate endpoints in clinical trials. Stat. Med. 31, 2973–2984.
2. Medeiros, F.A., 2015. Biomarkers and surrogate endpoints in glaucoma clinical trials. Br. J. Ophthalmol. 99, 599–603.
3. Samuels, J., 2016. Use of surrogate outcomes in nephrology research. Adv. Chronic Kidney Dis. 23, 363–366.
4. Svensson, S., Menkes, D.B., Lexchin, J., 2013. Surrogate outcomes in clinical trials: a cautionary tale. JAMA Intern. Med. 173, 611–612.
5. Grimes, D.A., Schulz, K.F., 2005. Surrogate end points in clinical research: hazardous to your health. Obstet. Gynecol. 105, 1114–1118.
6. Altman, D.G., 1994. The scandal of poor medical research. BMJ 308, 283–284.
7. von Elm, E., Egger, M., 2004. The scandal of poor epidemiological research. BMJ 329, 868–869.
8. Cefalu, C.A., 2004. Is bone mineral density predictive of fracture risk reduction? Curr. Med. Res. Opin. 20, 341–349.
9. Paschall, S., Kaunitz, A.M., 2008. Depo-Provera and skeletal health: a survey of Florida obstetrics and gynecologist physicians. Contraception 78, 370–376.
10. World Health Organization. WHO Statement on Hormonal Contraception and Bone Health. http://www.who.int/reproductivehealth/publications/family_planning/hc_bone_health/en/, accessed 27 March 2006.
11. Shulman, L.P., Bateman, L.H., Creinin, M.D., et al., 2006. Surrogate markers, emboldened and boxed warnings, and an expanding culture of misinformation: evidence-based clinical science should guide FDA decision making about product labeling. Contraception 73, 440–442.
12. Kaunitz, A.M., Grimes, D.A., 2011. Removing the black box warning for depot medroxyprogesterone acetate. Contraception 84, 212–213.
13. Cromer, B.A., Scholes, D., Berenson, A., et al., 2006. Depot medroxyprogesterone acetate and bone mineral density in adolescents—the Black Box Warning: a Position Paper of the Society for Adolescent Medicine. J. Adolesc. Health 39, 296–301.
14. Nissen, S.E., Wolski, K., 2007. Effect of rosiglitazone on the risk of myocardial infarction and death from cardiovascular causes. N. Engl. J. Med. 356, 2457–2471.
15. Avorn, J., 2013. Approval of a tuberculosis drug based on a paradoxical surrogate measure. JAMA 309, 1349–1350.
16. Ahuja, V., Sohn, M.W., Birge, J.R., et al., 2015. Geographic variation in rosiglitazone use surrounding FDA warnings in the Department of Veterans Affairs. J. Manag. Care. Spec. Pharm. 21, 1214–1234.
17. Gerstein, H.C., Miller, M.E., Byington, R.P., et al., 2008. Effects of intensive glucose lowering in type 2 diabetes. N. Engl. J. Med. 358, 2545–2559.
18. Geffen, N., 2016. Anything to Stay Alive: The challenges of a campaign for an experimental drug. Dev. World Bioeth. 16, 45–54.
19. Fleming, T.R., DeMets, D.L., 1996. Surrogate end points in clinical trials: are we being misled? Ann. Intern. Med. 125, 605–613.
20. Prentice, R.L., 1989. Surrogate endpoints in clinical trials: definition and operational criteria. Stat. Med. 8, 431–440.
21. Lassere, M.N., 2008. The Biomarker-Surrogacy Evaluation Schema: a review of the biomarker-surrogate literature and a proposal for a criterion-based, quantitative, multidimensional hierarchical levels of evidence schema for evaluating the status of biomarkers as surrogate endpoints. Stat. Methods Med. Res. 17, 303–340.
22. Biomarkers and surrogate endpoints: preferred definitions and conceptual framework, 2001. Clin. Pharmacol. Ther. 69, 89–95.
23. De Gruttola, V.G., Clax, P., DeMets, D.L., et al., 2001. Considerations in the evaluation of surrogate endpoints in clinical trials. summary of a National Institutes of Health workshop. Control Clin. Trials 22, 485–502.
24. IOM (Institute of Medicine). 2010. Evaluation of Biomarkers and Surrogate Endpoints in Chronic Disease. The National Academies Press, Washington, DC.

25. Robb, M.A., McInnes, P.M., Califf, R.M., 2016. Biomarkers and surrogate endpoints: developing common terminology and definitions. JAMA 315, 1107–1108.

26. FDA-NIH Biomarker Working Group. 2016. BEST (Biomarkers, EndpointS, and other Tools) Resource. U.S. Food and Drug Administration, Silver Spring, MD.

27. Grimes, D.A., Schulz, K.F., Raymond, E.G., 2010. Surrogate end points in women's health research: science, protoscience, and pseudoscience. Fertil. Steril. 93, 1731–1734.

28. Horton, R., 2000. From star signs to trial guidelines. Lancet 355, 1033–1034.

29. Stanczyk, F.Z., Grimes, D.A., 2008. Sex hormone-binding globulin: not a surrogate marker for venous thromboembolism in women using oral contraceptives. Contraception 78, 201–203.

30. Cordoba, G., Schwartz, L., Woloshin, S., Bae, H., Gøtzsche, P.C., 2010. Definition, reporting, and interpretation of composite outcomes in clinical trials: systematic review. BMJ 341, c3920.

31. Goldberg, R., Gore, J.M., Barton, B., Gurwitz, J., 2014. Individual and composite study endpoints: separating the wheat from the chaff. Am. J. Med. 127, 379–384.

32. Wittkop, L., Smith, C., Fox, Z., et al., 2010. Methodological issues in the use of composite endpoints in clinical trials: examples from the HIV field. Clin. Trials 7, 19–35.

33. Ross, S., 2007. Composite outcomes in randomized clinical trials: arguments for and against. Am. J. Obstet. Gynecol. 196, 119.e1–119.e6.

34. Tomlinson, G., Detsky, A.S., 2010. Composite end points in randomized trials: there is no free lunch. JAMA 303, 267–268.

35. Heddle, N.M., Cook, R.J., 2011. Composite outcomes in clinical trials: what are they and when should they be used? Transfusion (Paris) 51, 11–13.

36. Myles, P.S., Devereaux, P.J., 2010. Pros and cons of composite endpoints in anesthesia trials. Anesthesiology 113, 776–778.

37. Ferreira-Gonzalez, I., Permanyer-Miralda, G., Busse, J.W., et al., 2007. Methodologic discussions for using and interpreting composite endpoints are limited, but still identify major concerns. J. Clin. Epidemiol. 60, 651–657; discussion 8–62.

38. Crowther, C.A., Hiller, J.E., Doyle, L.W., Haslam, R.R., 2003. Effect of magnesium sulfate given for neuroprotection before preterm birth: a randomized controlled trial. JAMA 290, 2669–2676.

39. Ferreira-Gonzalez, I., Alonso-Coello, P., Sola, I., et al., 2008. Composite endpoints in clinical trials. Rev. Esp. Cardiol. 61, 283–290.

40. Gerstein, H.C., Yusuf, S., Bosch, J., et al., 2006. Effect of rosiglitazone on the frequency of diabetes in patients with impaired glucose tolerance or impaired fasting glucose: a randomised controlled trial. Lancet 368, 1096–1105.

41. Bin Abd Razak, H.R., Ang, J.E., Attal, H., Howe, T.S., Allen, J.C., 2016. P-hacking in orthopaedic literature: a twist to the tail. J. Bone Joint Surg. Am. 98, e91.

42. Lim, E., Brown, A., Helmy, A., Mussa, S., Altman, D.G., 2008. Composite outcomes in cardiovascular research: a survey of randomized trials. Ann. Intern. Med. 149, 612–617.

43. Freemantle, N., Calvert, M., Wood, J., Eastaugh, J., Griffin, C., 2003. Composite outcomes in randomized trials: greater precision but with greater uncertainty? JAMA 289, 2554–2559.

44. Montori, V.M., Permanyer-Miralda, G., Ferreira-Gonzalez, I., et al., 2005. Validity of composite end points in clinical trials. BMJ 330, 594–596.

CHAPTER 19

Multiplicity in Randomised Trials I: Endpoints and Treatments

Multiplicity problems emerge from investigators looking at many additional endpoints and treatment group comparisons. Thousands of potential comparisons can emanate from one trial. Investigators might only report the statistically significant comparisons, an unscientific practice if unwitting and fraudulent if intentional. Researchers must report all the endpoints analysed and treatments compared. Some statisticians propose statistical adjustments to account for multiplicity. Simply defined, they test for no effects in all the primary endpoints undertaken versus an effect in one or more of those endpoints. In general, statistical adjustments for multiplicity provide crude answers to an irrelevant question. However, investigators should use adjustments when the clinical decision-making argument rests solely on one or more of the primary endpoints being significant. In these cases, adjustments somewhat rescue scattershot analyses. Readers need to be aware of the potential for underreporting of analyses.

Many analytical problems in trials stem from issues related to multiplicity. Investigators sometimes address the issues responsibly; however, others ignore or remain oblivious to their ramifications. Put colloquially, some researchers torture their data until they speak. They examine additional endpoints, manipulate group comparisons, do many subgroup analyses, and undertake repeated interim analyses. Difficulties usually manifest at the analysis phase because investigators add unplanned analyses. Literally thousands of potential comparisons can emanate from one trial, in which case many statistically significant results would be expected by chance alone. Some statisticians propose adjustments in response, but unfortunately those adjustments frequently create more problems than they solve.[1,2]

Multiplicity problems stem from several sources. Here we address multiple endpoints and multiple treatments. In the next chapter, we address subgroup and interim analyses (Chapter 20).[3] The perspectives on multiplicity are contentious and complex.[4-7] In proposing approaches to handle multiplicity, any position alienates many (Panel 19.1).[1,5,8-10] Multiplicity issues stir hot debates.[11]

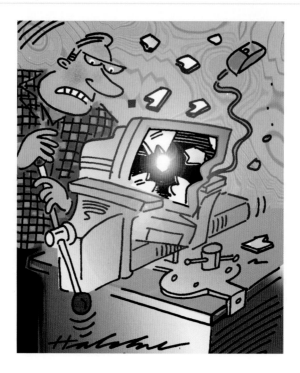

The Issue

Multiplicity portends troubles for researchers and readers alike for two main reasons. First, investigators should report all analytical comparisons implemented. Unfortunately, they sometimes hide the complete analysis, handicapping the reader's understanding of the results. Second, if researchers properly report all comparisons made, statisticians proffer statistical adjustments to account for multiple comparisons. Investigators need to know whether they should use such adjustments, and readers need to know whether to expect them.

Multiplicity can increase the overall error in significance testing. The type I error (α), under the hypothesis of no association between two factors, indicates the probability of the observed association from the data at hand being attributable to chance. It advises the reader of the likelihood of a false-positive conclusion.[12] (Chapter 11) The problem emerges when multiple independent

---

PANEL 19.1 ■ Divergent Views on Statistical Adjustments for Multiplicity
Some statisticians favour adjustments for multiple comparisons, whereas others disagree.

Several recent publications show that the multiple comparisons debate is alive and well. I . . . observe that it is hard to see views such as the following being reconciled . . .[8]

No adjustments are needed for multiple comparisons.[5]

Bonferroni adjustments are, at best, unnecessary and, at worst, deleterious to sound statistical inference.[1]

. . . Type I error accumulates with each executed hypothesis test and must be controlled by the investigators.[9]

Methods to determine and correct type 1 errors should be reported in epidemiologic and public health research investigations that include multiple statistical tests.[10]

associations are tested for significance. If d is the number of comparisons, then the probability that at least one association will be found significant is $(1 - [1 - \alpha]^d)$. Frequently, investigators in medical research set α at 0.05. Thus, if they test 10 independent associations, assuming the universal null hypothesis of no association in all 10, the probability of at least one significant result is 0.40 (i.e., $1 - [1 - 0.05]^{10}$. Stated alternatively the cumulative chance of at least one false-positive result out of the 10 comparisons is 40%. Nevertheless the probability of a false positive for every single comparison remains 0.05 (5%) whether one or a million are tested.[5]

A Proposed Statistical Solution

Most statisticians would recommend reducing the number of comparisons as a solution to multiplicity. Given many tests, however, some statisticians recommend making adjustments such that the overall probability of a false-positive finding equals α after making d comparisons in the trial. Authors usually attribute the method to Bonferroni and simply state that to test comparisons in a trial at α, all comparisons should be performed at the α/d significance level, not at the α level.[6,13] Thus, for an α of 0.05, with 10 comparisons, every test would have to be significant at the 0.005 level. Analogously, some investigators retain the same individual α threshold but multiply every observed p value by d.[11,14] Thus, with 10 comparisons, an observed $p = 0.02$ from a trial would yield an adjusted $p = 0.20$. Of note, the Bonferroni adjustment inflates β error, thereby reducing statistical power.[1]

Bonferroni adjustment, however, usually addresses the wrong hypothesis.[1,7] It assumes the universal null hypothesis which, simply defined, tests that two groups are identical for all the primary endpoints investigated versus the alternative hypothesis of an effect in one or more of those endpoints. That usually poses an irrelevant question in medical research. Clinically, a similar idea would be: 'the case of a doctor who orders 20 different laboratory tests for a patient, only to be told that some are abnormal, without further detail'.[1] 'Controlling the probability that at least one component is rejected is usually too restrictive and rarely of interest to the researcher'.[15] Indeed, Rothman wrote: 'To entertain the universal null hypothesis is, in effect, to suspend belief in the real world, and thereby to question the premises of empiricism'.[5]

Drug regulation with the need for clear dichotomous answers appropriately drives much of the activity in multiplicity adjustments. Adjustments fit the hypothesis-testing paradigm—approval or no approval—needed for drug regulation. In most published medical research, however, we encourage the presentation of interval estimation (e.g., relative risks with confidence intervals) for effects rather than just hypothesis testing (just a p value).[16] Moreover, we suggest that the decision-making intent in most medical research discourages multiplicity adjustments.

Multiple Endpoints

Although the ideal approach for the design and analysis of randomised controlled trials relies on one primary endpoint, investigators frequently examine more than one.[17] The most egregious abuse with multiplicity arises in the data-dredging that happens behind the scenes and remains unreported. Investigators analyse many endpoints but only report the favourable statistically significant comparisons. Failure to note all the comparisons made is unscientific if unwitting and fraudulent if intentional. 'Post hoc selection of the endpoint with the most significant treatment difference is a deceitful trick that invariably overemphasises a treatment difference.'[14] Investigators must halt this deceptive practice.

Researchers should restrict the number of primary endpoints tested. They should specify a priori the primary endpoint or endpoints in their protocol. Focusing their trial increases the simplicity of implementation and the credibility of results. Furthermore, they should follow their protocol for their analysis. Deviations for data-dredging can be condoned but should be clearly labelled as explorations and fully reported. Disappointingly, trial reports frequently contain examinations of endpoints not included in the trial protocol but ignore planned primary analyses from the protocol.[18] Safeguards to ensure that investigators have followed the protocol (such as *The Lancet*'s protocol acceptance track and asking for protocols for all randomised controlled trials) provide assistance, but more extensive registering and publishing of protocols make sense. Lastly, investigators must report all the comparisons made.[19-22]

Some authors have suggested that statistical adjustments for multiplicity should be applied much more frequently.[17] They stated that up to 75% of trials with multiple primary outcomes should have adjusted for multiplicity in their analyses. However, they did not appear to have evidence that the investigators analysing the multiple outcomes were using a decision-making criterion (i.e., testing the universal null hypothesis) that would require adjustment.

Statistical adjustments for multiple endpoints might sabotage interpretation. For example, suppose investigators undertook a randomised controlled trial of a new antibiotic compared with a standard antibiotic for prevention of febrile morbidity after hysterectomy. They designated fever the primary outcome, and the results showed a 50% reduction (relative risk 0.50 [95% CI 0.25–0.99]; $p = 0.048$). Note the statistically significant result. Alternatively, suppose they had designated two primary endpoints: wound infection and fever. As typically happens in trials, the endpoints are highly correlated. So in addition to the 50% reduction in fever, the trial also found a 52% decrease in wound infection (0.48 [0.24–0.97]; $p = 0.041$). From some statisticians' viewpoints, investigators should correct for multiple comparisons. As described earlier, the Bonferroni adjustment approach for multiple comparisons entails evaluating each primary endpoint at an adjusted statistical significance level boundary of α divided by the number of comparisons made. In this example with two comparisons (wound infection and fever), α would be divided by 2 or 0.05/2 = 0.025 for the 0.05 level of significance. Thus with adjustment, both endpoint comparisons become nonsignificant at the conventional 0.05 level and thus indeterminate ('negative'). Seasoned clinical trialists, however, look at these results quite differently. The wound infection result enhances rather than debases the first result on fever. Clinicians understand biologically that the two endpoints are highly related. Adding the second endpoint on wound infection and observing similar results lends credence to the observed reduction in febrile morbidity. That adjustments would abolish the basic finding defies logic.[1] Doing so would somewhat resemble a doctor finding an abnormally low haemoglobin level in a patient but no longer judging it worthy of treatment because the patient also had an abnormally low packed-cell volume (haematocrit).

Indeed, some statisticians would agree with not using formal adjustments for multiplicity in the aforementioned example. Even those predisposed to such adjustments recommend against them under certain delineated clinical decision-making scenarios.[4] For example, if an investigator proposes to claim treatment effect if all the endpoints are significant or if most (defined in the protocol) are significant, then they assert that no adjustment for multiple endpoints is necessary.[4]

Furthermore, the Bonferroni adjustment, advocated most frequently for multiplicity, is an overcorrection at best. Moreover, it can be a severe overcorrection when the endpoints are associated with one another,[4,14] which is frequently the case. Overcorrecting for p values hampers interpretation of results. The adjustment for multiple comparisons 'mechanizes and thereby trivialises the interpretive problem, and it negates the value of much of the information in large bodies of data'.[5] Clinical insights remain important. Investigators need to focus on the smallest number of endpoints that makes clinical sense and then report results on all endpoints tested. If more than one primary endpoint exists, investigators should address in their discussion whether additional endpoints reinforce or detract from the core findings. Formal adjustments for multiplicity frequently obscure rather than enhance interpretation.

Composite Endpoints

Composite endpoints (outcomes) alleviate multiplicity concerns.[23] A composite endpoint happens if any one of the prospectively defined components of the composite takes place (Chapter 18). For example, a composite cardiovascular endpoint would happen if myocardial infarction, stroke, or cardiovascular death arose. If designated *a priori* as the primary outcome, the composite obviates the multiple comparisons associated with testing of the separate components. Moreover, composite outcomes usually increase event rates, thereby increasing power or reducing sample size requirements. Not surprisingly, investigators frequently use composite endpoints.[23]

However, interpretational difficulties sometimes arise. For example, aspirin produced an 18% reduction (relative risk 0.82 [95% CI 0.70–0.96]) in the previously defined composite endpoint of cardiovascular events (myocardial infarction, stroke, or cardiovascular death), a seemingly worthwhile result.[24] However, a secondary look at the separate components revealed a 44% decrease in myocardial infarction, a 22% increase in stroke, and virtually no effect on cardiovascular death. That 18% reduction seems meaningless in view of the lack of beneficial effect on the more important outcomes of death and stroke.[24] Composite endpoints frequently lack clinical relevancy[25] (Chapter 18). Thus, composite endpoints address multiplicity and generally yield statistical efficiency at the risk of creating interpretational difficulties.

Multiple Treatments (Multiarm Trials)

Addressing multiplicity from multiple treatments is a more tractable problem than from multiple endpoints. First, investigators can avert multiple tests by one global test of significance across comparison groups[14] (e.g., comparing A versus B versus C in a three-arm trial) or by modelling a dose–response relationship.[26] Second, and perhaps most importantly, researchers have less opportunity to data-dredge on many treatments and not report them. Although they easily can add more endpoints for analysis, they would have difficulty adding treatments in a trial. They theoretically could implement a multigroup trial and then only report the favourable group comparisons, but little evidence exists for that practice. We suspect that readers of a trial report usually see all the treatments implemented. Indeed, multiarm trials have an important role in medical research (Panel 19.2).

However, the situation is not entirely sanguine. What readers of a journal article might not see are all the different comparisons among the treatment groups. For example, with a three-arm trial, at least seven possible analyses emerge (Fig. 19.1). With more than three arms, the potential comparisons explode. Obviously, investigators should specify *a priori* the comparisons intended.

PANEL 19.2 ■ A Role for Multiarm Trials in Medical Research

Multiarm trials are fairly common in the medical literature. A search of randomised controlled trials indexed on PubMed revealed that 78% of trials used a parallel design.[33] Of these, 22% had more than two arms—15% having three arms, 4% four arms, and 3% more than four arms.[33] From this broad slice of all medical research, these results display that multiarm trials occur more frequently than generally recognised; of all the parallel-designed randomised trials, over one in five employ a multiarm design.

The preponderance of material in clinical trial textbooks addresses two-arm trials. Furthermore, eminent researchers have strongly recommended against more than two arms: 'A positive result is more likely, and a null result is more informative, if the main comparison is of only two treatments, these being as different as possible'.[34] The argument against multiarm trials mainly centres on trial power. Published trials typically have inadequate power.[35] Given a finite number of potential participants, the argument holds that adding arms only further dilutes power. Although we sympathise with this argument, multiarm trials might not only be attractive in some circumstances but also be more efficient.

For example, imagine an instance whereby a standard treatment exists and two new potentially effective therapies have materialised. A two-arm approach dictates a comparison of a new with standard and then probably an additional trial of the other new with the preferred treatment from the first trial. In general, the overall study size and cost would be greater with this sequential two-arm approach than with one multiarm trial. Multiarm trials sometimes make sense.

Furthermore, multiarm trials do not necessarily raise methodological concerns. They can eliminate selection bias just like two-arm trials. Although they tend to be more complex to undertake and analyse, that complexity frequently yields commensurate gains in information.

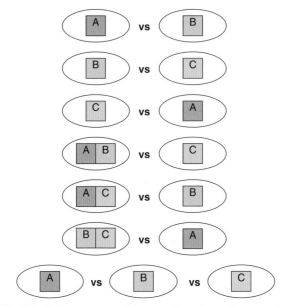

Fig. 19.1   At least seven possible comparisons from a three-arm trial.

With multiarm trials, as mentioned earlier, a frequently recommended approach entails undertaking one global test across all treatments. However, some methodologists believe such tests are of limited use because they do not identify which treatments are different and because of limited power to detect genuine differences.[14,27] Many multiarm trials are designed for direct comparison with controls.[14] Thus, investigators should plan the comparisons intended, limit the number, and document them in the protocol.

THE ISSUE OF MULTIPLICITY ADJUSTMENT IN MULTIARM TRIALS

Multiplicity adjustment for multiple comparisons among groups in a multiarm randomised trial is a debatable topic. Its complexity lies in the numerous matters having an effect on the need for adjustment. 'There are many issues that either separately or in combination may make a coherent case for multiplicity adjustment. These include the relatedness of the questions being considered, the number of comparisons, the degree of controversy, who stands to benefit, and the nature of the study/ alternative hypothesis'.[28] We will offer our distillation of the appropriateness of multiplicity adjustments for multiarm trials.

Many investigators conduct multiarm trials for reasons of efficiency. They evaluate distinct treatment arms versus a control arm, which could simply have been done in multiple separate trials rather than a single multiarm trial. Indeed, for a multiarm randomised trial design in which multiple treatment arms share a control arm, the trial design aims to assess the research question for each treatment separately. The understanding of the results of one treatment comparison has no direct connection to the understanding of the others. Many trialists and methodologists contend that multiplicity adjustments would not be needed in such instances because adjustments would not be needed if the treatments were compared in those separate trials.[29-31]

Some multiarm randomised trials compare several different doses of the same treatment (frequently a drug) against a treatment control arm. These characterise related comparisons. In such situations, methodologists tend to advise using multiplicity adjustments.[28-30]

An obvious instance transpires with specific decision-making criteria in submissions to a regulatory agency for drug approval. If the sponsor stipulates multiple treatment comparisons and intends to declare a treatment effect if one or more of the doses are statistically significant (test of the universal null hypothesis), most methodologists strongly advocate an adjustment for multiplicity.[28-32]

The need in that instance for multiplicity adjustment in multiarm trials with related comparisons demonstrates the complexity of this issue. First, the common method for adjustment (Bonferroni) becomes increasingly erroneous (too conservative) as the association among the comparisons becomes higher.[4] Thus, in situations where multiplicity adjustments are recommended, the adjustment method performs poorly.

Second, most medical research does not operate on the decision-making criteria of a regulatory framework. Medical researchers often evaluate different doses as if they had conducted multiple independent trials of those doses. They frequently discover that including more arms in a trial augments information, but the use of a multiplicity adjustment might detract from that improvement. Indeed, adjustments can obscure findings when a drug is effective at multiple doses. For example, in comparing a new antibiotic with standard antibiotic treatment for prevention of fever after hysterectomy, investigators might compare a 2-g dose and a 1-g dose of the new drug with the standard drug. The results show a 40% reduction for the 1-g dose (relative risk 0.60 [95% CI 0.37–0.98]; $p = 0.044$). Note the statistically significant result. The 2-g dose yields a similar result, a 45% decrease in fever (0.55 [0.31–0.98]; $p = 0.041$). As described earlier, the Bonferroni adjustment approach for multiple comparisons entails evaluating each dose level at an adjusted statistical significance level boundary of α divided by the number of comparisons made. In this example with two comparisons (2-g dose and 1-g dose), α would be divided by 2 or $0.05/2 = 0.025$ for the 0.05 level of significance. Thus with adjustment, both dose effects become nonsignificant at the conventional 0.05 level and thus indeterminate ('negative').

Clinicians interpret these results quite differently. The result for the 2-g dose augments rather than degrades the result for the 1-g dose on fever. Clinicians expect similar results biologically. They would utterly distrust an adjustment that abolishes those significant results. Adjusting p values in this example does not aid in interpreting the results of the trial. Thus frequently, multiplicity adjustment is unsuitable even in situations of related treatments in multiarm trials. Indiscriminate assertions of 'always' or 'never' needing to adjust for multiple testing should be disregarded. The need depends on the design and analysis. Usually in medical research, where the clinical decision-making approach resembles analysing two independent trials as opposed to a regulatory framework, adjustment is inappropriate. Adjustments for multiple comparisons generally need not play a role in multigroup trials.

With regard to reporting, agreement emerges on major matters. Authors should transparently and fully report all the comparisons emanating from their multiple groups. Perhaps no adjustments for multiplicity were needed. However, if they did use multiplicity adjustments, they should describe them.

With multiple treatments, investigators sometimes use a prioritised sequence of tests.[36] For example, investigators might decide on the 2-g new antibiotic versus standard treatment as the priority test and, if that comparison is significant, only then proceed to the 1-g comparison. Such procedures address multiplicity without adjustments.[36] Again, formal adjustments for multiplicity usually complicate rather than enlighten.

The Role of Adjustments for Multiplicity

Sometimes formal adjustments for multiplicity are inescapable. An obvious example would arise with certain decision-making criteria in submissions to a regulatory agency for drug approval. If the sponsor specifies more than one primary endpoint and proposes to claim treatment effect if one or more are significant, investigators should adjust for multiplicity.[4,31] Furthermore, the same principle extends to all investigators whose decision-making intent is to claim an effect based on any one of a number of endpoints being positive.

Adjustments might also be indicated in a multiarm trial in which investigators plan a scattershot analysis. For example, in a four-arm trial (treatments A, B, C, and D), they intend to claim an effect for A if any one of the following comparisons yielded significant results: A versus B, A versus C, A versus D, A versus B + C, A versus B + D, A versus C + D, or A versus B + C + D. Another example emanates from decision-making criteria in a multiarm trial for submissions to a regulatory agency for drug approval. If the sponsor proposes to claim a drug effect if one or more of the drug doses in a multiarm trial are statistically significant, investigators should adjust for multiplicity.

In general, when prudence indicates multiplicity adjustments, trials tend to be poorly and diffusely designed. An adjustment for multiplicity merely partly salvages credibility. Moreover, even when adjustment becomes appropriate, implementation becomes difficult. Bonferroni adjustments are frequently used, usually because of their simplicity. However, other adjustment strategies sometimes perform better.[4,15,32,37] Depending on the correlation among the endpoints, simulation experiments display wide variability in α error and power of various multiplicity adjustment strategies.[4] These comparative assessments help, but still clear-cut choices prove elusive.

What Readers Should Look for

Readers should expect the researchers to report all the endpoints analysed and treatments compared. Assessing whether they reported them all is usually difficult. Access to the protocol would be helpful but is usually impossible. We urge greater access to protocols. Poor, incomplete reporting, however, frequently renders readers helpless to know the complete analysis undertaken by the investigators. Reporting according to the CONSORT statement obviates these difficulties.[19-22]

Readers should expect the primary endpoint or endpoints to be specified, with other analyses being labelled as exploratory. Lacking direct statements, search for indirect indications. If the primary endpoint remains unclear, hopefully the authors provided a statistical power analysis that indicates the primary endpoint.

Readers should expect some interpretation if authors make multiple comparisons. If authors went overboard and reported results on 15 endpoints with one being significant, they should display appropriate caution. If multiple comparisons yield multiple effects, authors should address the internal consistency of the results. Most importantly, transparent reporting of all comparisons allows readers to come to their own interpretations.

If a trial report specifies a composite endpoint, the components of the composite should be in the well-known pathophysiology of the disease. The researchers should interpret the composite endpoint in aggregate rather than as showing efficacy of the individual components. However, the components should be specified as secondary outcomes and reported beside the results of the primary analysis.[23]

In general, readers need not expect corrections for multiplicity. For most trials, adjustments for multiplicity lack substance and prove unhelpful. An exception might include a medical research article with an argument that rests solely on one or more of the primary comparisons being statistically significant, essentially the test of the universal null hypothesis. An adjustment for multiplicity somewhat rescues such scattershot analyses.

Conclusion

Multiplicity problems emerge from investigators looking at many additional endpoints and treatment group comparisons. Readers need to be aware of the potential for under-reporting of these analyses in the literature. Indeed, researchers must report all the endpoints analysed and treatments compared.

Some statisticians propose statistical adjustments to account for multiplicity. In general, statistical adjustments for multiplicity provide crude answers to an irrelevant question. However, investigators should use adjustments when the clinical decision-making argument rests solely on one or more of the primary endpoints being significant.

References

1. Perneger, T.V., 1998. What's wrong with Bonferroni adjustments. BMJ 316, 1236–1238.
2. Perneger, T.V., 1999. Adjusting for multiple testing in studies is less important than other concerns. BMJ 318, 1288.
3. Schulz, K.F., Grimes, D.A., 2005. Multiplicity in randomised trials II: subgroup and interim analyses. Lancet 365, 1657–1661.
4. Sankoh, A.J., D'Agostino, R.B.S., Huque, M.F., 2003. Efficacy endpoint selection and multiplicity adjustment methods in clinical trials with inherent multiple endpoint issues. Stat. Med. 22, 3133–3150.
5. Rothman, K.J., 1990. No adjustments are needed for multiple comparisons. Epidemiology 1, 43–46.
6. Westfall, P., Bretz, F., 2003. Multiplicity in clinical trials. In: Encyclopedia of Biopharmaceutical Statistics, second ed. Marcel Dekker, Inc, New York, pp. 666–673.
7. Savitz, D.A., Olshan, A.F., 1995. Multiple comparisons and related issues in the interpretation of epidemiologic data. Am. J. Epidemiol. 142, 904–908.
8. Altman, D.G., 2000. Statistics in medical journals: some recent trends. Stat. Med. 19, 3275–3289.
9. Moye, L.A., 1998. P-value interpretation and alpha allocation in clinical trials. Ann. Epidemiol. 8, 351–357.
10. Ottenbacher, K.J., 1998. Quantitative evaluation of multiplicity in epidemiology and public health research. Am. J. Epidemiol. 147, 615–619.
11. Altman, D., 1991. Practical Statistics for Medical Research. Chapman and Hall, London.
12. Schulz, K.F., Grimes, D.A., 2005. Sample size calculations in randomised trials: mandatory and mystical. Lancet 365, 1348–1353.
13. Friedman, L., Furberg, C., DeMets, D., 1996. Fundamentals of Clinical Trials. Mosby, St. Louis.
14. Pocock, S., 1983. Clinical Trials: A Practical Approach. Wiley, Chichester, UK.
15. Glickman, M.E., Rao, S.R., Schultz, M.R., 2014. False discovery rate control is a recommended alternative to Bonferroni-type adjustments in health studies. J. Clin. Epidemiol. 67, 850–857.
16. Sterne, J.A., Davey Smith, G., 2001. Sifting the evidence-what's wrong with significance tests? BMJ 322, 226–231.
17. Vickerstaff, V., Ambler, G., King, M., Nazareth, I., Omar, R.Z., 2015. Are multiple primary outcomes analysed appropriately in randomised controlled trials? A review. Contemp. Clin. Trials 45, 8–12.
18. Chan, A.W., Hrobjartsson, A., Haahr, M.T., Gøtzsche, P.C., Altman, D.G., 2004. Empirical evidence for selective reporting of outcomes in randomized trials: comparison of protocols to published articles. JAMA 291, 2457–2465.
19. Schulz, K.F., Altman, D.G., Moher, D., 2010. CONSORT 2010 statement: updated guidelines for reporting parallel group randomised trials. BMJ 340, c332.
20. Schulz, K.F., Altman, D.G., Moher, D., 2010. CONSORT 2010 statement: updated guidelines for reporting parallel group randomized trials. Ann. Intern. Med. 152, 726–732.
21. Moher, D., Hopewell, S., Schulz, K.F., et al., 2010. CONSORT 2010 explanation and elaboration: updated guidelines for reporting parallel group randomised trials. J. Clin. Epidemiol. 63, e1–37.
22. Moher, D., Hopewell, S., Schulz, K.F., et al., 2010. CONSORT 2010 explanation and elaboration: updated guidelines for reporting parallel group randomised trials. BMJ 340, c869.
23. Freemantle, N., Calvert, M., Wood, J., Eastaugh, J., Griffin, C., 2003. Composite outcomes in randomized trials: greater precision but with greater uncertainty? JAMA 289, 2554–2559.
24. Pocock, S.J., 1997. Clinical trials with multiple outcomes: a statistical perspective on their design, analysis, and interpretation. Control. Clin. Trials 18, 530–545; discussion 46–49.
25. Meinert, C., 1986. Clinical Trials: Design, Conduct, and Analysis. Oxford University Press, New York.
26. Senn, S., 1997. Statistical Issues in Drug Development. John Wiley & Sons Ltd, Chichester.
27. Pocock, S.J., Shaper, A.G., Walker, M., et al., 1983. Effects of tap water lead, water hardness, alcohol, and cigarettes on blood lead concentrations. J. Epidemiol. Community Health 37, 1–7.
28. Proschan, M.A., Waclawiw, M.A., 2000. Practical guidelines for multiplicity adjustment in clinical trials. Control. Clin. Trials 21, 527–539.

29. Wason, J.M., Stecher, L., Mander, A.P., 2014. Correcting for multiple-testing in multi-arm trials: is it necessary and is it done? Trials 15, 364.
30. Freidlin, B., Korn, E.L., Gray, R., Martin, A., 2008. Multi-arm clinical trials of new agents: some design considerations. Clin. Cancer Res. 14, 4368–4371.
31. Schulz, K.F., Grimes, D.A., 2005. Multiplicity in randomised trials I: endpoints and treatments. Lancet 365, 1591–1595.
32. Howard, D.R., Brown, J.M., Todd, S., Gregory, W.M., 2018. Recommendations on multiple testing adjustment in multi-arm trials with a shared control group. Stat. Methods Med. Res. 27, 1513–1530.
33. Hopewell, S., Dutton, S., Yu, L.M., Chan, A.W., Altman, D.G., 2010. The quality of reports of randomised trials in 2000 and 2006: comparative study of articles indexed in PubMed. BMJ 340, c723.
34. Peto, R., Pike, M.C., Armitage, P., et al., 1976. Design and analysis of randomized clinical trials requiring prolonged observation of each patient. I. Introduction and design. Br. J. Cancer 34, 585–612.
35. Moher, D., Dulberg, C.S., Wells, G.A., 1994. Statistical power, sample size, and their reporting in randomized controlled trials. JAMA 272, 122–124.
36. Bauer, P., Chi, G., Geller, N., et al., 2003. Industry, government, and academic panel discussion on multiple comparisons in a "real" phase three clinical trial. J. Biopharm. Stat. 13, 691–701.
37. Hsu, J., 1996. Multiple Comparisons—Theory and Methods. Chapman & Hall, New York.

CHAPTER 20

Multiplicity in Randomised Trials II: Subgroup and Interim Analyses

Subgroup analyses can pose serious multiplicity concerns. By testing enough subgroups, a false-positive result will probably emerge by chance alone. Investigators might undertake many analyses but only report the significant effects, distorting the medical literature. In general, we discourage subgroup analyses. However, if they are necessary, researchers should do statistical tests of interaction, rather than analyse every separate subgroup. Investigators cannot avoid interim analyses when data monitoring is indicated. However, repeatedly testing at every interim analysis raises multiplicity concerns, and not accounting for multiplicity escalates the false-positive error. Statistical stopping methods must be used. The O'Brien–Fleming and Peto group sequential stopping methods are easily implemented and preserve the intended α level and power. Both adopt stringent criteria (low nominal p values) during the interim analyses. Implementing a trial under these stopping rules resembles a conventional trial, with the exception that it can be terminated early should a treatment prove greatly superior. Investigators and readers, however, need to grasp that the estimated treatment effects are prone to exaggeration, a random high, with early stopping.

Subgroup analyses have specious appeal. They seem logical and intuitive and even fun—to both investigators and readers. However, this insidious appeal causes important problems. Multiplicity and naivety combine to encourage interpretational missteps in trial conduct and reporting. The subgroup treatment effects revealed in many reports might be illusory.

By contrast, investigators cannot avoid interim analyses if data monitoring is indicated. Neither can they use their normal statistical approaches at interim analyses. Statistical stopping methods, essentially statistical adjustments for warning rather than stopping, must be used in support of data monitoring. Unfortunately, those methods baffle investigators and readers alike. Statistics frequently proves confusing anyway without throwing in second-order complications of stopping methods.

Multiplicity issues from subgroup and interim analyses pose similar problems to those from multiple endpoints and treatment groups[1] (Chapter 19). Investigators frequently data-dredge by doing many subgroup analyses and undertaking repeated interim analyses. Also, researchers conduct unplanned subgroup and interim analyses. Yet some of the approaches to multiplicity problems from subgroup and interim analyses differ from those for endpoints and treatments.

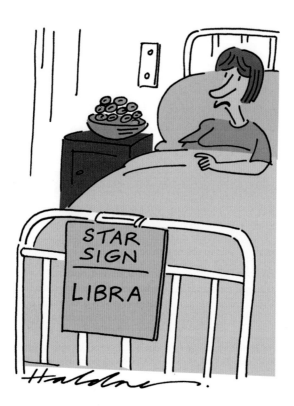

Subgroup Analyses

Indiscriminate subgroup analyses pose serious multiplicity concerns. Problems reverberate throughout the medical literature. Even after many warnings,[2] some investigators doggedly persist in undertaking excessive subgroup analyses.

Investigators define subgroups of participants by characteristics at baseline. They then do analyses to assess whether treatment effects differ in these subgroups. The major problems stem from investigators undertaking statistical tests within every subgroup examined. Combining analyses of multiple subgroups with multiple outcomes leads to a profusion of statistical tests.

Seeking positive subgroup effects (data-dredging), in the absence of overall effects, could fuel much of this activity. If enough subgroups are tested, false-positive results will arise by chance alone.

> *The answer to a randomized controlled trial that does not confirm one's beliefs is not the conduct of several subanalyses until one can see what one believes. Rather, the answer is to re-examine one's beliefs carefully.*[3]

Similarly, in a trial with a clear overall effect, subgroup testing can produce false-negative results due to chance and lack of power.

The Lancet published an illustrative example.[4] Aspirin displayed a strongly beneficial effect in preventing death after myocardial infarction ($p < 0.00001$, with a narrow confidence interval). The editors urged the researchers to include nearly 40 subgroup analyses.[2] The investigators reluctantly agreed under the condition that they could provide a subgroup analysis of their own to illustrate their unreliability. They showed that participants born under the astrological signs Gemini or

Libra had a slightly adverse effect on death from aspirin (9% increase, SD 13; not significant), whereas participants born under all other astrological signs reaped a strikingly beneficial effect (28% reduction, SD 5; $p < 0.00001$).[4]

Anecdotal reports of support from astrologers to the contrary, this chance zodiac finding has generated little interest from the medical community. The authors concluded from their subgroup analyses that

> All these subgroup analyses should, perhaps, be taken less as evidence about who benefits than as evidence that such analyses are potentially misleading.

These and other thoughtful investigators stress that usually the most reliable estimate of effect for a particular subgroup is the overall effect (essentially all the subgroups combined) rather than the observed effect in that subgroup.[4,5] We agree.

Proper analysis dissipates much of the multiplicity problem with subgroup analyses. Frequently, investigators improperly test every subgroup, which opens the door to chance findings. For example, breaking down age at baseline into four categories yields four tests just on that characteristic (Panel 20.1). A proper analysis uses a statistical test of interaction, which involves assessing whether the treatment effect on an outcome depends on the participant's subgroup. A test of interaction assesses whether the observed differences in outcome effects across subgroups could be ascribed to chance variation.[6] That not only tests the proper question but also produces a single test instead of four, substantially addressing the multiplicity problem. Investigators have questioned interaction tests based on lack of power. However, interaction tests provide proper caution. They recognise the

---

PANEL 20.1 ■ Effect of New Versus Standard Antibiotic on Febrile Morbidity in Four Age Strata and Overall

	Febrile Morbidity			
	Yes	No	Total	Rate Ratio (95% CI)
Age 20–24 Years				
New antibiotic	11	84	95	1.4 (0.6–3.2)
Standard antibiotic	8	86	94	
Age 25–29 Years				
New antibiotic	8	69	77	1.2 (0.4–3.1)
Standard antibiotic	7	72	79	
Age 30–34 Years				
New antibiotic	3	48	51	0.3 (0.1–0.9)
Standard antibiotic	11	38	49	
Age 35–39 Years				
New antibiotic	10	32	42	1.1 (0.5–2.5)
Standard antibiotic	9	33	42	
Total				
New antibiotic	32	233	265	0.9 (0.6–1.4)
Standard antibiotic	35	229	264	

The test for statistical interaction (Breslow–Day) is nonsignificant ($p = 0.103$), suggesting that a statistically significant subgroup finding in the 30–34 years age stratum is attributable to chance. However, that result, if inappropriately highlighted, would be an example of a superfluous subgroup salvage of an otherwise indeterminate (neutral) trial.

limited information available in the subgroups and have emerged as the most effective statistical method to restrain inappropriate subgroup findings while still having the ability to detect interactive effects, if present.[7,8]

Another problem with subgroup analyses is that investigators can do many analyses and only report the significant ones, which bestows more credibility on them than they deserve—a misleading practice and, if intentional, unethical. This situation is analogous to what we judge a major problem with multiple endpoints.

Subgroup analyses remain a problem in published work. In a review of 50 reports from general medical journals (*New England Journal of Medicine, The Lancet, JAMA,* and *BMJ*), 70% reported subgroup analyses.[9] Of those in which the number of analyses could be established, almost 40% did at least six subgroup analyses—one reported 24. Fewer than half used statistical tests of interaction. Furthermore, the reports did not provide information on whether the subgroup analyses were predefined or *post hoc.* The authors of the review suspected that 'some investigators selectively report only the more interesting subgroup analyses, thereby leaving the reader (and us) unaware of how many less-exciting subgroup analyses were looked at and not mentioned'.[9] Disappointingly, most trials reporting subgroup analyses noted a subgroup difference that was highlighted in the conclusions[9]—so much for cautious interpretation!

In general, we discourage subgroup analyses. If properly undertaken, they are not necessarily wrong.[10] Sometimes they make biological sense or are mandated by sponsors, both public and industry. Four clinical indications for subgroup analyses have been proposed: 'if there is a potentially large difference between groups in terms of harm that results from treatment; if pathophysiology makes patients from groups differ in their response to treatment; if there are clinically important questions relating to the practical application of treatment; and if there are doubts about the potential benefits of an intervention that results in underuse of this treatment in specific subgroups (for example in elderly patients)'.[10] If done, they should be confined to the primary outcome and a limited number of subgroups. Those planned should be prespecified in the protocol. Investigators must report all subgroup analyses done, not just the significant ones. Importantly, they should use statistical tests of interaction to assess whether a treatment effect differs among subgroups rather than individual tests within each subgroup.[6,10–12] This approach alleviates major concerns with multiple comparisons. Rarely should subgroup analyses affect the trial's conclusions.

Subgroup analyses are particularly prone to over interpretation, and one is tempted to suggest 'don't do it' (or at least 'don't believe it') for many trials, but this suggestion is probably contrary to human nature.[9,13]

Methodologists have been too restrained in criticising improperly undertaken subgroup analyses. Stronger denunciation is needed.

WHAT READERS SHOULD LOOK FOR WITH SUBGROUP ANALYSES

Readers should be wary of trials that report many subgroup analyses, unless the investigators provide valid reasons. Also, beware of trials that provide a small number of subgroup analyses. They might have done many and just cherry-picked the interesting and significant ones. Consequently, faulty reporting could mean that trials with few subgroup analyses are even worse than the trials with many. Investigators have more credence if they state that they reported all the analyses done. Furthermore, researchers should label nonprespecified subgroup analyses as hypothesis generating rather than confirming. Such findings should not appear in the conclusions.

Readers should expect interaction tests for subgroup effects. Discount analyses built on tests within subgroups. Even with a significant interaction test, readers should base interpretation of the findings on biological plausibility, on prespecification of analyses, and on the statistical strength of the information. Generally, adjustments for multiplicity are unnecessary when investigators use interaction tests. However, in view of the frequently frivolous data-dredging pursuits involved, the argument for statistical adjustments is stronger than that for multiple endpoints. Moreover, if investigators do not use interaction tests and report tests on every individual subgroup, multiplicity adjustments are appropriate.[14] Most subgroup findings tend to exaggerate reality. Be especially suspicious of investigators highlighting a subgroup treatment effect in a trial with no overall treatment effect.[15] They are usually superfluous subgroup salvages of otherwise indeterminate (neutral) trials (see Panel 20.1).[9] 'When the overall result of a major RCT is neutral, it is tempting to search across subgroups to see if there is a particular subgroup in which the treatment effect is favorable. In this context, subgroup claims require an especially cautious interpretation in a journal publication'.[6]

Readers should be the most suspicious of results in which the primary comparison is neutral, the interaction test is statistically significant, and the treatment effects in the subgroups are in opposite directions. This situation is described in a drug versus placebo RCT where the overall result is neutral.[6] 'Against a background of low-dose aspirin, 15,603 patients at high risk of atherothrombotic events were randomized to clopidogrel or placebo. Over a median 28 months, incidence of the primary endpoint (CV death, MI, or stroke) was 6.8% versus 7.3% ($p = 0.22$). But, in symptomatic patients (78% of all patients), the findings for clopidogrel looked better: 6.9% versus 7.9% ($p = 0.046$). In contrast, the results trended in the opposition [sic] direction in asymptomatic patients: 6.6% versus 5.5% ($p = 0.02$). The interaction test had $p = 0.045$, and the authors' conclusions included a claim of benefit for clopidogrel in symptomatic patients'.[6] Such qualitative interactions, where the treatment effects are in opposite directions among subgroups, are usually biologically implausible and seldom occur in clinical medicine.[6] An editorial stated that 'the charisma of extracting favourable subgroups should be resisted',[16] and the *New England Journal of Medicine* stiffened its policy on reporting subgroup analyses.[17]

Interim Analyses

Many randomised trials require interim analyses of the accumulating outcome data by treatment group. An independent statistician should generate those analyses and an independent data monitoring committee (DMC) should evaluate them.[18] Usually, several clinicians and a statistician comprise a DMC.[18]

Indeed, an ethics review board may require that investigators establish an independent DMC. The use of DMCs is increasing and, fortunately, a review of DMC recommendations has found, reassuringly, that most were made in the interest of participant safety.[19] However, the findings were not all sanguine in that some DMC recommendations may have lead to potentially biased trials.[19]

Appropriate monitoring of trials involves more than statistical warnings for stopping. Indeed, the superiority or inferiority of the studied treatment has a major role. However, slow accrual, poor data quality, poor adherence, resource deficiencies, unacceptable adverse effects, fraud, and emerging information that make the trial irrelevant, unnecessary, or unethical, all could lead to stopping a trial. The decision process is clearly complex. It best resides with an independent DMC.[20,21] The committee's task becomes manageable with a prespecified statistical stopping method. Yet investigators and readers frequently remain oblivious to these statistical issues.

In practice, the predominant reasons for stopping randomised trials early have not been based on preplanned interim analyses or stopping guidelines. In a review of randomised trials, 249 of 894 RCTs (27.9%) were stopped early (prematurely discontinued).[22] Forty-six of 249 RCTs (18%) were discontinued due to early benefit or futility, in other words, based on efficacy; of those, 80% were stopped outside a formal interim analysis or stopping guideline.[22] Most stopping, almost two-thirds, was due to poor recruitment, administrative reasons, or unexpected harm.[22] In another review including 102 stopped-early trials, 56% were discontinued for poor recruitment, financial

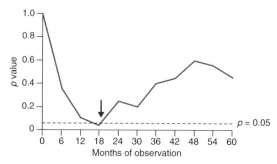

Fig. 20.1   Interim analyses done every 6 months for 5 years. The *p* value is shown for the comparison between the treatment group and control group.

issues, or various administrative topics, while 32% were discontinued due to early benefit or futility. In a separate review in which 32 trials were stopped early, 22 (69%) did not report predefined stopping guidelines and 15 (47%) did not provide information on statistical monitoring methods.[23]

Accumulating data in trials tempt investigators to do analyses on the main endpoint. If they seek $p < 0.05$ at the end of the study, they might still undertake all the interim analyses at $\alpha = 0.05$. That is wrong.

A graphical depiction of an example perhaps clarifies the issue (Fig. 20.1). A DMC does an interim analysis every 6 months for 5 years. At 18 months, the analysis slips under $p < 0.05$, but never again attains significance at that level. An early decision by the committee to stop the trial based on this result might have led to an incorrect conclusion about the effectiveness of the intervention.

Intuitively, undertaking many interim analyses at $p < 0.05$ should inflate the false-positive error rate (α). Indeed, if an investigator looks at the accumulating data at $\alpha = 0.05$ at every interim, then the actual overall α level rises with the number of challenges (e.g., overall $\alpha = 0.08$ after two challenges, $\alpha = 0.11$ after three, and $\alpha = 0.19$ after ten).[13,21] This multiplicity problem dictates the need for statistical adjustment: scientific credibility depends on it.

Methodologists have developed many statistical stopping (actually, warning) procedures, sometimes called data-dependent stopping rules or guidelines.[21] If investigators undertake interim analyses, they must use one of these procedures. The group sequential designs have garnered perhaps the most attention. They tend to be easier to understand, construct, and apply.[24] On the basis of the number of interim analyses planned, the methods define p values for considering trial stoppage at an interim look while preserving the overall type I error (α; Panel 20.2).

The fixed nominal level approach (Pocock approach) proves simple and allows fairly early termination of trials. However, it suffers from the final test of significance being at a smaller p value than that of a regular fixed-sample trial. For example, to yield an overall $\alpha = 0.05$ with three interim analyses, investigators would have to test at 0.022 at each analysis, including the final one (see Panel 20.2). If the final test yielded $p = 0.03$, then the trial would be deemed not significant by this group sequential approach, but it would have been significant if the group sequential approach had not been used. This approach is mainly of historical interest because other methods incorporate its advantages without this disadvantage.[24]

We favour two other procedures: O'Brien–Fleming and Peto.[20,21,24,25] Both adopt stringent criteria (low nominal p values) during the interim analyses (Panel 20.2). If the trial continues until the planned sample size, then all analyses proceed as if basically no interim analyses had taken place. The procedures preserve not only the intended α level but also the power.[26] Data are obtained in essentially the same way as in a fixed-sample design. Their beauty is in simplicity. Implementation of a trial under these stopping rules mirrors that of a conventional trial, with the exception that the

PANEL 20.2 ■ Interim Stopping Levels (p Values) for Different Numbers of Planned Interim Analyses by Group Sequential Design[24,25]

No. of Planned Interim Analyses	Interim Analysis	Pocock	Peto	O'Brien–Fleming
2	1	0.029	0.001	0.005
	2 (final)	0.029	0.05	0.048
3	1	0.022	0.001	0.0005
	2	0.022	0.001	0.014
	3 (final)	0.022	0.05	0.045
4	1	0.018	0.001	0.0001
	2	0.018	0.001	0.004
	3	0.018	0.001	0.019
	4 (final)	0.018	0.05	0.043
5	1	0.016	0.001	0.00001
	2	0.016	0.001	0.0013
	3	0.016	0.001	0.008
	4	0.016	0.001	0.023
	5 (final)	0.016	0.05	0.041

Overall $\alpha = 0.05$.

trial can be terminated early should a treatment prove greatly superior. As a general rule, investigators gain little by doing more than four or five interim analyses during a trial.[13,27] Usually, two or three interim looks should suffice.[18] Thus, with minimal additional effort, researchers address the ethical need to monitor for substantial treatment effects, positive or negative.

The Peto (or Haybittle–Peto) approach is simpler to understand, implement, and describe. It uses constant but stringent stopping levels until the final analysis (see Panel 20.2). For some trials, however, investigators believe that early termination of a trial is too difficult with Peto.

The O'Brien–Fleming approach appeals intuitively to many investigators because the stopping criteria are conservative early on, when everyone should be dubious of unstable results, and they successively ease as the results become more reliable and stable. Unlike the Peto approach, the O'Brien–Fleming stopping criteria vary with every interval look at the data.

If investigators plan interim analyses, they should prespecify the statistical stopping approach.[28] Furthermore, an independent trial statistician, rather than the researchers, should do the analyses for the DMC.[21] The interim analysis plan could be in the protocol, in a separate statistical analysis plan, or in a DMC charter. The analysis plan and charter, if appropriate, can be appendices to the protocol. Having them as appendices keeps the protocol more approachable to the implementation staff undertaking the trial.[21]

Many trials probably do not need an interim analysis and independent monitoring.[29] Indeed, most reports of trials do not describe the practice. Of 662 eligible trials identified in 2000, 24% mentioned use of a DMC, interim analyses, or both.[30] Of 648 paediatric trials, 17% mentioned a DMC, interim analysis, or early stopping.[23]

EARLY TERMINATION AND BIASED ESTIMATES OF TREATMENT EFFECTS

If a DMC stops a trial early on the basis of a group sequential stopping procedure, the estimates of treatment effect are biased. That remains a shortcoming of these procedures. Moreover, trials stopping early for benefit seem to be occurring more frequently.[31] As explanation, suppose the investigators did the same trial many times. Random fluctuations towards greater treatment effects would more probably result in early termination than random fluctuations towards lesser treatment effects. Thus when a trial is stopped early, readers need to grasp that the estimated treatment effects are prone to exaggeration (i.e., a random high).[20,24] Indeed, in a large systematic review and metaregression analysis, estimates of treatment effects were larger in those randomised trials that stopped early compared with those that did not stop early.[32] The authors concluded that 'In this empirical study including 91 truncated RCTs and 424 matching nontruncated RCTs addressing 63 questions, we found that truncated RCTs provide biased estimates of effects on the outcome that precipitated early stopping'.[32] When an unbiased estimate is paramount, investigators should focus on a fixed-sample design.

STOPPING FOR HARM OR FUTILITY

Stopping for harm or futility occurs more commonly than stopping for early efficacy benefit (demonstrated superiority). In a review of randomised trials, 249 were stopped (prematurely discontinued).[22] Of those, 15% were discontinued due to demonstrated futility, 4% due to demonstrated early benefit, and 10% due to unexpected harm.[22] Another review of randomised trials found 102 out of 574 stopped early.[33] Of the 102 discontinued trials, 30% stopped for demonstrated futility, only 2% for demonstrated superiority (early benefit), and 14% for harm (called 'safety signals' in this review).[33]

Thus far in our discussion of stopping guidelines, we have implied the same level of evidence to terminate early irrespective of whether for benefit or harm. Methodologists call such a strategy 'symmetrical stopping boundaries with group sequential methods', analogous to two-sided hypothesis testing.

Some investigators or DMCs, however, desire asymmetrical stopping boundaries.[28] These allow for a lower level of evidence to terminate for harm than for benefit. For example, O'Brien–Fleming sequential boundaries might be used in monitoring for benefit, whereas Pocock-type sequential boundaries could be used when monitoring for harm.[21]

Sometimes researchers or a DMC do not want to establish harm. Alternatively, they desire to denote trends that are sufficiently unfavourable, such that completion of the trial is unlikely to yield a significant beneficial effect. That facilitates stopping for futility (or lack of benefit), which only permits an assertion of inability to establish benefit. Some researchers argue that certain clinical settings require an aggressive monitoring for futility, whereas other clinical settings require a conservative approach to monitoring.[34] The determination depends on the disease severity, the toxicity of treatments, and whether reliable evidence of treatment benefit exists. Discussing these issues in detail is beyond the scope of this chapter, but we suggest a useful reference.[34]

Stopping for futility incorporates two general types of statistical approaches. The first approach evaluates whether the confidence interval (usually 95%) for the primary endpoint effect estimate excludes a predetermined (and documented) minimum benefit. If the interval does exclude it, then the indication is to stop the trial early for futility.[18]

The second approach engenders fancy terminology: conditional power and stochastic curtailment. With conditional power, investigators design trials with a stated power[35] (Chapter 11). However, once investigators start the trial, sustained data accumulation enriches knowledge (shielded from the investigators, of course). With accumulating data, the power can be recalculated. For example, an emerging trend towards treatment efficacy increases power, whereas an unfavourable trend reduces power. Conditional power describes this evolving power estimate.

DMCs use conditional power most frequently with trends unfavourable to treatment. If the conditional power calculations yield low power for various assumed treatment effects, including the assumed treatment effect in the trial protocol, then a monitoring group might consider continuation of the trial as futile and recommend stopping. The process of implementation of conditional power to discontinue a trial early breeds what some investigators call stochastic curtailment. These methods have been used effectively in monitoring trials.[18,21,24]

OTHER STATISTICAL STOPPING METHODS

Other statistical stopping methods also have appeal. Lan–DeMets (alpha spending function) developed a more flexible adaptation of group sequential methods.[36,37] It controls the false-positive error used at every interim analysis as a function of the proportion of total information observed, which allows the number and exact timing of the interim analyses to change after the trial has started.[21,24] The DMC begins with a schedule that could change on the basis of emerging data. Thus an alpha spending approach allows for unplanned looks.

We find Bayesian approaches helpful in clinical decision making[38] (see Chapter 9) but remain sceptical about their use in interim analyses. Bayesian approaches represent a separate branch of statistics. Correctly implemented, they can be useful for monitoring.[39–42] Readers, however, have little need to understand them, because they are used sparingly. Moreover, they elicit concerns. For example, every interim challenge might be at the 0.05 level, seriously escalating the overall false-positive error rate (α).[21] Unfortunately, some sponsors might take a keen interest in this higher likelihood of finding a significant effect.

WHAT READERS SHOULD LOOK FOR WITH INTERIM ANALYSES

Readers should remain alert for unreported interim analyses. If they find a statement from the researchers that no interim analyses were done, multiplicity is probably not a problem. However, such transparent reporting rarely happens. Poor reporting might camouflage the interim looks that the investigators did. Admittedly, detection of such interim analyses poses problems for readers. One clue is that the calculated p value is slightly less than 0.05, which could mean the researchers repeatedly tested and stopped the trial just when $p < 0.05$ was attained. Another clue might be if the completed trial size is less than that planned. One reason that sample size calculations are desired in the methods section is to indicate whether the trial stopped early. Readers should be wary if the trial stopped early and no statistical stopping rule was described.

Randomised trial registries could provide useful information on stopping. However, less than half of published trials that stopped early (prematurely discontinued) were properly labelled in registry records.[43] Moreover, only one-third of registry records provided a reason for stopping early. Unfortunately, at this writing, investigators cannot expect much help from registries.[43]

If researchers describe a statistical stopping rule, readers should evaluate its appropriateness. Peto and O'Brien–Fleming methods accomplish the goals of interim analyses without detracting from the trial. The other statistical approaches to interim analyses, most of which sport fancy names such as alpha spending function and conditional power, usually are appropriate, but Bayesian approaches can provoke concerns.

Conclusion

In reports of randomised trials, readers should cautiously interpret the results of subgroup analyses. If investigators test enough subgroups, a false-positive result will probably emerge by chance alone. Moreover, they might undertake many analyses but only report the statistically significant effects, distorting the medical literature. In general, we discourage subgroup analyses. However, if they are necessary, researchers should do, and readers should expect, statistical tests of interaction, rather than separate analyses of every subgroup.

Data monitoring activities in randomised trials often indicate interim analyses. However, repeatedly testing at every interim analysis raises multiplicity concerns, and not accounting for multiplicity escalates the false-positive error. Statistical stopping rules (essentially warning rules) must be used. We recommend group sequential stopping methods, which are easily implemented and preserve the intended α level and power. Implementing a trial under these stopping rules resembles a conventional trial, with the exception that it can be terminated early should a treatment prove greatly superior.

References

1. Schulz, K.F., Grimes, D.A., 2005. Multiplicity in randomised trials I: endpoints and treatments. Lancet 365, 1591–1595.
2. Horton, R., 2000. From star signs to trial guidelines. Lancet 355, 1033–1034.
3. Oei, S.G., Helmerhorst, F.M., Keirse, M.N.C., 1999. In: Cohlen, B.J., te Velde, E.R., Habbema, J.D. Postcoital test should be performed as routine infertility test. BMJ 318, 1008–1009.
4. ISIS-2 (Second International Study of Infarct Survival) Collaborative Group, 1988. Randomised trial of intravenous streptokinase, oral aspirin, both, or neither among 17,187 cases of suspected acute myocardial infarction: ISIS-2. Lancet 2, 349–360.
5. Yusuf, S., Wittes, J., Probstfield, J., Tyroler, H.A., 1991. Analysis and interpretation of treatment effects in subgroups of patients in randomized clinical trials. JAMA 266, 93–98.
6. Pocock, S.J., McMurray, J.J.V., Collier, T.J., 2015. Statistical controversies in reporting of clinical trials: part 2 of a 4-part series on statistics for clinical trials. J. Am. Coll. Cardiol. 66, 2648–2662.
7. Pocock, S.J., Assmann, S.E., Enos, L.E., Kasten, L.E., 2002. Subgroup analysis, covariate adjustment and baseline comparisons in clinical trial reporting: current practice and problems. Stat. Med. 21, 2917–2930.
8. Altman, D.G., Bland, J.M., 2003. Interaction revisited: the difference between two estimates. BMJ 326, 219.
9. Assmann, S.F., Pocock, S.J., Enos, L.E., Kasten, L.E., 2000. Subgroup analysis and other (mis)uses of baseline data in clinical trials. Lancet 355, 1064–1069.
10. Guillemin, F., 2007. Primer: the fallacy of subgroup analysis. Nat. Clin. Pract. Rheumatol. 3, 407–413.
11. Sun, X., Briel, M., Busse, J.W., et al., 2012. Credibility of claims of subgroup effects in randomised controlled trials: systematic review. BMJ 344, e1553.
12. Schulz, K.F., Grimes, D.A., 2005. Multiplicity in randomised trials II: subgroup and interim analyses. Lancet 365, 1657–1661.
13. Pocock, S., 1983. Clinical Trials: A Practical Approach. Wiley, Chichester, UK.
14. Perneger, T.V., 1998. What's wrong with Bonferroni adjustments. BMJ 316, 1236–1238.
15. Dyson, D.C., Crites, Y.M., Ray, D.A., Armstrong, M.A., 1991. Prevention of preterm birth in high-risk patients: the role of education and provider contact versus home uterine monitoring. Am. J. Obstet. Gynecol. 164, 756–762.
16. Pfeffer, M.A., Jarcho, J.A., 2006. The charisma of subgroups and the subgroups of CHARISMA. N. Engl. J. Med. 354, 1744–1746.
17. Wang, R., Lagakos, S.W., Ware, J.H., Hunter, D.J., Drazen, J.M., 2007. Statistics in medicine—reporting of subgroup analyses in clinical trials. N. Engl. J. Med. 357, 2189–2194.
18. Pocock, S.J., Clayton, T.C., Stone, G.W., 2015. Challenging issues in clinical trial design: part 4 of a 4-part series on statistics for clinical trials. J. Am. Coll. Cardiol. 66, 2886–2898.
19. Tharmanathan, P., Calvert, M., Hampton, J., Freemantle, N., 2008. The use of interim data and Data Monitoring Committee recommendations in randomized controlled trial reports: frequency, implications and potential sources of bias. BMC Med. Res. Methodol. 8, 12.
20. Pocock, S.J., 1992. When to stop a clinical trial. BMJ 305, 235–240.
21. Ellenberg, S.S., Fleming, T.R., DeMets, D.L., 2002. Data Monitoring Committees in Clinical Trials. John Wiley & Sons Ltd, Chichester.
22. Stegert, M., Kasenda, B., von Elm, E., et al., 2016. An analysis of protocols and publications suggested that most discontinuations of clinical trials were not based on preplanned interim analyses or stopping rules. J. Clin. Epidemiol. 69, 152–160.
23. Fernandes, R.M., van der Lee, J.H., Offringa, M., 2009. A systematic review of the reporting of Data Monitoring Committees' roles, interim analysis and early termination in pediatric clinical trials. BMC Pediatr. 9, 77.

24. Piantadosi, S., 1997. Clinical Trials: A Methodologic Perspective. John Wiley & Sons, New York.
25. Geller, N.L., Pocock, S.J., 1987. Interim analyses in randomized clinical trials: ramifications and guidelines for practitioners. Biometrics 43, 213–223.
26. O'Brien, P.C., Fleming, T.R., 1979. A multiple testing procedure for clinical trials. Biometrics 35, 549–556.
27. McPherson, K., 1990. Sequential stopping rules in clinical trials. Stat. Med. 9, 595–600.
28. Tyson, J.E., Pedroza, C., Wallace, D., D'Angio, C., Bell, E.F., Das, A., 2016. Stopping guidelines for an effectiveness trial: what should the protocol specify? Trials 17, 240.
29. Sydes, M.R., Spiegelhalter, D.J., Altman, D.G., Babiker, A.B., Parmar, M.K.B., DAMOCLES Group, 2004. Systematic qualitative review of the literature on Data Monitoring Committees for randomized controlled trials. Clin. Trials 1, 60–79.
30. Sydes, M.R., Altman, D.G., Babiker, A.B., Parmar, M.K.B., Spiegelhalter, D., DAMOCLES Group, 2004. Reported use of data monitoring committees in the main published reports of randomized trials: a cross-sectional study. Clin. Trials 1, 48–59.
31. Montori, V.M., Devereaux, P.J., Adhikari, N.K., et al., 2005. Randomized trials stopped early for benefit: a systematic review. JAMA 294, 2203–2209.
32. Bassler, D., Briel, M., Montori, V.M., et al., 2010. Stopping randomized trials early for benefit and estimation of treatment effects: systematic review and meta-regression analysis. JAMA 303, 1180–1187.
33. van den Bogert, C.A., Souverein, P.C., Brekelmans, C.T.M., et al., 2017. Recruitment failure and futility were the most common reasons for discontinuation of clinical drug trials. Results of a nationwide inception cohort study in the Netherlands. J. Clin. Epidemiol. 88, 140–147.
34. Freidlin, B., Korn, E.L., 2009. Monitoring for lack of benefit: a critical component of a randomized clinical trial. J. Clin. Oncol. 27, 629–633.
35. Schulz, K.F., Grimes, D.A., 2005. Sample size calculations in randomised trials: mandatory and mystical. Lancet 365, 1348–1353.
36. Lan, K.K.G., DeMets, D.L., 1983. Discrete sequential boundaries for clinical trials. Biometrika 70, 659–663.
37. DeMets, D.L., Lan, K.K., 1994. Interim analysis: the alpha spending function approach. Stat. Med. 13, 1341–1352 discussion 1353–1356.
38. Grimes, D.A., Schulz, K.F., 2005. Refining clinical diagnosis with likelihood ratios. Lancet 365, 1500–1505.
39. Spiegelhalter, D.J., Freedman, L.S., Parmar, M.K., 1993. Applying Bayesian ideas in drug development and clinical trials. Stat. Med. 12, 1501–1511; discussion 1513–1517.
40. Freedman, L.S., Spiegelhalter, D.J., Parmar, M.K., 1994. The what, why and how of Bayesian clinical trials monitoring. Stat. Med. 13, 1371–1383; discussion 1385–1389.
41. Parmar, M.K., Spiegelhalter, D.J., Freedman, L.S., 1994. The CHART trials: Bayesian design and monitoring in practice. CHART Steering Committee. Stat. Med. 13, 1297–1312.
42. Parmar, M.K., Griffiths, G.O., Spiegelhalter, D.J., Souhami, R.L., Altman, D.G., van der Scheuren, E., 2001. Monitoring of large randomised clinical trials: a new approach with Bayesian methods. Lancet 358, 375–381.
43. Alturki, R., Schandelmaier, S., Olu, K.K., et al., 2017. Premature trial discontinuation often not accurately reflected in registries: comparison of registry records with publications. J. Clin. Epidemiol. 81, 56–63.

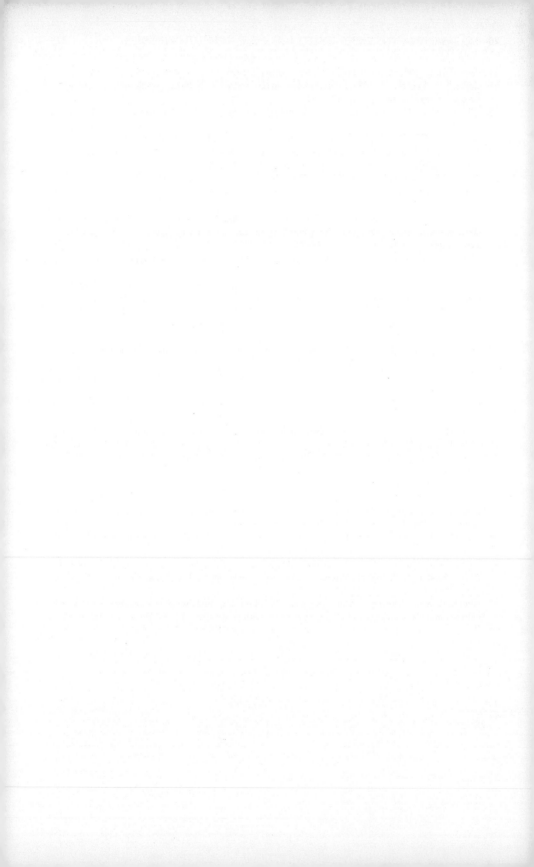

CHAPTER 21

Conducting a Randomised Trial as Part of a Prospective Meta-Analysis

A prospective meta-analysis (PMA) conducts single-site randomised trials in conjunction with an active, contemporaneous approach to a meta-analysis. This contrasts with the common approach of investigators designing, conducting, and publishing a trial without any further plan. Frequently, they passively wait for the results to be combined with other similar randomised trials in a traditional, retrospective meta-analysis as part of a systematic review. Alternatively, they may eventually plan a traditional meta-analysis that includes their trial. However, in a PMA, an investigator designs a meta-analysis while planning and conducting a component trial that will contribute to the PMA.

A prospective meta-analysis (PMA) circumvents some of the challenges to traditional, retrospective meta-analyses. A PMA is a meta-analysis of randomised trials that were recognised and determined to be appropriate for the meta-analysis before the findings of any of those trials are known. Unaware of the findings of individual trials, investigators stipulate hypotheses *a priori* and establish prospective application of study selection criteria. Moreover, PMAs allow *a priori* declarations of planned analyses, including any subgroup analyses, before the findings of the individual component trials are known. Thus PMAs skirt potential problems in interpretation related to *post hoc*, data-dependent analyses in traditional meta-analyses.

In addition, all of the sites contributing to a PMA must agree on the intervention and outcomes. Thus problems are averted compared with retrospective meta-analyses with discrepancies in interventions being combined and disparities in outcomes being measured. Without the collective determinations of the PMA collaborative process, the independent sites might generate irreconcilable data that could not be combined in a scientifically acceptable meta-analysis.

PMAs are commonly implemented by a collaborative group, and they usually collect and analyse individual patient data (IPD). Unlike traditional multicentre trials, they allow variation in the protocols of the included trials, while maximising power in the preplanned meta-analyses. A PMA would usually require fewer resources than a multicentre randomised trial while cultivating opportunities for research participation. Thus PMAs may foster increased research capacity through collaboration.

Moreover, PMAs expand opportunities for authorship of peer-reviewed publications. With a PMA, contributing institutions can publish their own trial results. Indeed, the PMA methodology enables several investigators at each site to qualify for authorship of their site report.

PMAs present a host of efficiencies and opportunities. Clinical researchers need to be familiar with the concepts behind a PMA and, when appropriate, capitalise on its advantages. We encourage interested readers to consider the approach.

Introduction

In planning a randomised trial, investigators frequently discover that they have low power with their anticipated sample size. They lack a sufficient number of potentially available participants at their institution. In these situations, some methodologists and ethicists will advise those investigators to abandon such an apparent 'low-power' trial.[1] Some ethics review boards (ERBs) deem low-power trials as unethical.[1] However, we take a different view as described in Chapter 11. We believe, with three caveats, that these so-called underpowered trials can be acceptable because they can ultimately be combined in a traditional, retrospective meta-analysis. Traditional meta-analysis is not, however, the only option for addressing low power.

MULTICENTRE RANDOMISED CONTROLLED TRIAL

Another solution to low power is a multicentre randomised controlled trial (MCRCT). Essentially, it replicates a single-site randomised controlled trial; extra sites add numbers of participants and thus statistical power. This usually involves a collective protocol, standard eligibility criteria, standard interventions, shared randomisation procedures, common data-collection forms, shared data management, standard operational procedures, collective data analysis, and centralised oversight. We deliberately avoid discussion of issues of the design and planning of MCRCTs in this book for several reasons. First, good descriptions are found elsewhere.[2,3] Second, novice investigators may not have the resources necessary to initiate an MCRCT. They may have the opportunity to respond to a funder's solicitation, but the design and planning will likely have been done by that funding source. Third, some potential disadvantages make MCRCTs less attractive to single-site investigators who are interested in collaborative trials.

PROSPECTIVE META-ANALYSIS

A PMA is a planned, active approach to a meta-analysis. It conducts single-site randomised trials in conjunction with an active, contemporaneous approach to a meta-analysis. This contrasts with the common approach of investigators designing, conducting, and publishing a trial without any further plan. Frequently, they passively wait for their results to be combined with other similar randomised trials in a traditional, retrospective meta-analysis as part of a systematic review. However, in a PMA, investigators design a meta-analysis while planning and conducting a component trial that will contribute to the PMA.

This chapter provides a primer on PMAs and familiarises readers with the concept. We discuss some of the disadvantages of MCRCTs, which remain the main alternative scientific study design to a PMA. Next, we review the advantages and disadvantages of PMAs vis-à-vis MCRCTs, retrospective meta-analyses, and single-site RCTs. Finally, we describe the basic steps in a PMA and encourage readers to consider this approach. We will not provide comprehensive, detailed methods for planning and conducting a PMA.

Some Disadvantages of Multicentre Randomised Trials

Well-conducted, multicentre randomised trials are the gold standard for evidence-based medicine. Yet they can be expensive, cumbersome, and unrewarding for individual investigators. Disadvantages can emerge in the design, conduct, and reporting of an MCRCT.

The need for a uniform data-collection form, or case report form (CRF), in an MCRCT can pose logistical challenges. In a multicentre trial, one centre may consent to inclusion of another centre's desired data-collection items if that other centre consents to its own desired data-collection items. When many centres are involved, these multiple *quid pro quo* negotiations frequently yield a long and unwieldy CRF. These negotiations may delay implementation, increase the cost of the trial, and potentially decrease the quality of the data gathered. Moreover, long CRFs unnecessarily burden participants, which discourages participant retention.

The requirement for approvals by multiple institutional ERBs in an MCRCT creates more hurdles. Usually an ERB for one centre will not allow the trial to begin at that centre until all the other ERBs involved in the multicentre trial also approve the trial at their respective centres. Thus an individual centre may have all its own approvals and be ready to begin enrolling, but be prohibited from doing so because it awaits ERB approvals from all the contributing centres. This consequently delays commencement and increases the cost of the MCRCT due to 'treading water' or idling trial costs. Also, the delays can frustrate the research staff. The slowest ERB becomes the 'rate-limiting enzyme' for starting the trial.

The most industrious and efficient investigators can suffer further disadvantages in an MCRCT. If investigators at an individual centre proficiently and promptly complete their enrolment and follow-up, their rewards will be delayed. With other centres lagging, analysis and manuscript activities must wait for those other centres to complete their data-collection activities. Thus costs are increased, and time to publication is delayed while waiting on the slowest centre to finish.

Investigators may be less invested in an MCRCT than in a trial done only at their institution. First, they probably are not as intimately involved in the analysis and manuscript writing as they would have been had they conducted a single-site RCT. Second, in multicentre trials, authorship is often limited to the principal investigators at each site. Investigators may only be identified in group authorship in the final manuscript (often represented by an asterisk and each author's name in small font at the end of the paper). Group authorship does not carry the same weight as having one's name in the byline. Although it certainly counts as being a valid author, many find it a bit anticlimactic after the long, hard, arduous tasks of recruitment, data collection, and follow-up. Indeed, some hardworking investigators involved in MCRCTs are frustrated by the lack of recognition.

When the resources are available and investigators accept the challenges, we certainly encourage the conduct of large multicentre randomised trials. However, in many circumstances, PMAs may be a less costly, more efficient, faster, and more satisfying approach to gathering evidence (Panel 21.1).[4-8]

PANEL 21.1 ■ Some Potential Advantages of Prospective Meta-Analyses (PMAs) vis-à-vis Multicentre Randomised Controlled Trials

- With a PMA, individual contributing sites will have a more concise and focused data-collection form.
- Only one ethical review board approval is needed before a site starts its trial.
- With a PMA, the individual contributing institutions can publish their own results, which expands opportunities in institutions for authorship of peer-reviewed publications.
- PMAs expedite time to a peer-reviewed publication for individual contributing institutions.
- The individual trials contributing to a PMA may yield improved trial conduct, coming as a by product of separate, individual trial authorship.
- A PMA expands opportunities for research participation through research mentoring.
- PMAs would generally require fewer resources than a multicentre randomised controlled trial.

With a PMA, individual contributing sites can have a more concise and focused data-collection form. All the sites in a PMA must agree upon the intervention groups and the measurement of the primary and secondary outcomes, along with perhaps some baseline measurements. Other than those uniform data requirements, individual sites are free to collect only information of interest to them. Unlike in an MCRCT, they do not have to collect data of interest to other sites. Thus their data collection becomes more specific, and their trial, in general, is more streamlined. That leads to lower costs, quicker completion, and potentially better data quality. The shorter data-collection form is beneficial to participants. Treating them responsibly by being parsimonious with data gathering will likely improve follow-up and retention of participants.

PMAs simplify the role of an institutional ethical review board (ERB). Instead of waiting for all the other ERBs to approve the trial, as in a multicentre trial, a contributing institution in a PMA simply secures approval from their institution's ERB. That can remove exogenous obstacles, reduce costs, and hasten completion.

PMAs expedite time to publication for a contributing institution. A multicentre trial must wait for the slowest centre to finish their data collection before the team begins to analyse the results and write their report. However, a PMA is more expeditious. When a contributing institution completes its data collection, researchers can analyse their own data, write the manuscript, and then submit it for publication. Therefore results reach the medical literature more quickly from their single-site trial than if they had been part of a multicentre trial.

PMAs can expand opportunities for authorship of peer-reviewed publications.[6] With a PMA, contributing institutions can publish their own results. Indeed, several investigators at each site conduct the trial and qualify for authorship of the individual site publication. Typically, with a PMA, an individual institution publishes their results in a journal and then also contributes, through group authorship, to the publication of the eventual PMA. This bestows byline authorship benefits to the contributing investigators at each site. That visible authorship at the front of the paper, immediately following the title, is an immensely satisfying reward for their efforts.

The individual trials contributing to a PMA may yield improved trial conduct as a byproduct of separate, individual trial authorship. Some investigators have speculated that this responsibility of authorship may improve study conduct because it 'may optimize individual site protocol execution (proper administration of medications, maximizing participant retention, and collecting all data points) and motivate individual sites to conclude the project in a timely fashion'.[6]

A PMA expands opportunities for research mentoring. The PMA may foster increased research capacity through collaboration. PMAs can involve both senior and novice researchers. Novice researchers from smaller sites can benefit from involvement in a PMA by gaining access to well-developed protocols and the opportunity to recruit smaller numbers of participants. Thus the PMA provides a vehicle for mentorship from senior researchers and allows multiple sites the opportunity to gain experience and scientific expertise in the conduct of randomised trials. Indeed, a primary aim of one PMA was to create the opportunity for mentorship to new investigators and to promote more 'rapid and effective growth of the ... research community'.[6]

A PMA requires fewer resources than an MCRCT. When sites conduct their own trials, they develop protocols that best match their interests, the accessibility of trial participants, and the availability of institutional resources. This decentralisation lowers cost by avoiding centralised oversight. Furthermore, individual site investigators can seek smaller grants for their sites rather than attempting to pursue 'a large, less readily obtainable grant for an unwieldy and costly multi-center trial'.[6]

PANEL 21.2 ■ Some Potential Advantages of Prospective Meta-Analyses (PMAs) vis-à-vis Traditional, Retrospective Meta-Analyses

- PMAs allow investigators to stipulate hypotheses *a priori* and to facilitate prospective application of study selection criteria.
- PMAs allow *a priori* declarations of planned analyses, including any subgroup analyses, before the findings of the individual component trials are known. This avoids inherent data-dependent analyses in retrospective meta-analyses.
- With common intervention groups and outcomes, a PMA obviates problems in traditional meta-analyses with different interventions being combined and disparate outcomes being measured.
- A PMA increases the likelihood that an eventual meta-analysis on the topic will be conducted, which addresses power concerns.
- The process of a PMA may recruit investigators who may not have otherwise contemplated conducting a trial on their own of the proposed topic.
- A PMA easily facilitates an individual patient data (IPD) analysis.

A PMA circumvents some of the challenges to traditional, retrospective meta-analyses (Panel 21.2).[9,10] Because they are prospective, PMAs allow investigators, unaware of the findings of individual trials, to stipulate hypotheses *a priori* and to facilitate prospective application of study selection criteria. Moreover, PMAs allow *a priori* declarations of planned analyses, including any subgroup analyses, before the findings of the individual component trials are known. Thus PMAs avoid potential problems in interpretation related to the *post hoc*, data-dependent analyses in retrospective meta-analyses.[11]

In addition, all of the sites contributing to a PMA must approve uniform interventions and outcomes. This avoids problems found in traditional meta-analyses which often encounter discrepancies in interventions and outcomes being measured. These discrepancies sometimes preclude aggregation of data, as we often found in conducting Cochrane systematic reviews of randomised trials.

A PMA provides a higher likelihood that an eventual meta-analysis will be conducted. If an investigator conducts and reports a single-site trial, the prospect for a future meta-analysis is unknown. That can be a concern, particularly if it is a low-power trial. A PMA planned in concert with a single-site trial alleviates, but may not eliminate, this concern.

A PMA provides additional encouragement for sites to contribute. The actual process of a PMA reaches out to potential investigators for contribution. That process enlists investigators who may not have otherwise contemplated conducting a trial on their own.

Finally, a PMA facilitates an individual patient data (IPD) analysis. Many meta-analyses pool aggregate data from the component trials, because the process of acquiring IPD from investigators of completed trials ranges from difficult to impossible. With a PMA, individual patient data, by definition, are easily available for the pooled analysis.

Some Potential Disadvantages of PMAs

Although a PMA offers important advantages, it still suffers from real or perceived disadvantages. Compared with typical single-site RCTs, PMAs require increased time and effort.[5] Of course, in both instances, the investigators conduct an individual trial. However, when a contributing site is part of a PMA, investigators have additional organisation and collaboration activities. That increased effort is heavily front-loaded, with much occurring at the beginning but usually continuing throughout the PMA process. Notably, the increased work effort could be substantial, especially for the coordinating centre.

Compared with an MCRCT, a PMA might be less likely to be completed and published. If resources are secured from a funding source for an MCRCT and commitments obtained from individual trial sites for participation, that process generally assures analysis and publication of the pooled results. We suspect that the likelihood of publication of an MCRCT surpasses that of a comparable PMA. Suppose that reports from individual sites in a PMA begin to be published. Suppose further that the results are not as favourable as envisioned. As a number of sites finish and publish, the unfavourable results of the pooled analysis become preordained. The motivation of the PMA collaborators to conduct the analysis and publish the pooled PMA results may decrease.

Basic Steps in a PMA

We will summarise the steps in a PMA. If you find the concept interesting, references are available elsewhere.[6,7,12] In particular, the Cochrane Collaboration provides excellent guidance and support.[11] Here are some important elements of a PMA:

- Search computerised databases to assure that trials are not already published that answer the questions proposed by the PMA.
- Develop a preliminary PMA protocol.
- Identify potential collaborating sites by such methods as contacting professional colleagues, searching clinicaltrials.gov for ongoing similar research, and recruiting while presenting at regional and national scientific meetings.
- Agree on the PMA coinvestigators and the PMA coordinating centre.
- Achieve collaborative judgements with coinvestigators on a common PMA protocol and site responsibilities.
  - Determine the uniform intervention and control groups to be compared.
  - Determine the uniform measurement of primary and secondary outcomes.

PANEL 21.3 ■ The Cochrane Prospective Meta-Analysis Methods Group Recommendations for a PMA Protocol

Each protocol should contain
1. The specific hypotheses/objectives.
2. Eligibility criteria for trial design (e.g., requirements for randomisation, minimum follow-up).
3. Eligibility criteria for the patient population.
4. Eligibility criteria for the treatment comparisons.
5. Definition of outcomes.
6. Details of subgroups.
7. Analysis plan. This should include details of sample size calculations (for the PMA), interim analyses, subgroup analyses, etc.
8. Details of trials identified for inclusion, including (a) efforts made to identify ongoing trials, (b) a statement confirming that at the time of submission for registration any trial results were unknown (to anyone outside the trial's own data-monitoring committee); trials should be included only if their results were unknown at the time they were identified and added to the PMA, and (c) agreement of each of the trial groups to collaborate.
9. Management and coordination, including (a) details of management committee, (b) data management (data to be collected, format required, when required, quality assurance procedures, etc.), and (c) statistical analyses (who performs these, will the statisticians be blinded to treatment group, etc.).
10. Publication policy, including (a) policy regarding authorship (e.g., will publications be in 'group' name?), (b) writing committee (membership, responsibilities), and (c) policy regarding manuscript (e.g., drafts to be circulated to all trialists for comment).

Source: http://methods.cochrane.org/pma/how-plan-and-execute-pma; accessed 6 August 2017

- Determine the uniform baseline variables to measure.
- Consider if uniform eligibility criteria will be used and, if so, agree on them.
- Develop a PMA protocol and submit the protocol for review to a journal or to The Cochrane Prospective Meta-Analysis Methods Group of the Cochrane Collaboration, which has a detailed list of what the protocol should include (Panel 21.3).
- Obtain approval independently from the ERBs at each contributing site.
- Initiate the trial conduct independently at each contributing site after ethical approval is granted.
- Analyse data independently at each site when that site completes enrolment, follow-up, and data collection activities.
- Write, submit, and publish a manuscript from each contributing site.
- Provide IPD to the PMA coordinating centre for aggregation and the eventual pooled analysis.
- Collaborate with the coordinating centre and the other contributing centres on the analysis and manuscript preparation for the PMA.
- Submit the final PMA manuscript for publication.

Conclusion

The PMA approach offers advantages over MCRCTs and traditional, retrospective meta-analyses. PMAs encourage trials that, when pooled, answer research hypotheses that necessitate larger sample sizes. The wider adoption of PMAs would facilitate more and better-designed randomised controlled trials while building increased research capacity.

PMAs offer flexibility. For example, a site not accruing participants as fast as expected will not delay other sites. Slow-recruiting sites can, of course, delay the PMA aggregate analysis and publication. Slow recruitment at sites can be addressed by having other sites enrol additional participants or by adding additional sites.

Submitting the PMA protocol for review to the Cochrane Collaboration is an important consideration. Although not mandatory, we recommend doing so for two reasons. First, if the investigators meticulously follow their PMA protocol, that almost guarantees publication of their completed PMA manuscript in the Cochrane Library. Second, and even more importantly, the PMA protocol will be reviewed at an early stage by expert meta-analysts. That critique can be invaluable, especially for beginning researchers.

References

1. Halpern, S.D., Karlawish, J.H., Berlin, J.A., 2002. The continuing unethical conduct of underpowered clinical trials. JAMA 288, 358–362.
2. Pocock, S., 1983. Clinical Trials: A Practical Approach. Wiley, Chichester, UK.
3. Meinert, C., 1986. Clinical Trials: Design, Conduct, and Analysis. Oxford University Press, New York.
4. Tavernier, E., Trinquart, L., Giraudeau, B., 2016. Finding alternatives to the dogma of power based sample size calculation: is a fixed sample size prospective meta-experiment a potential alternative? PLoS One 11, e0158604.
5. Walker, D.M., 2010. Prospective meta-analysis within complementary medicine research. J. Altern. Complement. Med. 16, 1249.
6. Turok, D.K., Espey, E., Edelman, A.B., et al., 2011. The methodology for developing a prospective meta-analysis in the family planning community. Trials 12, 104.
7. Askie, L.M., Baur, L.A., Campbell, K., et al., 2010. The Early Prevention of Obesity in CHildren (EPOCH) Collaboration—an individual patient data prospective meta-analysis. BMC Public Health 10, 728.
8. Valsecchi, M.G., Masera, G., 1996. A new challenge in clinical research in childhood ALL: the prospective meta-analysis strategy for intergroup collaboration. Ann. Oncol. 7, 1005–1008.

9. Simes, R.J., Prospective meta-analysis of cholesterol-lowering studies: the Prospective Pravastatin Pooling (PPP) Project and the Cholesterol Treatment Trialists (CTT) Collaboration, 1995. Am. J. Cardiol. 76, 122c–126c.

10. Reade, M.C., Delaney, A., Bailey, M.J., et al., 2010. Prospective meta-analysis using individual patient data in intensive care medicine. Intensive Care Med. 36, 11–21.

11. Ghersi, D., Berlin, J., Askie, L., 2011. Chapter 19: Prospective meta-analysis. In: Higgins, J.P.T., Green, S. (Eds.), Cochrane Handbook for Systematic Reviews of Interventions Version 5.1.0 (updated March 2011). Available from www.handbook.cochrane.org: The Cochrane Collaboration.

12. Baigent, C., Keech, A., Kearney, P.M., et al., 2005. Efficacy and safety of cholesterol-lowering treatment: prospective meta-analysis of data from 90,056 participants in 14 randomised trials of statins. Lancet 366, 1267–1278.

CHAPTER 22

Reporting Studies in Medical Journals: CONSORT and Other Reporting Guidelines

Medical research seeks to expand scientific understanding and guide clinical care. However, poor scientific reporting of research, including nonreporting, hinders understanding and impedes the potential benefits to clinicians, researchers, and patients.

Deficient reporting is widespread. It ensues when a key aspect of the methods or results is omitted, incomplete, or vague. Selective reporting results from publication bias or biased reporting within publications. Unfortunately, investigators of many research studies, including randomised controlled trials (RCTs), never publish their findings. Indeed, if a study is not published, it did not happen in the eyes of the research community. Publication bias results from the preferential publication of studies with statistically significant outcomes. Biased reporting within publications appears when outcomes that were statistically significant were more likely to be reported, regardless of their status in the original trial protocol ('cherry picking').

We focus on reporting of randomised trials because of their importance to medical research and because most of the early work on improving reporting related to randomised trials. In the early 1990s, a group of researchers and editors started a guideline process that ended with the CONsolidated Standards Of Reporting Trials (CONSORT) Statement. The CONSORT Statement includes a checklist and a flow diagram. CONSORT enables the accurate, complete, and transparent reporting of a trial that facilitates critical appraisal and interpretation.

The CONSORT 2010 Statement provides guidance for reporting all RCTs, regardless of design. It pertains fundamentally to all randomised trials. However, it concentrates on the most common design type, individually randomised, two-group, parallel trials.

Investigators should use a reporting guideline for both planning and reporting all types of studies, not just randomised trials. Usually, as a rule of thumb, a reporting guideline that also has an explanation and elaboration (E&E) paper for support will be more useful. We recommend STARD for diagnostic test accuracy studies, STROBE for observational epidemiological studies, and PRISMA for systematic reviews including meta-analyses of randomised trials (Panel 22.1).

Continued

Empirical investigations substantiate that CONSORT leads to improved reporting in medical journals. However, the improvements appear moderate, and substantial room for improvement remains. CONSORT has spawned other useful guidelines for studies besides randomised trials. Authors should utilise appropriate reporting guidelines. Such use aids in study design and manuscript writing, and, in the end, likely leads to a higher probability of publication success.

Introduction

Medical research seeks to expand scientific understanding and guide clinical care. However, poor scientific reporting, including nonreporting, hinders understanding and impedes the potential benefits to clinicians, researchers, and patients.

Principally, medical journals convey research results. The report in a journal of a research study is almost always the only documentation of the study results. Indeed, if a study is not published, it remains invisible to the research community. Unfortunately, many investigators never publish their findings.[1,2]

Published articles of research studies offer potential benefits to multiple audiences. For example, other researchers use the methods and results of articles to guide their forthcoming research. Clinicians use journal articles to choose the treatment of patients. Systematic reviewers examine journal articles for inclusion in their reviews. They also need sufficiently detailed information on methods and results for potential integration into a meta-analysis. Many patients access the medical literature to guide their treatment decisions.

Publication is necessary but not sufficient. A journal article must contain full descriptions of the methods used and the results found. Readers need clear, accurate, complete, and transparent reporting. Only then can they correctly interpret the study findings.[3,4]

These general reporting principles pertain basically to all types of healthcare research. However, in this chapter we focus on reporting of RCTs for three reasons. First, one of us (K.F.S.) has been involved in setting the standards for reporting trials.[5-12] Second, throughout this book we intentionally devote more attention to trials. Third, the reports of randomised trials have the highest likelihood of all published research of having an immediate effect on patient care.[13] Indeed, as noted by a famous editor, 'The whole of medicine depends on the transparent reporting of clinical trials'.[14] Nevertheless, in a later section, we will recommend reporting guidelines for studies other than RCTs.

Reporting of Randomised Controlled Trials

RCTs, when appropriately designed, conducted, and reported, embody the gold standard in evaluating healthcare interventions. That distinguished position in the medical research taxonomy does not mean, however, that readers should uncritically accept the results of all RCTs. Indeed, randomised trials can yield biased results if they lack methodological rigour.[15,16] Although readers of journal articles need complete, clear, and transparent information on their methodology and findings, many authors fail to report critical information.

DEFICIENT REPORTING

Deficient reporting ensues when a key aspect of the methods or results is vague, incomplete, or omitted. Certainly, some overlap occurs among all these terms. For example, a description of a trial only as 'randomised' is vague, incomplete, and omits critical information. Clearly, critical information on the details of the randomisation methods is missing.

Deficient reporting is common. For example, one group of investigators found 177 reviews assessing the quality or reporting of RCTs published just between 1987 and 2007.[17] The consistent theme from this enormous body of research is that the reporting of RCTs in the literature is greatly deficient.

To exemplify the level of poor reporting, two of the more recent studies provide the best general estimates.[18,19] These two studies examine trial reports indexed in PubMed. As such, they provide information on all journals indexed in PubMed, including the most elite weekly general medical journals as well as the less recognised, lower-impact-level specialty journals. Overall, the level of reporting was dismal with only some small improvement over time.

The glaring deficiency was that authors omitted critical information. For example, information on random sequence generation and allocation concealment, arguably the most important ingredients in a randomised trial,[16] was not described in about two-thirds and three-quarters, respectively, of trial reports.

Unfortunately, the true state of conduct was even more dire. One would reasonably expect that when allocation concealment was reported in about one-fourth of the reports, it was an acceptable approach. That represents a rational expectation. Not so. Another study found the same level of good reporting but then further examined the quality of the method described.[20] More than half the authors described an inadequate approach to allocation concealment.[20] In other words, when the reporting was good, the actual method revealed was frequently bad. That sad fact further illustrates the need for good reporting for two reasons. First, with good reporting, the reader at least can identify a trial with poor methods and thereby properly interpret the results. Second, trials that report well but reveal poor methods provide an indication of the poor methods likely used in all those trials that report no information on allocation concealment.

Poor reporting extends beyond trial design and statistical methods. Medical research publications guide clinical practice. Published articles on randomised trials should provide adequate details of treatments studied such that they could be used by clinicians upon reading the article. That seems a minimum expectation. However, when investigators assessed descriptions of treatments in 80 published articles, critical elements of the treatments were not described in 41 of those studies.[21] Readers would not be able to replicate the treatments.

SELECTIVE REPORTING

The most recognised form of selective reporting is termed 'publication bias'. This bias results from authors of completed trials preferentially not publishing the trials with statistically nonsignificant findings. Extensive investigations support the existence of publication bias.[22] A large review that assessed study publication bias found persuasive support that trials with statistically significant results were more likely to be published.[1] Of note, some maintain that the term 'publication bias' is confusing and prefer the term 'nonpublication bias'.[3]

Another form of selective reporting, biased reporting within publications, is gaining recognition. It might be the most insidious form of selective reporting. The culprit appears to be that outcomes that were statistically significant were more likely to be reported, regardless of their status in the original trial protocol ('cherry picking').[3] Moreover, other investigations have demonstrated that the primary outcome described in the trial protocol frequently is not necessarily the primary outcome reported in the trial publication.[23,24] Indeed, 40%–62% of studies had at least one primary outcome changed, newly introduced, or excluded.[23,24]

The CONSORT Statement: A Reporting Guideline for Randomised Trials

As the burgeoning evidence pointed to the poor reporting of RCTs, investigators considered solutions. Poor reporting may simply signify ignorance on the vital information that must be included in the report of an RCT. Naivety may be more responsible than malevolence.[25] A reporting guideline could provide insight to that vital information, and, thus, theoretically help improve reporting.

However, not all reporting guidelines are created equal.[3] Early guidelines for RCT publications seemed to have minimal effect.[26,27] In the early 1990s, a group of researchers and editors started a guideline process that resulted in the CONsolidated Standards Of Reporting Trials (CONSORT) Statement.[28] The CONSORT Statement includes a checklist and a flow diagram. CONSORT enables the accurate, complete, and transparent reporting of a trial. It was designed to help authors, peer reviewers, and editors, and facilitates critical appraisal and interpretation.[3]

All the information required to evaluate a trial guided the reasoning for including items in the checklist.[7] The checklist ensures provision of the basic information that readers need to appraise the validity of the findings. Inclusion of items was based on relevant empirical evidence, whenever possible. The flow diagram (Fig. 22.1) depicts the movement of trial participants from recruitment to final analysis. The checklist (Table 22.1) and flow diagram form the CONSORT Statement.[7]

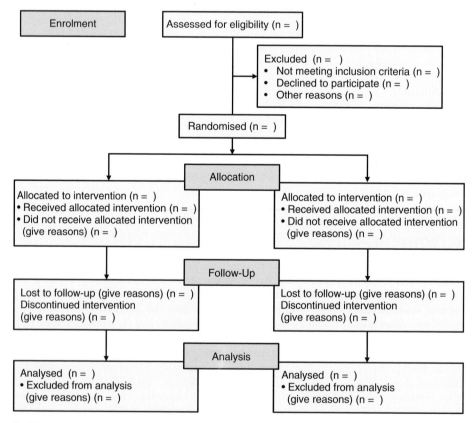

Fig. 22.1 Flow diagram of the progress through the phases of a parallel randomised trial of two groups (that is, enrolment, intervention allocation, follow-up, and data analysis).

TABLE 22.1 ■ CONSORT 2010 Checklist of Information to Include When Reporting a Randomised Trial*

Section/Topic	Item No	Checklist Item	Reported on Page Number
Title and Abstract			
	1a	Identification as a randomised trial in the title	_____
	1b	Structured summary of trial design, methods, results, and conclusions (for specific guidance see CONSORT for abstracts)[51,52]	_____
Introduction			
Background and objectives	2a	Scientific background and explanation of rationale	_____
	2b	Specific objectives or hypotheses	_____
Methods			
Trial design	3a	Description of trial design (such as parallel, factorial) including allocation ratio	_____
	3b	Important changes to methods after trial commencement (such as eligibility criteria), with reasons	_____
Participants	4a	Eligibility criteria for participants	_____
	4b	Settings and locations where the data were collected	_____
Interventions	5	The interventions for each group with sufficient details to allow replication, including how and when they were actually administered	_____
Outcomes	6a	Completely defined prespecified primary and secondary outcome measures, including how and when they were assessed	_____
	6b	Any changes to trial outcomes after the trial commenced, with reasons	_____
Sample size	7a	How sample size was determined	_____
	7b	When applicable, explanation of any interim analyses and stopping guidelines	_____
Randomisation: Sequence generation	8a	Method used to generate the random allocation sequence	_____
	8b	Type of randomisation; details of any restriction (such as blocking and block size)	_____
Allocation concealment mechanism	9	Mechanism used to implement the random allocation sequence (such as sequentially numbered containers), describing any steps taken to conceal the sequence until interventions were assigned	_____
Implementation	10	Who generated the random allocation sequence, who enrolled participants, and who assigned participants to interventions	_____
Blinding	11a	If done, who was blinded after assignment to interventions (for example, participants, care providers, those assessing outcomes) and how	_____
	11b	If relevant, description of the similarity of interventions	_____
Statistical methods	12a	Statistical methods used to compare groups for primary and secondary outcomes	_____
	12b	Methods for additional analyses, such as subgroup analyses and adjusted analyses	_____

TABLE 22.1 ▦ CONSORT 2010 Checklist of Information to Include When Reporting a Randomised Trial (Continued)

Section/Topic	Item No	Checklist Item	Reported on Page Number
Results			
Participant flow (a diagram is strongly recommended)	13a	For each group, the numbers of participants who were randomly assigned, received intended treatment, and were analysed for the primary outcome	_____
	13b	For each group, losses and exclusions after randomisation, together with reasons	_____
Recruitment	14a	Dates defining the periods of recruitment and follow-up	_____
	14b	Why the trial ended or was stopped	_____
Baseline data	15	A table showing baseline demographic and clinical characteristics for each group	_____
Numbers analysed	16	For each group, number of participants (denominator) included in each analysis and whether the analysis was by original assigned groups	_____
Outcomes and estimation	17a	For each primary and secondary outcome, results for each group, and the estimated effect size and its precision (such as 95% confidence interval)	_____
	17b	For binary outcomes, presentation of both absolute and relative effect sizes is recommended	_____
Ancillary analyses	18	Results of any other analyses performed, including subgroup analyses and adjusted analyses, distinguishing prespecified from exploratory	_____
Harms	19	All important harms or unintended effects in each group (for specific guidance see CONSORT for harms)[50]	_____
Discussion			
Limitations	20	Trial limitations, addressing sources of potential bias, imprecision, and, if relevant, multiplicity of analyses	_____
Generalisability	21	Generalisability (external validity, applicability) of the trial findings	_____
Interpretation	22	Interpretation consistent with results, balancing benefits and harms, and considering other relevant evidence	_____
Other Information			
Registration	23	Registration number and name of trial registry	_____
Protocol	24	Where the full trial protocol can be accessed, if available	_____
Funding	25	Sources of funding and other support (such as supply of drugs), role of funders	_____

*We strongly recommend reading this statement in conjunction with the CONSORT 2010 Explanation and Elaboration[37] for important clarifications on all the items. If relevant, we also recommend reading CONSORT extensions for cluster randomised trials,[38] noninferiority and equivalence trials,[39] nonpharmacological treatments,[45] herbal interventions,[49] and pragmatic trials.[40] Additional extensions are forthcoming: for those and for up-to-date references relevant to this checklist, see www.consort-statement.org.

The CONSORT Statement was always intended to be a living document in that it would be updated as needed. The CONSORT Group is an international and eclectic group of clinical trialists, statisticians, epidemiologists, and biomedical editors. They have published two updates. In 2001, the second version was published simultaneously in three prominent general medical journals (seemingly without precedent).[29-31] The third version was published in 2010 and eight journals published it simultaneously.[5-11,32] Additional journals have subsequently published it.[12,33,34]

The original CONSORT Statement in 1996 neglected explanations or justifications for most of the items in the checklist.[28] The CONSORT Group decided to produce a paper to provide the scientific rationale, detail the importance, and describe the implementation of each item on the CONSORT checklist. The ensuing E&E document was published simultaneously with the second version of the CONSORT Statement.[35] For each item in the checklist, the essential methodological issues were clarified and a synopsis of the empirical evidence was provided. Also, at least one example of adequate reporting was provided for each checklist item.

REPORTING USING THE CONSORT STATEMENT

Courtesy of the CONSORT Group, we have reproduced in this chapter the 25-item checklist (Table 22.1) and flow diagram (Fig. 22.1) from the CONSORT 2010 Statement (also referred to as the Statement or CONSORT 2010) from the CONSORT website (www.consort-statement.org/). We recommend that the checklist and flow diagram be read in conjunction with the CONSORT 2010 Explanation and Elaboration (E&E) for crucial support. [36,37] All of the original CONSORT Statement papers and the E&E can be found on the aforementioned CONSORT website.

The CONSORT Group regards their checklist as a minimum provision of trial information. However, for some trials, other information might also be relevant. Obviously, any essential information about a trial should be included, regardless of whether it is explicitly in the checklist.

OTHER THAN A TWO-GROUP, PARALLEL RANDOMISED TRIAL

The CONSORT 2010 Statement provides guidance for reporting all RCTs, regardless of design. It pertains fundamentally to all randomised trials. However, it concentrates on the most common design type, individually randomised, two-group, parallel trials. Other trial designs—such as cluster randomised trials, noninferiority trials, pragmatic trials, and N-of-1 trials—and trials that involve specialised interventions—such as nonpharmacological treatment interventions or herbal interventions—may necessitate supplementary information.[38-49] These and other extensions can be accessed through the CONSORT website (www.consort-statement.org). Moreover, other extensions, for example on multiarm parallel randomised trials, are being developed.

Two additional CONSORT extensions pertain to a broad cross section of all trials. They address the reporting of harms[50] and the content of abstracts of reports of trial findings.[51,52] Authors should probe the CONSORT website for new or updated CONSORT publications.

Studies Other Than RCTs

Investigators should use a reporting guideline for both planning and reporting all types of studies, not just randomised trials. However, not all published reporting guidelines are good and accepted by journals.

The CONSORT approach has led to a veritable explosion of reporting guidelines. Many groups have embraced the CONSORT model for developing a reporting guideline. Indeed, the CONSORT originators developed and published recommendations for future guideline developers.[53,54] Currently, hundreds of reporting guidelines have been recognised and compiled on

PANEL 22.1 ■ Recommended Reporting Guidelines by Types of Research Study Other Than RCTs

Type of Research Study	Year of Publication	Reporting Guideline
Diagnostic test accuracy studies	2015	STARD[57,58]
Observational epidemiological studies	2007	STROBE[55,59]
Systematic reviews/meta-analyses of randomised trials	2009	PRISMA[56,60]

the EQUATOR (Enhancing the QUAlity and Transparency Of Research Network website (www. equator-network.org)). Moreover, some reporting guideline developers followed the CONSORT model to generate long E&E papers.[55-57] Usually, as a rule of thumb, a reporting guideline that also has an E&E paper for support will be a better and more useful guideline.

Using that rule of thumb, along with our involvement in and use of guidelines, we recommend a few specific reporting guidelines for consideration. Fortunately, these few listed later, along with CONSORT, should satisfy most investigators reporting guideline needs. Certainly, consult the reporting guideline website (www.equator-network.org) for any additional, new, or updated guidelines.

Conclusion

The reporting of biomedical research is often of poor quality. Deficiencies include nonreporting of completed studies, absence of vital information in the description of research methods and interventions, and selective reporting or switching of outcomes. These reporting flaws can lead to severe consequences for medical practice, research, clinical care guidelines, and eventually patient care.[61] Reporting guidelines aspire to guide researchers towards presenting adequate descriptions of their research. Some actually do.

The first broadly recognised reporting guideline was the CONSORT Statement, offering recommendations for reporting of randomised trials. It was initially published in 1996 with the most recent revision published in 2010.[7] Assiduous adherence by authors to the checklist items promotes clarity, completeness, and transparency of reporting. Explicit descriptions, not abstruseness or omission, best satisfy the needs of all readers.

Of note, the CONSORT 2010 Statement does not contain recommendations for designing, conducting, and analysing trials. It exclusively tackles reporting. Guidance for randomised trial protocol development is available elsewhere.[62-64] Yet the CONSORT 2010 Statement ultimately influences design and conduct via an indirect pathway. Transparent reporting exposes deficiencies in medical research, if indeed problematic. Thus researchers who conduct deficient trials, but who must transparently report, will not traverse the publication process without revealing whatever deficiencies exist. 'That emerging reality should provide impetus to improved trial design and conduct in the future, a secondary indirect goal of our work'.[7] Indeed, illustratively stated by an editor of the *Annals of Internal Medicine*:

> By itself, accurate, transparent reporting does not make good science. Knowing that editors expect a high standard of accuracy and transparency in reports of finished research can, however, encourage researchers do a better job in planning and carrying out the research in the first place. Accurate, transparent reporting is like turning the light on before you clean up a room: It doesn't clean it for you, but does tell you where the problems are.[65]

PANEL 22.2 ■ Good Research Practices for Randomised Trials (Adapted From Altman et al.[66])

Protocol
- Must have a protocol.
- Should consult the SPIRIT guideline for protocols.[62–64]
- Should be publicly available (e.g., in a journal article or on a trial website).
- Should be updated as necessary, with dates and rationale for changes.
- Should address items in CONSORT 2010 that will have to be reported in the publication.

Registration
- The trial should be registered before the start of recruitment.*
- The information entered in the registry should match what is in the protocol.
- The registry entry should be updated as necessary, with dates and rationale for changes.

Publication
- The main report of trial findings should follow the CONSORT 2010 Statement.
- The site of the trial protocol should be given (or should be published as a web appendix).
- The discrepancies, if any, from the protocol or registry entry should be declared and explained.

---

*Registration after starting enrolment is poor practice but better than nonregistration.

The CONSORT 2010 Statement forms a critical part of good research practices for an RCT. (Panel 22.2). A reasonable question is whether reporting guidelines work. The first and oldest guideline, CONSORT, has elicited the most evidence. Indeed, a systematic review from a few years ago found 50 studies that evaluated the effect of CONSORT on the quality of reporting of RCTs.[67] The results substantiate that CONSORT leads to improved reporting. It works. However, the improvements appear modest, and substantial room for improvement remains. Moreover, CONSORT as a reporting guideline has negligible influence on publication bias (preferably referred to as 'nonpublication bias') because the trials are never published.

CONSORT has broad support from medical journals. More than 600 have explicitly supported the Statement. Furthermore, thousands more have implicitly supported it with the endorsement of the Statement by the International Committee of Medical Journal Editors (www.icmje.org). Other prominent editorial groups, the Council of Science Editors and the World Association of Medical Editors, officially support CONSORT.

Although the attention given to CONSORT by medical journals reaches impressive levels, they broadly endorse CONSORT but often do not enforce compliance. In 165 high-impact-factor journals, only 38% mentioned CONSORT in their 'Instructions to Authors' in 2007, and just 37% of those stated that adhering was compulsory.[68] For CONSORT to have its full effect, it must be used by authors and editors. Currently, the CONSORT Group is focusing on endorsement and adherence. They devote less attention to the checklist and more to a knowledge translation strategy to attempt to recognise the barriers and facilitators to implementing CONSORT in journals.

The CONSORT 2010 Statement is a reporting guideline and should not be used to construct a 'quality score'.[7] Nevertheless, we suggest that investigators design trials with their primary reporting publication in mind. 'Poor reporting allows authors, intentionally or inadvertently, to escape scrutiny of any weak aspects of their trials. However, with wide adoption of CONSORT by journals and editorial groups, most authors should have to report transparently all important aspects of their trial. The ensuing scrutiny rewards well conducted trials and penalises poorly conducted trials. Thus investigators should understand the CONSORT 2010 reporting guidelines before starting a trial as a further incentive to design and conduct their trials according to rigorous standards'.[7]

In sum, authors should utilise appropriate reporting guidelines. CONSORT has spawned other useful guidelines for studies besides randomised trials. The appropriate reporting guideline aids in study design and manuscript writing, and, in the end, its use leads to a higher probability of publication success.

References

1. Dwan, K., Altman, D.G., Arnaiz, J.A., et al., 2008. Systematic review of the empirical evidence of study publication bias and outcome reporting bias. PLoS One 3, e3081.
2. Dwan, K., Altman, D.G., Cresswell, L., Blundell, M., Gamble, C.L., Williamson, P.R., 2011. Comparison of protocols and registry entries to published reports for randomised controlled trials. Cochrane Database Syst. Rev., MR000031.
3. Altman, D.G., Moher, D., Schulz, K.F., 2012. Improving the reporting of randomised trials: the CONSORT Statement and beyond. Stat. Med. 31, 2985–2997.
4. Chalmers, I., Glasziou, P., 2009. Avoidable waste in the production and reporting of research evidence. Obstet. Gynecol. 114, 1341–1345.
5. Schulz, K.F., Altman, D.G., Moher, D., 2010. CONSORT 2010 statement: updated guidelines for reporting parallel group randomised trials. PLoS Med 7, e1000251.
6. Schulz, K.F., Altman, D.G., Moher, D., 2010. CONSORT 2010 statement: updated guidelines for reporting parallel group randomised trials. J. Clin. Epidemiol. 63, 834–840.
7. Schulz, K.F., Altman, D.G., Moher, D., 2010. CONSORT 2010 statement: updated guidelines for reporting parallel group randomised trials. BMJ 340, c332.
8. Schulz, K.F., Altman, D.G., Moher, D., 2010. CONSORT 2010 statement: updated guidelines for reporting parallel group randomized trials. Obstet. Gynecol. 115, 1063–1070.
9. Schulz, K.F., Altman, D.G., Moher, D., 2010. CONSORT 2010 statement: updated guidelines for reporting parallel group randomized trials. Ann. Intern. Med. 152, 726–732.
10. Schulz, K.F., Altman, D.G., Moher, D., 2010. CONSORT 2010 statement: updated guidelines for reporting parallel group randomised trials. BMC Med. 8, 18.
11. Schulz, K.F., Altman, D.G., Moher, D., 2010. CONSORT 2010 statement: updated guidelines for reporting parallel group randomised trials. Trials 11, 32.
12. Schulz, K.F., Altman, D.G., Moher, D., 2011. CONSORT 2010 statement: updated guidelines for reporting parallel group randomised trials. Int. J. Surg. 9, 672–677.
13. Dancey, J.E., 2010. From quality of publication to quality of care: translating trials to practice. J. Natl. Cancer Inst. 102, 670–671.
14. Rennie, D., 2001. CONSORT revised—improving the reporting of randomized trials. JAMA 285, 2006–2007.
15. Jüni, P., Altman, D.G., Egger, M., 2001. Systematic reviews in health care: assessing the quality of controlled clinical trials. BMJ 323, 42–46.
16. Schulz, K.F., Chalmers, I., Hayes, R.J., Altman, D.G., 1995. Empirical evidence of bias. Dimensions of methodological quality associated with estimates of treatment effects in controlled trials. JAMA 273, 408–412.
17. Dechartres, A., Charles, P., Hopewell, S., Ravaud, P., Altman, D.G., 2011. Reviews assessing the quality or the reporting of randomized controlled trials are increasing over time but raised questions about how quality is assessed. J. Clin. Epidemiol. 64, 136–144.
18. Chan, A.W., Altman, D.G., 2005. Epidemiology and reporting of randomised trials published in PubMed journals. Lancet 365, 1159–1162.
19. Hopewell, S., Dutton, S., Yu, L.M., Chan, A.W., Altman, D.G., 2010. The quality of reports of randomised trials in 2000 and 2006: comparative study of articles indexed in PubMed. BMJ 340, c723.
20. Dickinson, K., Bunn, F., Wentz, R., Edwards, P., Roberts, I., 2000. Size and quality of randomised controlled trials in head injury: review of published studies. BMJ 320, 1308–1311.
21. Glasziou, P., Meats, E., Heneghan, C., Shepperd, S., 2008. What is missing from descriptions of treatment in trials and reviews? BMJ 336, 1472–1474.
22. Song, F., Parekh, S., Hooper, L., et al., 2010. Dissemination and publication of research findings: an updated review of related biases. Health Technol. Assess. 14, 1–193, iii, ix–xi.
23. Chan, A.W., Hrobjartsson, A., Haahr, M.T., Gøtzsche, P.C., Altman, D.G., 2004. Empirical evidence for selective reporting of outcomes in randomized trials: comparison of protocols to published articles. JAMA 291, 2457–2465.

24. Chan, A.W., Krleza-Jeric, K., Schmid, I., Altman, D.G., 2004. Outcome reporting bias in randomized trials funded by the Canadian Institutes of Health Research. CMAJ 171, 735–740.

25. Grimes, D.A., Schulz, K.F., 1996. Methodology citations and the quality of randomized controlled trials in obstetrics and gynecology. Am. J. Obstet. Gynecol. 174, 1312–1315.

26. Grant, A., 1989. Reporting controlled trials. Br. J. Obstet. Gynaecol. 96, 397–400.

27. Squires, B.P., Elmslie, T.J., 1990. Reports of randomized controlled trials: what editors want from authors and peer reviewers. CMAJ 143, 381–382.

28. Begg, C., Cho, M., Eastwood, S., et al., 1996. Improving the quality of reporting of randomized controlled trials. The CONSORT statement. JAMA 276, 637–639.

29. Moher, D., Schulz, K.F., Altman, D.G., 2001. The CONSORT statement: revised recommendations for improving the quality of reports of parallel-group randomised trials. Lancet 357, 1191–1194.

30. Moher, D., Schulz, K.F., Altman, D., 2001. The CONSORT statement: revised recommendations for improving the quality of reports of parallel-group randomized trials. JAMA 285, 1987–1991.

31. Moher, D., Schulz, K.F., Altman, D.G., 2001. The CONSORT statement: revised recommendations for improving the quality of reports of parallel-group randomized trials. Ann. Intern. Med. 134, 657–662.

32. Schulz, K.F., Altman, D.G., Moher, D., 2010. CONSORT 2010 statement: updated guidelines for reporting parallel group randomized trials. Open Med. 4, e60–e68.

33. Schulz, K.F., Altman, D.G., Moher, D., 2010. CONSORT 2010 statement: updated guidelines for reporting parallel group randomised trials. J. Pharmacol. Pharmacother. 1, 100–107.

34. Schulz, K.F., Altman, D.G., Moher, D., 2010. CONSORT 2010 statement: updated guidelines for reporting parallel group randomised trials (Chinese version). Zhong Xi Yi Jie He Xue Bao 8, 604–612.

35. Altman, D.G., Schulz, K.F., Moher, D., et al., 2001. The revised CONSORT statement for reporting randomized trials: explanation and elaboration. Ann. Intern. Med. 134, 663–694.

36. Moher, D., Hopewell, S., Schulz, K.F., et al., 2010. CONSORT 2010 explanation and elaboration: updated guidelines for reporting parallel group randomised trials. J. Clin. Epidemiol. 63, e1–e37.

37. Moher, D., Hopewell, S., Schulz, K.F., et al., 2010. CONSORT 2010 explanation and elaboration: updated guidelines for reporting parallel group randomised trials. BMJ 340, c869.

38. Campbell, M.K., Piaggio, G., Elbourne, D.R., Altman, D.G., 2012. CONSORT 2010 statement: extension to cluster randomised trials. BMJ 345, e5661.

39. Piaggio, G., Elbourne, D.R., Pocock, S.J., Evans, S.J., Altman, D.G., 2012. Reporting of noninferiority and equivalence randomized trials: extension of the CONSORT 2010 statement. JAMA 308, 2594–2604.

40. Zwarenstein, M., Treweek, S., Gagnier, J.J., et al., 2008. Improving the reporting of pragmatic trials: an extension of the CONSORT statement. BMJ 337, a2390.

41. Shamseer, L., Sampson, M., Bukutu, C., et al., 2016. CONSORT extension for reporting N-of-1 trials (CENT) 2015: explanation and elaboration. J. Clin. Epidemiol. 76, 18–46.

42. Shamseer, L., Sampson, M., Bukutu, C., et al., 2015. CONSORT extension for reporting N-of-1 trials (CENT) 2015: explanation and elaboration. BMJ 350, h1793.

43. Vohra, S., Shamseer, L., Sampson, M., et al., 2016. CONSORT extension for reporting N-of-1 trials (CENT) 2015 statement. J. Clin. Epidemiol. 76, 9–17.

44. Vohra, S., Shamseer, L., Sampson, M., et al., 2015. CONSORT extension for reporting N-of-1 trials (CENT) 2015 statement. BMJ 350, h1738.

45. Boutron, I., Altman, D.G., Moher, D., Schulz, K.F., Ravaud, P., 2017. CONSORT statement for randomized trials of nonpharmacologic treatments: a 2017 update and a CONSORT extension for nonpharmacologic trial abstracts. Ann. Intern. Med. 167, 40–47.

46. Boutron, I., Moher, D., Altman, D.G., Schulz, K.F., Ravaud, P., 2008. Extending the CONSORT statement to randomized trials of nonpharmacologic treatment: explanation and elaboration. Ann. Intern. Med. 148, 295–309.

47. Boutron, I., Moher, D., Altman, D.G., Schulz, K.F., Ravaud, P., 2008. Methods and processes of the CONSORT group: example of an extension for trials assessing nonpharmacologic treatments. Ann. Intern. Med. 148, W60–W66.

48. Gagnier, J.J., Boon, H., Rochon, P., Moher, D., Barnes, J., Bombardier, C., 2006. Recommendations for reporting randomized controlled trials of herbal interventions: explanation and elaboration. J. Clin. Epidemiol. 59, 1134–1149.

49. Gagnier, J.J., Boon, H., Rochon, P., Moher, D., Barnes, J., Bombardier, C., 2006. Reporting randomized, controlled trials of herbal interventions: an elaborated CONSORT statement. Ann. Intern. Med. 144, 364–367.

50. Ioannidis, J.P., Evans, S.J., Gøtzsche, P.C., et al., 2004. Better reporting of harms in randomized trials: an extension of the CONSORT statement. Ann. Intern. Med. 141, 781–788.

51. Hopewell, S., Clarke, M., Moher, D., et al., 2008. CONSORT for reporting randomised trials in journal and conference abstracts. Lancet 371, 281–283.

52. Hopewell, S., Clarke, M., Moher, D., et al., 2008. CONSORT for reporting randomized controlled trials in journal and conference abstracts: explanation and elaboration. PLoS Med 5, e20.

53. Moher, D., Schulz, K.F., Simera, I., Altman, D.G., 2010. Guidance for developers of health research reporting guidelines. PLoS Med 7, e1000217.

54. Moher, D., Weeks, L., Ocampo, M., et al., 2011. Describing reporting guidelines for health research: a systematic review. J. Clin. Epidemiol. 64, 718–742.

55. Vandenbroucke, J.P., von Elm, E., Altman, D.G., et al., 2007. Strengthening the Reporting of Observational Studies in Epidemiology (STROBE): explanation and elaboration. Ann. Intern. Med. 147, W163–W194.

56. Liberati, A., Altman, D.G., Tetzlaff, J., et al., 2009. The PRISMA statement for reporting systematic reviews and meta-analyses of studies that evaluate health care interventions: explanation and elaboration. J. Clin. Epidemiol. 62, e1–e34.

57. Bossuyt, P.M., Reitsma, J.B., Bruns, D.E., et al., 2015. STARD 2015: an updated list of essential items for reporting diagnostic accuracy studies. BMJ 351, h5527.

58. Bossuyt, P.M., Reitsma, J.B., Bruns, D.E., et al., 2015. STARD 2015: an updated list of essential items for reporting diagnostic accuracy studies. Radiology 277, 826–832.

59. von Elm, E., Altman, D.G., Egger, M., Pocock, S.J., Gøtzsche, P.C., Vandenbroucke, J.P., 2007. The Strengthening the Reporting of Observational Studies in Epidemiology (STROBE) statement: guidelines for reporting observational studies. Lancet 370, 1453–1457.

60. Moher, D., Liberati, A., Tetzlaff, J., Altman, D.G., 2009. Preferred reporting items for systematic reviews and meta-analyses: the PRISMA statement. BMJ 339, b2535.

61. Simera, I., Altman, D.G., 2009. Writing a research article that is "fit for purpose": EQUATOR network and reporting guidelines. Evid. Based Med. 14, 132–134.

62. Chan, A.W., Tetzlaff, J.M., Altman, D.G., Dickersin, K., Moher, D., 2013. SPIRIT 2013: new guidance for content of clinical trial protocols. Lancet 381, 91–92.

63. Chan, A.W., Tetzlaff, J.M., Altman, D.G., et al., 2013. SPIRIT 2013 statement: defining standard protocol items for clinical trials. Ann. Intern. Med. 158, 200–207.

64. Chan, A.W., Tetzlaff, J.M., Gøtzsche, P.C., et al., 2013. SPIRIT 2013 explanation and elaboration: guidance for protocols of clinical trials. BMJ 346, e7586.

65. Davidoff, F., 2000. News from the International Committee of Medical Journal Editors. Ann. Intern. Med. 133, 229–231.

66. Altman, D.G., Moher, D., Schulz, K.F., 2017. Harms of outcome switching in reports of randomised trials: CONSORT perspective. BMJ 356, j396.

67. Turner, L., Shamseer, L., Altman, D.G., et al., 2012. Consolidated standards of reporting trials (CONSORT) and the completeness of reporting of randomised controlled trials (RCTs) published in medical journals. Cochrane Database Syst. Rev. 11, MR000030.

68. Hopewell, S., Altman, D.G., Moher, D., Schulz, K.F., 2008. Endorsement of the CONSORT statement by high impact factor medical journals: a survey of journal editors and journal 'Instructions to Authors'. Trials 9, 20.

Note: Page numbers followed by f indicate figures, t indicate tables, and b indicate boxes.